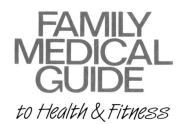

FAMILY MEDICAL GUIDE
to Health & Fitness

Volume 2

Family Health and General Diseases

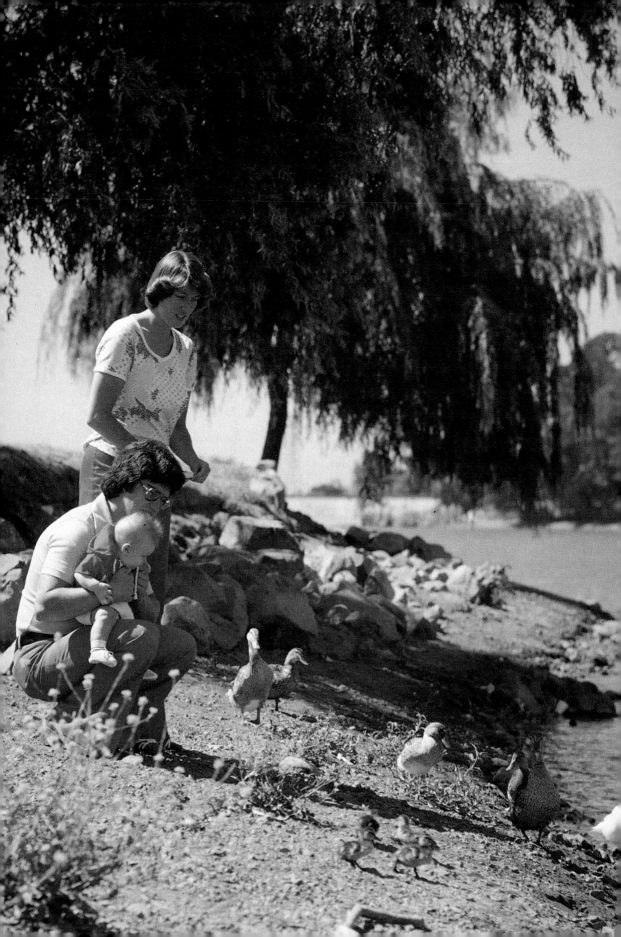

Volume **2**

Family Health and General Diseases

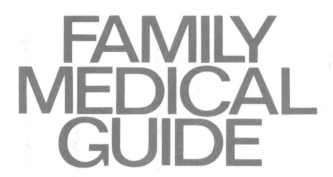

FAMILY MEDICAL GUIDE

to Health & Fitness

in three volumes, illustrated

Mervyn G. Hardinge, M.D., Dr.P.H., Ph.D.
Harold Shryock, M.A., M.D.

In collaboration with 28 leading medical specialists

Published jointly by

Pacific Press Publishing Association
Boise, ID 83707
Oshawa, Ontario, Canada

Review and Herald Publishing Association
Washington, D.C. 20039-0555
Hagerstown, MD 21740

PHOTO AND ILLUSTRATION CREDITS:

Pages 362, 368, 370, 416, 419, 496, 504, 506, 602, 604, 738, 740, 742 by Betty Blue.
Pages 382, 538, 701 by Lucille Innes.
Pages 397, 522, 523 by Duane Tank.
Pages 423, 475, 724 by Loma Linda University School of Medicine.
Page 463 by Eli Lilly and Company.
Page 463 by Elias Papazian.
Pages 465, 471, 489, 700, 706, 724, 727, 728, 729, 736, 760, 764 by Public Health Service Audiovisual Facility.
Pages 362, 527, 565, 568, 591 by Duane Tank/Betty Blue.
Pages 534, 535, 731 by Joe Maniscalco.
Page 608 by The Photo Department, Meylan C. Thoreson.
Page 716 by Clay Adams.
Page 746 by © CIBA.
Pages 753, 754, 755, 759 by Chas. Pfizer and Co., Inc.
Page 758 by James Converse.

Edited by Marvin Moore
Designed by Ira Lee
Cover photo by Duane Tank and Betty Blue
Inside art by Kim Justinen
Typeset in 11/13 Century Old Style

Copyright © 1991 by
Pacific Press Publishing Association
Printed in United States of America
All Rights Reserved
Revised Edition 1994

Library of Congress Catalog Number: 90-60852

ISBN 0-8163-0846-2: Volume 2
ISBN 0-8163-0926-4: Volumes 1-3

94 95 96 97 98 ● 6 5 4 3 2

Contents

Volume 1—Lifestyle

Section 1—A healthy lifestyle

Section 2—Mental and spiritual health

Section 3—Nutrition: Charts and recipes, disorders

Section 4—Things to avoid

Section 5—Understanding medications

Volume 2—Family health and general diseases

Section 1—The stages of life

Section 2—Medical care at home

Section 3—General diseases

Volume 3—The systems of the body and their disorders

Section 1—The cardiovascular and lymphatic systems and their disorders

Section 2—The digestive and respiratory systems and their disorders

Section 3—The skeletal and cutaneous systems and their disorders

Section 4—The endocrine and nervous systems and their disorders

Section 5—The reproductive and urinary systems and their disorders

Section 6—The sense organs and their disorders

Introduction to volume 2

Volume 2 of the *Family Medical Guide* is divided into two parts: (1) Family health and (2) General diseases.

Family health

Health is not only an individual matter. It's just as much a family matter, because when one person is ill, the whole family is affected. The reproductive process, which in one sense is not a health *problem* at all, is what makes families possible in the first place. Also, some diseases and disorders of the body are especially typical of certain age groups, and thus are especially prone to affect families. That is why the first part of volume 2 of the *Family Medical Guide* is about family health.

The first section in volume 2, called "The stages of life," will be especially helpful to you as you deal with problems of reproduction, infancy, childhood, adolescence, and old age. Much of the advice in this section will help you to avoid problems in the first place, and it will give you good practical advice on questions such as, How much should I feed my baby, or How can I be sure my child is developing normally?

The section on "Medical care at home" will help you to avoid accidents and other emergencies, and it will help you to deal with them when they do occur. It will give you many practical suggestions on how to care for a sick person at home—the kinds of things nurses do when they care for patients in the hospital. And there is a chapter full of simple treatments you can give yourself at home that will speed recovery—and probably save you money.

And, of course, the authors also advise you when to consult a physician rather than trying to take care of problems yourself.

General diseases

The third section, called "General diseases," is one of the most practical in the entire three-volume *Family Medical Guide*. The first chapter, "Why disease?" will help you to understand why disease occurs in the first place, which will help you to keep from getting sick. When you do get sick, the next two chapters, "Common problems and symptoms" and "Ready diagnosis of common problems," will give you an idea of the possible causes of your illness even before you go see your family doctor. These two chapters will also help you to ask the right questions when you do consult him. The flowcharts in chapter 21 are a quick way to diagnose some of the problems and symptoms that people most often ask their doctors about.

Also in this section are several chapters on infectious diseases that include information on how to avoid them and what to do when you are overcome by them.

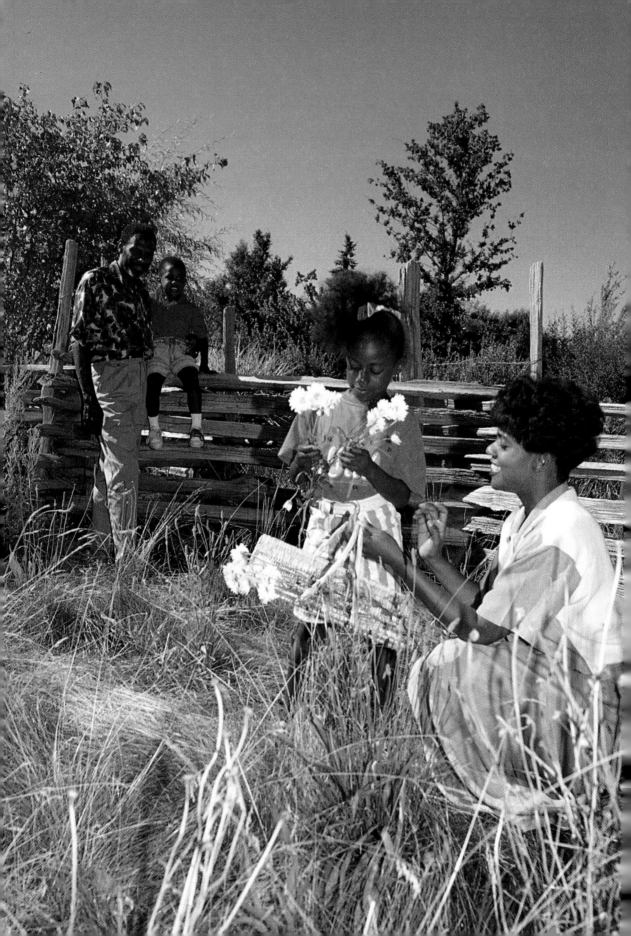

CHAPTER 1

Home and the family

A house is where a group of individuals live, but a home is much more. A home is where people live together and interrelate in an environment of mutual respect, understanding, and love for one another. This social unit forms a family, ideally made up of a father, mother, and children. The family may be enlarged to include one or more grandparents.

The family

Such a family unit or home starts when a couple—a young man and young woman—are first attracted to each other. As the attraction grows and deepens, strong emotional ties unite them in a bond of love. The couple yearn to be in each other's company as often as possible. Obstacles and hardships often appear trivial, and they face the future with glowing optimism. They look forward to a life together in which this loving relationship will never end, and their lives, filled with happiness, will be shared with children yet unborn.

In Western societies the choice of a mate is generally made by the young people themselves. In the past the choice was considered to be made for life, the marriage vows stating that their union was "until death do us part." Unfortunately, forces present in modern societies have caused frequent dissolution of the home, so that today, one or more of every two marriages end in divorce.

The causes for this are many and varied. Young people often marry while still in their teens. Though physically developed, their mental and emotional systems have not yet matured. The one they can't stand to be away from today they may not be able to tolerate tomorrow. Some young people marry too quickly, without allowing time to reveal the true characteristics of the other. Their dispositions may be quite different—one short-tempered, unreasonable, and selfish, the other self-centered, conceited, and jealous. It is often said that "opposites make successful marriages." This can be correct, but often it is far from the truth. The more a couple have in common in their likes and dislikes, the more likely they are to form a stable relationship.

With the erosion of moral standards and the almost universality of premarital sex, young people often live together without entering into any form of permanent relationship, and even when they do get married, they do so with the thought that "if it doesn't work, we'll divorce and try again." Such relationships are usually quite fragile, and when children are born, the woman is often left to fend for herself. The problems of divorce seem never to end, especially when children are involved. And experience shows that second marriages are less likely to be successful than first marriages.

A successful marriage and the establishment of a happy home are no mere accident. Both should be carefully planned. Young people should seek the counsel of those who are older, such as parents or teachers, as they can perhaps discern characteristics that would spell trouble. Unfinished education, lack of work or professional skills, differences in ethnic or religious backgrounds, personality differences—these and many other factors can complicate a marriage.

The economics of maintaining a home often cause stresses and strains in family relationships. When a single income is inadequate to support the desired lifestyle and both partners have to work, the conditions for dissension in the home are greatly multiplied. This is especially true after children have arrived. Sometimes there are no simple solutions to the problems. Here is where

careful consideration in advance might have avoided some of the perplexing situations.

In some cultures parents decide whom their children will marry. This is totally unacceptable in the Western world. However, the success rate of arranged marriages in those cultures where it is accepted is quite surprising. This suggests that adjustments in likes and dislikes can be made, and obstacles in relationships can be overcome even when they seem quite insurmountable—as long as both parties are of a mind to do so in a mutual give and take.

Single-parent homes are common today. Generally, such a family consists of the mother and one or more children. The mother is the breadwinner, and preschool children are left during much of the day with a baby sitter or in a day-care center. When the child reaches school age, school becomes the caring institution. The family gets together again at the end of the day and on weekends and holidays. Close interpersonal relationships are difficult to maintain at best.

Homes that are established by people who have been divorced introduce their own set of problems, especially where one or both have children. Among these are the acceptance by one parent of the other's children, frictions between the children of the two parents (often spilling over into conflicts between the adults), differences in norms of behavior, and the financial burdens of one or both spouses. These and other factors combine to make ideal relationships difficult, but not impossible, in second marriages.

The health of the adults as well as that of the children is an extremely important ingredient in maintaining a successful home. In the marriage ceremony it is common for the man and woman to promise to remain faithful to each other "in sickness and in health." Yet little do most people realize that illness is one of life's worst tragedies—a misfortune that all too often casts a cloud over the family's experience.

The health of the husband is vital if he is to be the wage earner. The wife's health is equally important, for she has the dual responsibility of homemaking and childbearing, along with, in many instances, earning a second income to maintain the desired lifestyle or even the basic needs. Many forms of illness cannot be predicted, even when healthful living is at its best. Infections do occur, and hereditary weaknesses become evident in a variety of diseases such as cancer, diabetes, allergies, and high blood pressure. These and other illnesses are discussed elsewhere in these volumes, and where possible, suggestions are made for avoiding them.

One of the most important considerations when contemplating the establishment of a home is lifestyle, for the lifestyle of each partner will play a major role in either maintaining health or predisposing to illness.

When the laws of health are disregarded and unhealthful habits and patterns of life are chosen, the immediate and long-term consequences are inevitable. Smoking, drinking, the use of nonmedicinal drugs, over-eating, carousing, and aberrant sexual habits are but a few of the many factors that can precipitate disease and put a strain on an otherwise stable home. It is for these reasons that volume 1 is devoted to presenting the advantages of a simple, healthful lifestyle. It is the authors' hope that many readers will learn from these pages how to avoid the physical and emotional suffering that inevitably accompany a disregard of nature's laws.

The children

A couple's decision to have a child is a serious matter that should not be entered into lightly. The habits and patterns of life of the mother, and even the father, will influence the child to be born. Some of these influences will be transmitted through the genes, while others will be communicated directly and indirectly by the environment in which the child is raised. From the earliest days the impact of the home, and later of the school, shape and form the character of the developing infant, child, and youth.

Unfortunately, and all too often, conception occurs without careful thought. The sexual act is entered into lightly by partners who have no intention to stay or live together. The transient physical pleasure is the sole motivation, rather than the union of a man and woman who love each other, and who hope, if given the opportunity, to raise a child that someday will make a contribution to society. Children born out of wedlock, sharing a place to live with brothers and sisters who have different fathers or different mothers, may never learn the feeling of being wanted and loved. Most unfortunate are those children who have no home at all, but who are cast upon society, raised in some institution. These are even more likely to grow up with no understanding of true love and affection.

Naturalists know that birds and animals are imprinted in some mysterious way to either one or both of their parents. The parent of a baby penguin, flamingo, or pelican can distinguish its youngster's call from hundreds of others all around.

As a boy growing up in the hills of northeast India, one of the authors was out for a walk with his father and brother. We passed a large flock of sheep, numbering two or three hundred. It was lambing season, and the air was filled by the bleating of both old and young.

About a half mile upstream from the flock, my brother and I found a newborn lamb lying in the grass by the bank of the river. Apparently the flock of sheep had passed that way, and the unknowing shepherd had hurried the mother on, leaving behind her tiny offspring. We picked it up and took turns carrying it back to the flock. About ten feet from the outer boundary of the flock, we put the wobbly-legged creature on the grass. It gave a plaintive bleat that to us seemed lost amid the hundred others. But immediately we saw a mother sheep in the middle of the flock raise her head. Moments later the little lamb gave another bleat. The mother turned, and with rapid bounds came in the direction of the

lamb. She nuzzled it, and together mother and lamb disappeared among the other sheep.

Human babies have an inborn attachment and loyalty to their parents that is weak at first, but that grows steadily stronger. This is as it should be, for the growing infant and child is completely dependent on its parent or parents for life. This relationship should never be broken, but cultivated and strengthened as the child becomes a youth, and the youth an adult. Early planning should forestall the developing of a so-called "generation gap." Until the age of reason, the child is *conditioned,* as it were, to the philosophy and lifestyle of the parents.

With the dawn of reason around the age of six, when permanent memory beings to develop, learned behavior gradually unfolds. Then, when youth seeks independence, the foundations of sound character development have been solidly laid. Obviously the home and its multitude of activities must be a school in which the child is trained for a useful future life.

It is in the home where children are taught, by hearing and seeing, to be obedient, sharing, caring, and loving members of the family. Responsibilities should be given, matched to the children's ages, so they can grow up prepared to carry the duties of life. In all this, the parents must be the pattern.

Grandparents can be a blessing in a home. Until reaching very advanced age, many can ease the burdens of mother or father. Children learn to care for the needs of those who are older, and perhaps dependent, and often can both bestow and receive loving attention that the pressures of the parents' time might not permit. Pets in the home may also serve a useful function. The care they require is generally bountifully returned by the affection the animals spontaneously give.

Like any successful society, a home requires an orderly conduct of its affairs. Children thrive in an environment of assurance. A reasonable schedule of activities, with assigned responsibilities for the day, removes uncertainty and misunderstandings. A sensible schedule is extremely helpful: when to get up and when to go to bed; when meals are served and duties performed; when to leave for school and when to play.

Illnesses

This volume discusses infectious diseases, which are the result of an invasion of the body. An infecting organism may be a bacteria, rickettsia, virus, spirochete, or parasite. The type of infection varies, depending on the agent, its virulence, the site of entry, and the level of resistance or immunity of the individual.

If the virulence of the organism is low and the resistance of the person is high, the infection may not occur or will be mild. On the other hand, if the organism is virulent and the person's resistance is low, the resulting infection may be severe and even fatal.

In recent years, numerous drugs, such as antibiotics, sulfas, and other anti-infective agents, have been developed to help combat infections, but these are not the whole answer. In fact, it has become evident that the maintenance of health, and thus the preservation of a strong, effective immune system, is indispensable in the fight against disease. While large sections of these volumes are devoted to explaining how to maintain and enhance health, a few of the main ingredients of a healthful lifestyle will be mentioned here.

Immunizations, discussed in detail elsewhere (see page 407), have proved to be a great blessing to humanity. By means of immunizations, *given at appropriate times,* most of the so-called childhood diseases have been largely brought under control.

In every home, the principles of health and hygiene should be practiced from childhood onward. Regularity in eating, working, playing, and sleeping, along with cleanliness of both body and home, should be routine. Healthful food, served at regular times in a pleasant atmosphere of happiness and love, will provide a physical, mental, and emotional environment in which both children and adults can thrive.

Religion

Religion, when believed and practiced, brings a stability that otherwise is difficult to attain. Standards of conduct and guidance for desirable interrelationships will go far in making the activities of a home successful. And, finally, trust in God gives comfort and assurance in times of uncertainty, illness, suffering, and death.

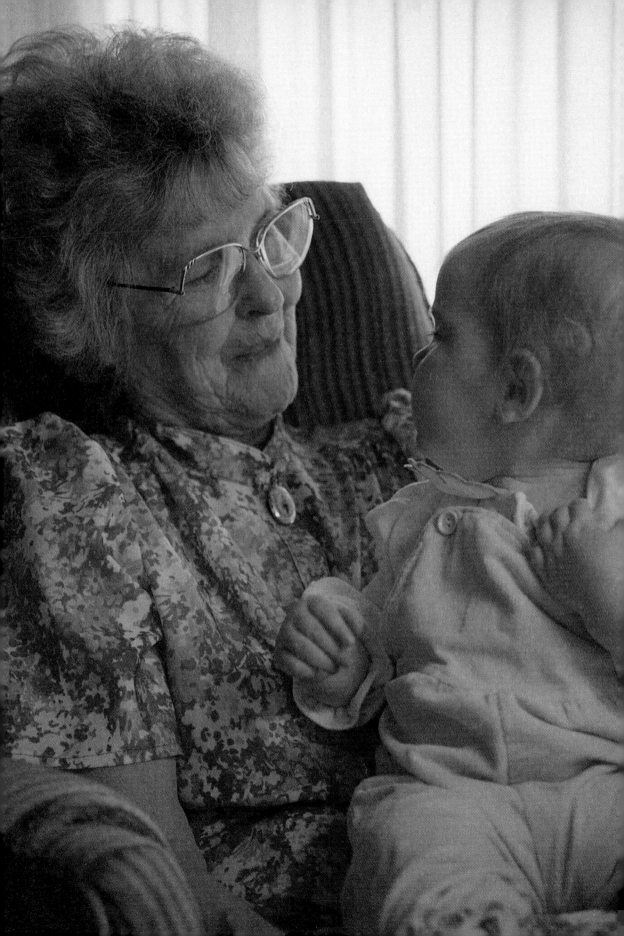

VOL. 2

SECTION 1

THE STAGES OF LIFE

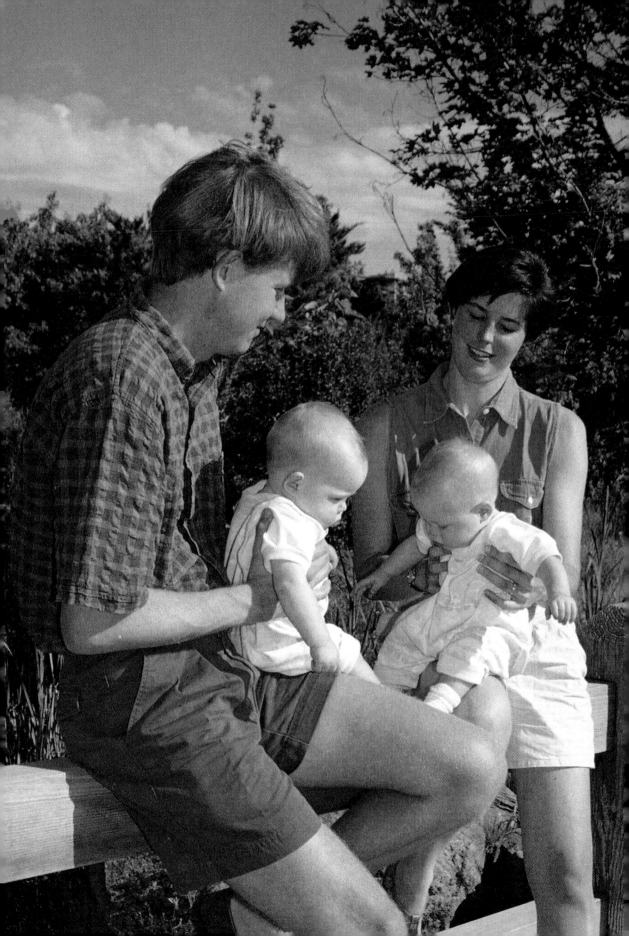

CHAPTER 2

Reproduction

While *lives* end, *life* goes on. Life is passed from one generation to the next, and children carry on after their parents have passed away. This passing on of life from parent to child is a great privilege, but with it comes a great responsibility for the child's physical, mental, emotional, and spiritual welfare. By heredity and the home environment, parents profoundly influence their children's well-being, and determine in large part their intellect and character.

The physical components of the passing on of life will be presented in this section. The reader is advised to read the chapter dealing with the normal reproductive organs of both sexes, and the sexual act by which the father and mother contribute the biological components from which a new human life is formed (see page 1085). This event transpires nine months before the birth of the baby.

The genetics of reproduction

Sex cells differ from the other cells contained within a person's body. The male sex cells, or sperm, are produced in the testes, while the woman's ovum develops within an ovary. During intercourse the sperm are deposited in the woman's vagina. From here they travel via the cervical canal and uterus to the oviducts.

Somewhere in the oviducts, if conception is to take place, a single sperm (a whole cell with only half the number of chromosomes found in a regular cell) enters an ovum (also a whole cell containing only half the chromosomes found in a regular cell), and the two cells combine to form a single cell or fertilized ovum. The fertilized ovum, now a single cell, slowly makes its way through the remainder of the oviduct into the uterus and lodges within the cavity of the uterus, at which point conception has occurred. Should all things proceed normally, nine months later a full-term baby will be born.

Should no male cells be available in the oviduct, or if none are able to penetrate the ovum, the unfertilized ovum will simply pass through the remainder of the oviduct, through the cavity of the uterus, and then perish. If a fertilized ovum is unable to

371

attach itself to the uterine wall, it, too, will be swept out of the uterus and conception will not ensue.

Every cell of the body contains in its nucleus (central portion) a group of twenty-three pairs of rod-shaped chromosomes—forty-six in all. One of each pair of chromosomes is contributed by the father, the other by the mother. Each chromosome, in turn, contains thousands of genes, which are the determiners of all hereditary characteristics such as the color of the eyes, the set of the jaw, and even the dimple in the cheek. Thus these forty-six chromosomes with their mix of thousands of genes hold complete within themselves a potential new human being.

The genes are composed of DNA (deoxyribonucleic acid), the marvelous giant protein molecules that control the form and function of every cell, tissue, and organ of the particular individual. The genes function as blueprints for every cell in the body. In this way every cell is regulated so that the myriads of cells composing the body function cooperatively.

At conception, the fertilized ovum grows by division. The single cell divides to form two, the two divide to form four, four make eight, eight make sixteen, and so on and on. Nine months later this one cell will have multiplied into countless cells to form an infant. The continuation of the growth process requires the continued multiplication of cells.

Every time a cell divides and produces two cells, the chromosomes split also, producing a double set of chromosomes—one for each

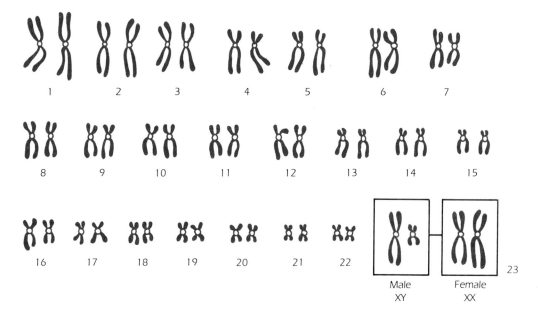

Human chromosomes. Each male and female sex cell has twenty-three pairs of chromosomes. The sex chromosomes are number 23. The males = X Y; the females = X X.

"daughter cell." Thus every cell in the human body contains its full quota of forty-six chromosomes that are an exact copy of the chromosomes in the original single cell. This is true even of the immature sex cells in the testes and the ovaries. However, a remarkable thing happens just before the sex cells mature. One member of each chromosome pair is eliminated. Which chromosome will be lost, whether from the father's or the mother's side, is a matter of chance. Because of this, it is most unlikely that any two sex cells produced by the same individual will have the same mix of chromosomes, whether a sperm or an ovum.

Geneticists estimate that 281 billion combinations of chromosomes are possible when the sex cells from a husband and a wife unite at the time of conception. No wonder, then, that no two brothers and sisters in the same family are exactly alike, with the exception of identical twins.

Defining the baby's sex— boy or girl?

One of the twenty-three pairs of chromosomes in each cell contains the sex chromosomes. In a female, the two members of this pair appear alike and are called X chromosomes. In the male the two members are different, one being an X chromosome and the other a Y chromosome. When a sex cell matures (either sperm or ovum), one member of the sex chromosome is eliminated. In the female sex cell or ovum, the one retained will always be an X chromosome since she only has X chromosomes, while in the male the

chromosome that disappears may be either an X or a Y. Thus a mature sperm may carry an X or a Y chromosome.

At conception, when a sperm carrying an X chromosome unites with an ovum, the fertilized egg will have two X chromosomes and the baby

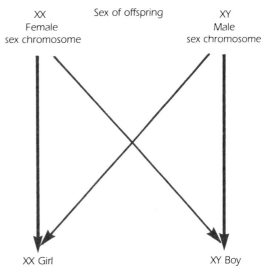

XX
Female
sex chromosome

Sex of offspring

XY
Male
sex chromosome

XX Girl

XY Boy

The sex of the offspring is determined by the contribution of the male sex chromosome. If X, the baby will be a girl; if Y, a boy.

will be a girl. When a sperm carrying a Y chromosome unites with an ovum, the fertilized egg will have one X and one Y chromosome, and the child will be a boy. From this it is obvious that sex determination is a matter of chance, just as are all other matters of heredity.

Twins

Twins are born in approximately one out of ninety births. Some are fraternal twins, others identical.

Fraternal twins, the most common type, result from two female sex cells (ova) being fertilized during the same month. Each of the ova are fertilized by a separate sperm, and thus two embryos are conceived at the same time. Fraternal twins, as far as their heredity is concerned, are no more alike than any other brothers or sisters in the same family. They are simply born at the same time. They may be both boys, both girls, or one boy and one girl.

Identical twins, on the other hand, are derived from a single fertilized ovum. In the early stages of development, within hours after conception, the dividing cells become separated into two identical groups, each of which forms a separate embryo. Since each embryo was derived from the same ovum and the same sperm, the hereditary characteristics are identical, and, of necessity, they are of the same sex—either both boys or both girls.

Heredity vs. environmental influences

Just as a child's sex is determined by chance, depending upon which chromosomes from the father and the mother happened to unite at conception, so the color of the hair, the shape of the face, the general body build, the color of the eyes, and even certain preferences and abilities are randomly determined.

However, not all traits of personality and character are the result of chance at the time of conception. Research is now providing evidence that both the father and the mother transmit to their offspring many of their own character traits, both good and bad. These provide the foundation and framework on which a person then builds his life.

The environment in which the child is reared—physical, intellectual, emotional, and spiritual—profoundly influences his developing personality and character. His home, parents, school, and associates play an important and continuing role in his life until he is an adult, fully responsible for making his own decisions.

A wise person evaluates the hereditary traits received from his parents. He strives to overcome those that are undesirable and to capitalize on those that are good. There is no time for regrets, for life moves steadily on.

What about deformities?

A congenital defect in a baby is a deep concern to its parents. When planning for a child, three circumstances need to be carefully evaluated. First, if a person contemplating marriage wants children and knows that he has a birth defect or that a serious defect has occurred in one of his close relatives or in the family of the person he or she would like to marry, he should ask whether it is advisable to marry.

Second, when a man and woman are already married and know that one of them or a close relative has a birth defect, they should ask whether it would be wise for them to have children. And third, the married couple that already has one child born with a defect should ask whether they ought to risk having another defective child.

Each of these questions is justified, and requires a physician's advice,

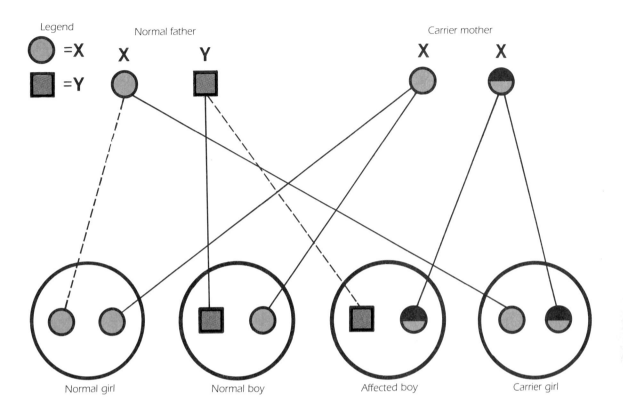

How a carrier mother transmits a sex-linked disease to her offspring.

preferably a specialist such as an obstetrician or a geneticist. The specialist will provide the information the couple needs as they consider the type of defect, the hereditary background, the possible environmental factors, and the possibility of having a second child with the same defect. If some causative factor can be avoided, the risk of having a deformed child will not be so great. If, however, a defect is likely to recur, the couple must decide whether the possibility of a second defective child is worth the risk.

Both parents contribute the genetic material that determines all the characteristics of their offspring—twenty-three pairs of chromosomes in every cell, half from the father, and half from the mother. The genes, with their DNA molecules, are the component parts of the chromosomes, and are actually responsible for transmitting inherited traits.

Inherited deformities occur when there is a flaw in the gene that controls the development of a particular part of the body. When the parents come from unrelated family lines, the defective gene donated in the sperm is not likely to match a similar faulty gene in the ovum. However, if the man and woman are related, as when first or second cousins marry, the probability of their contributing the same faulty gene is greatly increased.

Amniocentesis

Amniocentesis is a method for removing a small amount of amniotic fluid from the uterus with a needle that is directed into the amniotic sac under the guidance of ultrasound. A large variety of tests can be performed on both the amniotic fluid itself and on cells shed from the embryo that are contained in the amniotic fluid. These analyses are performed in a laboratory and require several weeks to complete. The test is usually performed during the first sixteen weeks of pregnancy. More than sixty fetal disorders can be detected or ruled out with an accuracy of over 99 percent.

Amniocentesis entails a small risk, so it is not performed routinely. However, it is recommended for women who become pregnant at or after the age of thirty-five; for women who have had three or more miscarriages; and where there is a history of Down's syndrome, spina bifida, hemophilia, and other genetic abnormalities in either parent. An example

of the test's usefulness is seen in detecting Down's syndrome. This inherited disorder occurs once in every 300 births in women in their mid-thirties; once in thirty births for women in their early forties; and once in ten births during the mid-forties. Certain other disorders also increase with the mother's age.

When a defect is found, depending on its nature, parents face crucial choices. Many have found that even a defective child enjoys a meaningful life and brings joy to the family. Allowing the pregnancy to proceed means, of course, making the appropriate adjustment in caring for a handicapped child. Fortunately, the vast majority of these tests show that fetal development is normal, which is very reassuring to concerned parents.

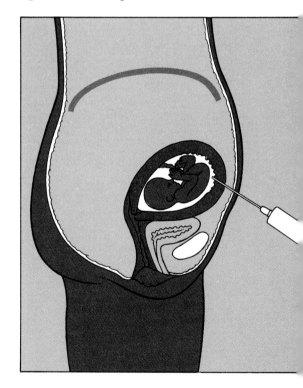

Amniocentesis: the withdrawal of amniotic fluid by needle.

Unfavorable environmental conditions

The cells that form the various specialized tissues of the developing baby's organs and body systems are especially vulnerable during the early weeks of embryonic life. At this time, anything that deprives these cells of their physiological needs can give rise to defects. Examples are a particular vitamin or mineral deficiency, and a reduction in the amount of oxygen delivered to the cells, such as when certain anesthetics are used during early pregnancy. Also, the fetus is endangered any time the attachment of the placenta to the mother's uterus is disturbed.

Carbon monoxide poisoning during early pregnancy can injure the cells of the fetus by reducing the amount of oxygen it receives. The presence of carbon monoxide in tobacco smoke is just one of the important reasons why smoking is harmful to the fetus. Alcohol, caffeine, and certain other drugs (see pages 263, 276, and 292) also have detrimental effects.

X-rays have been a great boon to mankind, especially in the diagnosis and treatment of injuries and disease, but an expectant mother must avoid all unnecessary exposure during the early months of pregnancy. Rapidly multiplying cells are more susceptible to the damaging effects of X-rays than at any other time of life, especially during the period of cell differentiation. And the damage may not be apparent until the deformed fetus is born. A pregnant woman should receive only the most essential X-rays, and these should be administered with the utmost caution. Every effort must be made to shield the developing fetus.

German measles (rubella) is a mild illness for a woman, but it is an extremely dangerous illness to a fetus. The virus is a common cause of deformity, with a 50 percent incidence of impairment if the disease occurs during the first month of pregnancy. Fortunately, the likelihood of an abnormality decreases when the illness occurs later than the first month, and is virtually nonexistent after the fourth month.

Public health organizations urge that children, especially girls under the age of twelve, be immunized against German measles. To delay such immunization until a girl becomes a wife and conceives is a needless danger to the life of her offspring, since a vaccination is in reality a mild form of the disease.

CHAPTER 3

Pregnancy

Motherhood provides one of the most intimate bonds that can exist between two human beings. Its closeness is rivaled only by that between husband and wife.

The role of parents

We hear much about planned parenthood, and this emphasis is well placed, for the future welfare of the child—physically, mentally, emotionally, and spiritually—depends in large part on the contribution *both* parents make to the child to be. The quality of sex cells (sperm and ovum) determines the hereditary endowment that father and mother bestow on their offspring.

The importance of the father's role has not been given the attention it deserves. Studies in many countries by numerous investigators have shown some startling findings. Alcoholic parents transmit their cravings to their children and grandchildren. Writing in the *Archives of General Psychiatry,* Dr. Donald A. Goodwin of Washington University, St. Louis, and his associates make this remarkable statement: "The 'father's sins' may in fact be visited on the sons without the father's presence."[1] Other research suggests that the transmission of a tendency to alcoholism occurs through a dominant gene.

It is well known that injurious chemicals (drugs or toxins) in the mother's blood adversely influence the development of the fetus. Infants born to smoking mothers have lower birth weights than do those born to nonsmoking women. Other problems in early development are also present. Thus, such a child fails to receive the good start in life that he deserves.

The quality of the sex cells that the father and the mother contribute and the mother's health during pregnancy are also important factors. The susceptibility to adverse influences on the sperm and ovum before conception is just as great as that on the fertilized ovum after conception. Preparation for pregnancy thus focuses on the quality of the sex cells contributed at the time of conception. Anyone can benefit from a program that promotes health, but this is particularly important for couples considering whether to have a child. They should adopt a strict health enhancement program at least three months before conception, and a longer period is better. (For details, see page 124 under "a healthful lifestyle.")

This health program should include the following: adequate exercise, preferably outdoors; a wholesome diet; adequate rest; and a calm, happy attitude. Overweight people should go on a weight-reduction program under the guidance of their physician. Alcohol, tobacco, and drinks that contain caffeine (coffee, tea, mate [mah-teh], and cola soft drinks) should be avoided, as caffeine adversely affects the fetus. Medications should only be taken on the advice of a physician.

Any couple contemplating having a family should be sure they want one. The demands on the wife are considerable, both physically and emotionally. Raising a child should involve both parents, for it takes many years and a great deal of money. Under no circumstances should a couple ever

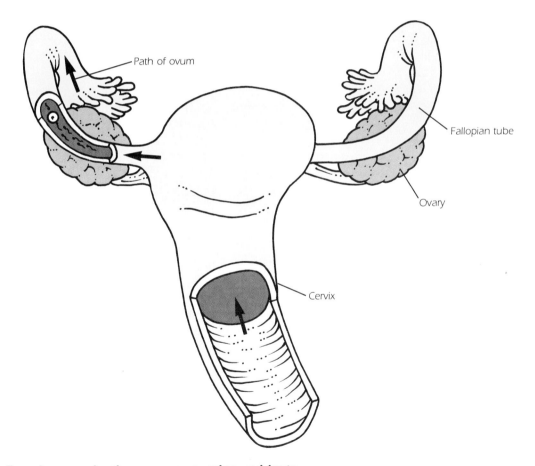

Female reproductive organs: ovaries, oviducts, uterus, cervix, and vagina.

Path of ovum

Fallopian tube

Ovary

Cervix

379

decide to have a child in order to save a tottering marriage or to give a parent the pleasure of a grandchild.

Evidences of pregnancy

During the early period of pregnancy, it is usually difficult to know whether conception has actually occurred. In fact, doubt may persist until the mother's **enlarging abdomen** makes the situation obvious.

The usual first clue is **missing a regular menstrual period.** Menstruation does not normally occur during pregnancy. If the menses have been regular, missing one is an important indicator, but the question is left open for women who experience irregular periods. A serious illness, excessive emotional strain, or disturbances of the endocrine organs can also interfere with the usual menstrual cycle.

Another common early clue of pregnancy is **morning sickness.** One out of two women experiences nausea and some vomiting soon after the beginning of pregnancy. The problem disappears spontaneously after the third month. This symptom is reason enough to see your physician. If the vomiting is severe, the doctor can prescribe a medication that will provide relief.

Another indicator of pregnancy is **tenderness and enlargement of the breasts.** This is a physiological response to the hormones controlling the events of pregnancy that begin preparing the glandular tissue of the breasts to provide milk after the child is born.

Pregnancy tests that are taken about two weeks after the first missed menstrual period are about 95 percent dependable. The test evaluates a small sample of the woman's urine. Serum pregnancy tests are reliable at the time of the first missed period.

The mother adapts

The development and growth of a new human that within nine months is sufficiently mature to get along nicely in the outside world is remarkable, but two other marvels are also associated with pregnancy. The first is the capacity of the mother's body to alter its structure and function to meet the new demands made upon it. The second, just as wonderful, is its capacity to return to its previous condition following the birth of the child.

The mother's body begins to alter its structure and function in response to the arrival within the uterus of the cells from which the fetus will develop. As already mentioned (see page 371), the union of the sperm and ovum takes place in the oviduct. Within the next thirty-six hours, the single cell will have divided to form two cells exactly alike. These, in turn, subdivide again and again, forming a small mass of cells.

It takes about three or four days for these cells to travel through the rest of the oviduct and reach the uterus. By this time the tiny clump of cells contains at least sixteen cells. During the first eight weeks, it is commonly called the **embryo.**

When the embryo reaches the uterus, it penetrates the cells lining the uterine wall (uterine mucosa),

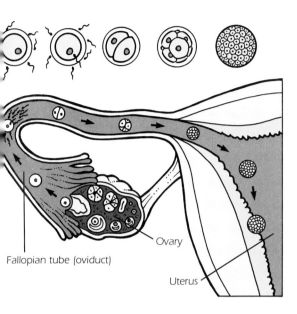

Fallopian tube (oviduct)

Ovary

Uterus

Fertilization of an ovum by a single sperm takes place within the fallopian tube (oviduct).

and becomes completely surrounded by them. As it develops, the embryo derives its nourishment from the mucosal cells, which produce what is known as "uterine milk." Within a few weeks the embryo continues enlarging till it completely fills the uterine cavity. From then on the wall of the uterus must continually stretch in order to accommodate the growing embryo (later called the **fetus**) and the fluid-filled membranes that surround it.

Two hormones, progesterone and estrogen (see page 1089), increase in concentration at this time and work together to bring about three changes: they stimulate the uterus to accommodate the increasing size of the embryo and the placenta; they promote the growth of the embryo; and they stimulate the development of the mother's breasts in preparation for the production of milk following childbirth.

Eventually the uterine "milk" becomes inadequate to meet the needs of the rapidly growing embryo, so a special organ called the **placenta** develops adjacent to the embryo. Attached to the uterus, it meets the embryo's need for nourishment. The placenta transfers oxygen and food from the mother's blood to the embryo, and transports carbon dioxide and other wastes from the embryo's blood to that of the mother. After the eighth week the embryo is called the **fetus**—a name that it carries until birth. An **umbilical cord** with connecting blood vessels attaches itself to the outer surface of the placenta and extends between it and the body of the fetus.

The placenta grows in proportion to the growth of the fetus, eventually reaching a diameter of about 7 inches (17.5 cm). Both the mother's blood and that of the fetus circulate within the placenta, separated from each other by a membrane so thin that substances easily pass from one bloodstream to the other in either direction.

The placenta makes it possible for the fetus to carry on its vital functions while still within its mother's uterus and surrounded by fluid. The fetus does not have to breathe, because it receives oxygen through the placenta. It does not have to eat, because the nutrients it needs are brought to it by the same route. And its waste materials are transferred through the placenta to the mother's blood and eliminated

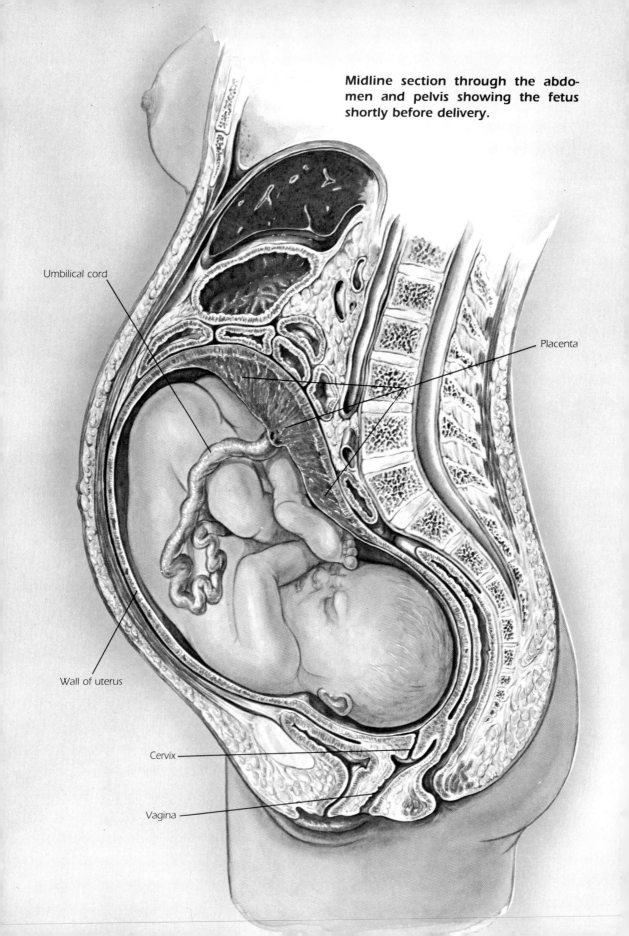

Umbilical cord

Placenta

Wall of uterus

Cervix

Vagina

Midline section through the abdomen and pelvis showing the fetus shortly before delivery.

through her organs of elimination. The fetus uses the mother's lungs, digestive organs, and kidneys in place of its own during this developmental period. Partly for this reason, the functions of all the mother's body organs must increase during pregnancy.

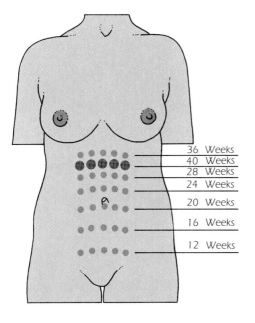

36 Weeks
40 Weeks
28 Weeks
24 Weeks
20 Weeks
16 Weeks
12 Weeks

The progress of pregnancy is estimated by the increasing height of the uterus.

See your physician

Pregnancy is a normal physiological occurrence rather than a disease. A normal pregnancy should terminate in a normal delivery at full term, with both mother and child in excellent health. If you are a prospective mother, you naturally want to do everything possible to ensure the birth of a normal child and give it the best possible start in life. It is wise, therefore, to see your physician as early as possible. Your doctor may

be a family physician, or he may be an obstetrician who specializes in this area. Some prospective mothers choose a licensed midwife who has adequate medical backup. The person you choose to assist you with the delivery of your baby will want to provide prenatal care as well, since he or she can best serve your needs by keeping informed of your progress as the time for delivery draws near. The entire service is included in a regular fee.

If you do not already have a physician and wish to make a wise selection, check with a local hospital, the health department in your county, the local medical society, or a public-health nurse.

Generally an expectant mother sees her physician every month for the first six months, every two weeks for the next two months, and every week during the last month of pregnancy.

At the time of your first visit, your physician will take a medical history. He will inquire regarding your past surgeries, illnesses, and pregnancies, your family's history of twins, and the father's health. He will also give you a physical examination to determine your pelvic measurements and general well-being. Laboratory tests generally include a Pap smear, blood count, blood type, Rh factor, and syphilis test. Especially if you are over the age of thirty, your physician may recommend additional tests, such as evaluation of your amniotic fluid (obtained through amniocentesis) for genetic abnormalities, or a maternal serum alpha-feto protein test, which detects neural tube defects.

383

Should you develop an infectious disease during your pregnancy or be exposed to one, report it to your physician immediately, or it may cause damage to your unborn child. The most serious of these diseases is German measles (see page 421).

Delivery date

Your physician will help you calculate the approximate time at which you may expect your baby to be born. Conception usually occurs about two weeks after the first day of the previous menstruation. From the day of conception to the day of delivery should be approximately 266 days (thirty-eight weeks or nine calendar months). On the other hand, if you estimate from the first day of your last menstrual period to term you should allow 280 days (forty weeks or ten lunar months).

One easy way to arrive at the probable date of childbirth is to count ahead nine months from the first day of the last menstruation and then add seven days. For example, if your last menstrual period began February 7, counting ahead nine months would bring you to November 7. Adding a week brings you to November 14, the expected delivery date. You can achieve the same thing by adding twelve months, subtracting three months, and adding one week. If your last menstrual period began February 7 of this year, twelve months later brings you to February 7 of next year. Subtract three months, add one week, and you come to the same November 14 delivery date.

This day is only an approximation and is by no means certain. A baby born three weeks before or two weeks after the calculated date is considered a normal, full-term infant. Many women have irregular monthly cycles, especially if they have been taking contraceptive medications. Calculating the birth date is even more difficult for these women.

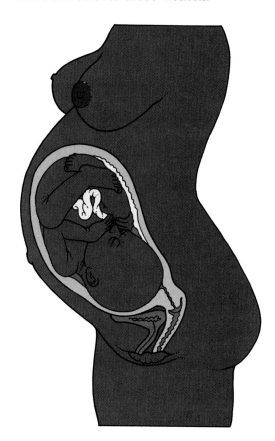

Late in pregnancy the head of the fetus lies low in the uterus.

Signs of progress

There are two common ways of measuring the progress of pregnancy. One is to divide the period of pregnancy into three periods of three months (thirteen weeks), each called a trimester, and the other is to count the number of weeks elapsed since the beginning of the last menstrual period.

At about five weeks the embryo should be about the size of a grain of wheat. At twelve weeks, when it is called a fetus, it is approximately 2.5 inches (6 cm) long. At sixteen weeks you may feel the baby move—a sort of delicate flutter. From this time to delivery is usually twenty-two to twenty-four weeks. Not all mothers experience this "quickening," and its absence does not indicate a problem. As the fetus grows, the movements become more vigorous and may even be observed through the abdominal wall.

Programs for mothers

Specially designed general classes and exercise programs are available in most communities for pregnant mothers. Inquire from your physician or health department about where you might enroll. Such classes are usually conducted by trained instructors. They will prepare you for delivery and for problems you might encounter when nursing your baby.

Diet and pregnancy

Pregnancy, as already pointed out, is not a disease but a normal physiological episode. Common sense, then, should tell you that drastic changes in your diet are not needed unless your diet before pregnancy has been unsatisfactory. Assuming that your diet before becoming pregnant was adequate, the customary recommendation of taking increased quantities of specific nutrients (vitamins, minerals, and protein) is unnecessary. A good diet before pregnancy will provide all essential elements during both pregnancy and lactation. The amount you eat may vary. You will very likely eat more toward the latter part of your pregnancy and during the time you nurse your baby. But it is not desirable for you to "eat for two" and gain weight, nor is a fat baby necessarily a healthy baby.

If your diet has been and is inadequate, you should make the appropriate changes. Follow the simple suggestions on page 237. The most critical time, when your need for nutrients is absolutely essential for the developing embryo inside of you, is during the first three to four months of pregnancy. Unfortunately, this is the time when many women suffer from morning sickness and do not handle food well, forcing their body to draw on its nutritional reserves. This is one situation in which your physician may recommend that you take food supplements. However, it is better to place yourself on a good diet some time before conception rather than trying to compensate for possible deficiencies after conception has occurred.

Exercise

A regular exercise program is important at all times, and this is especially true during pregnancy. Your baby's health depends on your health. Exercise will keep you fit and your muscles strong. Your food will digest better, and your sleep will be sounder. Walking (jogging if you have been doing it), swimming, gardening, and calisthenics are all ap-

385

propriate. However, you should avoid sports in which you might injure yourself or the baby, and avoid weight-lifting activities as term approaches.

Especially direct your exercises toward helping you to stand correctly and to strengthen the muscles of your abdominal wall, pelvic floor, and low back. Your local health department undoubtedly provides a pamphlet that tells you how to do these exercises.

Travel

In general, you do not need to restrict your travel because of pregnancy, except perhaps during the last few weeks as the delivery day nears. At this time you should be sure that you are reasonably close to a hospital and/or to your physician. Because sitting for prolonged periods, as in a car or bus, accentuates swelling in the ankles and feet, it is best, when traveling, to stop periodically and walk around. If you are in a plane, walk in the aisle if possible. Many planes will not accept passengers nearing delivery. Anytime you use a seat belt, whether riding in a car or plane, be sure to position the lower strap over your pelvis, not over your lower abdomen.

Sexual intercourse

Healthy couples can maintain normal sexual intercourse during the first six months of pregnancy. As the womb enlarges, intercourse should be done lying on the side to avoid undue pressure on the mother's abdomen. Your physician can advise you whether to discontinue intercourse during the last month of your pregnancy.

The desire for sexual activity during pregnancy varies from woman to woman. In some the desire increases, while in others it decreases. It would be desirable for your husband to accompany you now and then when you visit your physician. This will give him a better understanding of his role during your pregnancy. Should you experience any bleeding or discomfort (cramps) after intercourse, see your physician.

Personal hygiene

Daily baths or showers are even more advisable during pregnancy because the glands of the skin are now more active. During the last month, a shower is preferable to a bath because it reduces the possibility of germs entering the birth canal. For the same reason, it is advisable that a woman not douche at any time during her pregnancy. Consult your physician if you have a distressing discharge.

Body weight

It is not uncommon for a woman to lose a few pounds during the first three or four months of pregnancy. This is usually due to the nausea and vomiting of morning sickness. However, after that, an average gain of a pound a week (for a total of about 24 pounds or 11 kg) is normal. This extra weight comes from a number of sources, including the increasing size of the uterus, breasts, and muscles of the low back and pelvis; the enlarging placenta; the expanding membranes; the increasing amniotic fluid; the more dense bones; and, of course, the growing fetus. The approximate distribution of weight among the various structures is shown in the table below.

Women who lose significant weight during the first twelve weeks should gain this back in addition to the usual 24 pounds. If weight gain during pregnancy is excessive, childbirth may be more difficult because of an oversized baby, and the mother's weight will not return promptly to its former level after the baby is born. On the other hand, severe weight restriction during pregnancy interferes with normal development of the baby.

In addition to the gain in weight due to the growing fetus, the enlarging uterus, the developing membranes, and accumulating fluids, other profound changes are occurring in the woman's body. The volume of her blood doubles, and her tissues take on water. Her muscles enlarge to carry the increasing weight, and as a result, her bones become more dense. Many of these changes have a double role. They are essential both for fetal growth and development and for carrying the pregnancy successfully to term. But after the birth of the baby, as the uterus shrinks and the enlarged muscles and dense bones return to normal, the extra protein, calcium, and phosphorus stored in these structures are used by the lactating breasts to provide the infant with the milk it needs.

You should study carefully the details regarding a desirable diet during pregnancy (see page 385). Keep in mind, also, that any time a pregnant woman suffers a nutritional deficiency, she and the fetus compete for the available nutrients, and contrary to popular belief, the fetus usually suffers the loss.

After the first three months of pregnancy, a woman's weight gain should be steady. Abrupt changes are a danger signal that should be immediately reported to your physician. Rapid weight gain is a symptom

Weight gain in pregnant women		
Source	Pounds	Kilograms
Fetus	7.5	3.4
Uterus	2.0	0.9
Placenta	1.5	0.7
Amniotic fluid	2.0	0.9
Fetal membranes	0.5	0.2
Breasts	1.5	0.7
Blood and body fluids	6.0	2.7
Bones, muscles, and fat	3.0	1.4
TOTAL	24.0	10.9

of toxemia of pregnancy or pre-eclampsia, in which the body retains fluid (which causes the rapid weight gain), the blood pressure rises, and protein is lost in the urine. This is a serious situation. Sudden weight loss may also indicate a problem.

Mental attitudes

There is some evidence that the mother's attitudes during pregnancy may influence the attitudes of her developing child. Prospective mothers should be encouraged to have the most wholesome attitudes possible. If the child is not wanted, if the mother is afraid that the child might be abnormal, or if she dreads the experience of childbirth, these mental conflicts and fears can affect the fetus negatively. The hormonal mix in the mother's blood may influence the developing child.

It is certain that a mother's prevailing attitudes have their influence on her state of health. Other factors being equal, the woman who is optimistic, cheerful, and courageous will enjoy more abundant health than the one who harbors unpleasant and unwholesome mental attitudes. This principle applies at least as much during pregnancy as at other times of life.

Development before birth

Many things happen between the moment of conception and the time the infant takes its first breath. The hereditary ledger itself is closed nine months before the parents lay eyes on their child. The combination of chromosomes contributed by both father and mother determines whether the child will be a boy or girl, have dark hair or light, have brown eyes or blue, whether it will be of stocky build or slight, etc. Even the child's mental capacities—its inclination to be a scholar, tradesman, or artist—are largely determined by the genetic mix contributed by the union of the sperm and ovum.

However, during the next several months, this single microscopic cell will unfold into a trillion cells packaged in a 7 1/2-pound (3.5 kg) baby: a brain with its myriad sensors, a heart with its pulsating vessels, a stomach with its digestive organs, a kidney with its million filters, a lung with its tiny air sacs, skin, blood, bone, and muscle—all these and so much more, in just nine short months!

The nine-month period from conception to birth is roughly divided into three-month periods called **trimesters.** The characteristics of the growth of the embryo and fetus and the changes occurring in the mother are grouped under the events of the first, second, and third trimesters.

The first trimester

That wondrous cell. All cells in the human body descend from the one original cell composed of the united fractions of sperm and ovum.

The fertilized ovum promptly separates into two identical cells, and these keep on dividing until a small colony of cells is formed, each cell exactly like every other cell.

But then a wondrous thing occurs. Within a few days, certain of these cells begin to develop differently from others, some being modified to become the ancestors of all the muscle cells; others to form nerve cells; and still others to form bone, tendon, skin, and membrane cells.

As a cell specializes, its functions become limited and adapted in a way that best fits it to carry on its particular role. For example, muscle cells acquire the ability to shorten when stimulated, but they can no longer move from place to place as do blood cells or generate impulses as do nerve cells or produce secretions or hormones as can gland cells. Bone cells develop the ability to form fibers and interlace them with mineral salts to give rigid support to the body, but bone cells cannot contract as do muscle cells nor can they produce hydrochloric acid as do gland cells in the stomach wall.

The wall of the stomach is made of smooth muscle cells on the outside and gland cells on the inside, held together with fibers of connective tissue. Interspersed between them are blood vessels and nerves. Thus, by appropriately combining different specialized cells, all the structures and organs of the body are formed.

At one month. Four weeks after conception the tiny embryo is only 1/4 inch (0.6 cm) long, yet already there are the beginnings of a brain; signs of the eyes, ears, and nose; a heart that has begun to beat, pushing blood through minute blood vessels; lungs with tiny sacs; and a digestive tube with a beginning liver.

At two months. During the second month, the embryo increases 6 times in length and 500 times in weight. It now measures about 1-1/2 inches (4 cm). A face develops, with a mouth and nose, eyes that have lids, and ears. Arms and legs also appear, with joints and fingers. The miniature bones, composed primarily of cartilage, are soft and flexible, and lend some support to the miniature muscles attached to them. The heart, with its four chambers, is well established, rhythmically pumping blood through its expanding network of arteries and veins. Even the internal sex organs are formed, and if studied under a microscope, the ovaries of a girl can be distinguished from the testes of a boy.

Yet the expectant mother, having missed only two menstrual periods, is still unsure whether she is even pregnant! The changes within are not noticeable without.

At three months. The embryo is now called a fetus. By the end of the third month, the fetus weighs about an ounce (30 gm) and measures almost 4 inches (10 cm). The different organ systems are being established. The digestive tract emerges with its accessory glands, together with the kidneys and their filters. The different parts of the brain are also forming.

The second trimester

While differentiation of tissues continues, the second three-month period is primarily distinguished by the rapid growth of the fetus. It more than doubles its length, from 4 to 14 inches (10 to 25 cm), while increasing more than thirty-two-fold in weight, from 1 ounce to more than 2 pounds (900 gm).

The mother's pregnancy now becomes obvious. Her enlarging breasts and bulging abdomen can be observed by others, and before the trimester is over (at the twentieth week), she will be able to feel the fetus moving within her womb.

The third trimester

The last trimester is a period of weight gain for the now-maturing fetus. It will gain 1 pound during the first month, a pound and a half the second, and almost double its weight the last and final month, to about 7.5

pounds (3.4 kg). However, a weight range from 4.5 to 11 pounds (2 to 5 kg) is completely normal for a healthy full-term baby.

During the third trimester, the mother's uterus will enlarge to contain the rapidly growing fetus and its accumulating amniotic fluid, and her posture will change to help her cope with the increasing weight. Women tend to experience increasing discomfort during this time, both when standing and lying. The joints between the pelvic bones are loosening, making walking awkward. Two or more weeks before the onset of labor, the head of the fetus will "drop," or descend, into the lower pelvis. Urination may become frequent as the bladder is further compressed.

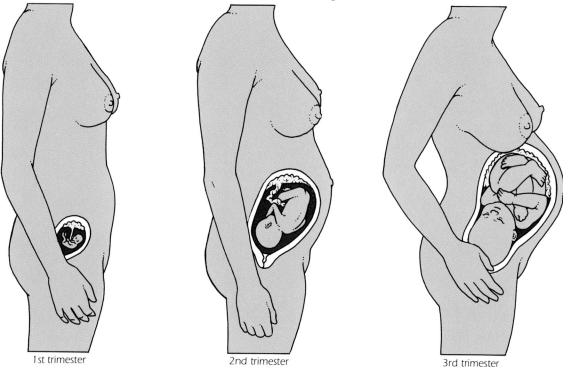

1st trimester   2nd trimester   3rd trimester

During the three trimesters of pregnancy, the size of the fetus changes, as does the posture of the mother.

Problems during pregnancy

Happiness and security mean more during pregnancy than at any other time. Use self-discipline, and cultivate optimism. This will help you personally, and will react favorably on your developing fetus. Make allowance for certain unavoidable discomforts and limitations, and do not allow yourself to become fretful and apprehensive. The following is a discussion of some of the problems that arise and some suggestions that may help you resolve them.

Medical and dental emergencies

Should you require medical or dental help, tell your physician (if he is not the physician who is caring for your pregnancy) or dentist that you are pregnant. Since virtually all medications taken by the mother pass from her blood to the blood of the fetus, seek the counsel of your physician or dentist before taking any medication. Should X-rays be required, they should be kept at a minimum, and the pelvic area should be carefully protected against unnecessary exposure. If they are available, other diagnostic procedures such as ultrasound are much preferred. If surgery is required, local anesthetics are less likely to affect the fetus than are general anesthetics.

Fatigue

It is normal to feel tired, especially during the first three months of pregnancy. At this time your body is making major adjustments. Make sure that you get adequate sleep each night, and if possible take a rest during the day, preferably in mid-afternoon.

Frequent urination

At certain times during pregnancy, the enlarging uterus or the head of the infant will exert pressure on the bladder, and the urge to urinate may occur even though there is little urine in the bladder. If this problem becomes extremely troublesome or is accompanied with burning, see your physician.

Swelling of the ankles

Pregnant women accumulate considerable quantities of fluid in their tissues (see page 387), some of which collects in the lower legs, ankles, and feet. The pressure on the veins in the pelvic area, retarding the return of blood to the heart, partially contributes to ankle swelling. Excessive salt intake and a decrease in physical activity may also be causes. You can relieve this problem somewhat by exercising more frequently, elevating your feet when sitting, and reducing your salt intake.

Should the swelling become severe, and should it also occur in the hands and face, see your physician immediately, since this may indicate that you have a serious condition (toxemia of pregnancy).

Food cravings

Many women develop a strong desire for certain foods during pregnancy, such as for confections, and even for unusual tastes. This does not mean that your body has a need for any particular food elements. A good, nutritious diet is all that is necessary.

Morning sickness

Almost all pregnant women experience some discomfort in their stomachs during early pregnancy. Most feel nauseated, and some vomit, especially on awakening in the morning. This condition disappears spontaneously by the third or fourth month. Dry toast the first thing in the morning may help. Small, low-fat meals are also helpful. If the condition becomes severe, see your physician, as you could become dehydrated and develop a mineral imbalance. Because of possible harm to your fetus, do not take any medications to relieve morning sickness without first consulting your physician.

Heartburn

Most pregnant women suffer heartburn, a burning sensation in the region of the lower breastbone or upper abdomen, during pregnancy. Contrary to its name, this condition has nothing to do with the heart, but results from stomach contents and acid flowing back into the lower esophagus or gullet. Late in pregnancy the enlarging womb often makes the condition worse. Small meals seem to help. Should the condition become intolerable, see your physician, who may recommend an acceptable antacid. Do not use soda, as it may upset your body's chemical balance.

Constipation

Women frequently experience constipation during pregnancy. As the womb enlarges, pressure is placed on the terminal colon, impeding the movements of the bowel. The tone of the muscles in the pelvic floor and lower abdomen is decreased, diminishing the usual propulsive strength. Fortunately, several simple but effective measures can help to eliminate the problem. These include drinking lots of water, regular exercise, and eating foods high in dietary fiber (fruits, vegetables, and whole grain cereals). If the condition persists, do not use laxatives unless your physician approves.

Hemorrhoids and varicose veins

Enlargement of the veins inside the anus (hemorrhoids) and in the legs (varicose veins) is more common during pregnancy than at other times. This occurs because the pressure of the uterus on the veins in the pelvis interferes with the return of blood from the lower parts of the body. Hemorrhoids may cause discomfort and pain, while varicose veins make the legs feel heavy and tired.

For hemorrhoids, avoid getting constipated or straining when you have a bowel movement. Increase the amount of fiber in your diet, drink plenty of water, place a little lubricant inside the anal canal, and possibly use a softening agent (see your pharmacist) for your bowel movements. For varicose veins, avoid wearing tight garments or crossing your legs when sitting. Use support hose on awakening in the morning, and whenever you rest, raise your feet above the level of your heart. If your work requires you to stand a lot, break it up with short walks. Both hemorrhoids and varicose veins will improve or disappear after delivery.

Backache

Backache is common in pregnant women. As the enlarging womb causes your center of gravity to shift, appropriate adjustments will occur in your posture. Later in the pregnancy, the joints of your pelvis will slacken, enlarging the pelvic opening for the passage of the infant during delivery. Good posture and appropriate exercises to strengthen the muscles of your abdomen and back (see under "posture," page 962) should help to ease the discomfort. Low-heeled shoes may also help. Backache usually disappears after childbirth.

Cramps

Some women experience cramps in their legs and, sometimes, in the area of the lower abdomen and groin. For suggestions on relief of **leg cramps,** see page 963.

Pain and spasm in the groin area may be due to stretching of either the right or left round ligament **(round ligament pain),** which holds the enlarging womb in position. Lying on your back and bringing your knees up toward your chest (knee-to-chest position) may give relief. A heating pad or hot-water bottle may also provide comfort. If the pains become intense and occur rhythmically, see your physician.

Nerve pains

The cause of nerve pain is similar to that of cramps. As the fetus grows it crowds the pelvis, and pressure is often applied to the nerves passing through the pelvic area. If the right or left sciatic nerve is involved, you will experience a sharp pain in your buttocks and down the back of your thigh. The treatment is the same as for cramps.

Some women experience a tingling ("pins-and-needles") sensation in the vaginal area. This is also due to pressure on the local nerves from the growing fetus. Such sensations may also be felt in the neck, shoulders, and arms. This is due to a pull on the nerves passing from the lower neck, across the shoulder, to the arms. The cause is the weight of the enlarging breasts. Swinging the arms and raising the shoulders should provide comfort.

Skin changes

Pale red streaks commonly appear in the skin of the abdomen and breasts as these parts enlarge during pregnancy. These **striae** are due to the stretching of the skin. This redness will fade after childbirth.

About two-thirds of Caucasian women develop a blotchy, browning pigmentation of the skin of the forehead, temples, nose, and cheekbone area during pregnancy. This condition is called **chloasma,** or "mask of pregnancy." It is a physiological response to the excess of hormones during pregnancy. The condition is aggravated by exposure to sunlight, but it fades after delivery.

Complications of pregnancy

More serious complications may also occur during pregnancy, and the most common of these will now be discussed.

Vaginal bleeding

Spotting or a brownish, discolored discharge is not uncommon during the early part of pregnancy, especially at the time the first two or three periods would have occurred. However, bright red blood that is flowing indicates a serious problem that you should report to your physician immediately, as it may threaten both your life and that of your child. Such bleeding may indicate a miscarriage, an ectopic pregnancy, or a separated placenta.

Miscarriage

Miscarriage is a spontaneous delivery of the fetus before it has developed sufficiently to survive in the outside world. Arbitrarily, it is the birth of the fetus before the fifth month of pregnancy. One in five of all pregnancies terminates in a miscarriage, and about half of those occurring during the first three months are due to an abnormality of the fetus (genetic defects) so severe that the child would not have survived even if it had been delivered at full term. A miscarriage does not mean that you can never have a baby, but you should consult with your physician before planning a future pregnancy.

Bleeding from the vagina during pregnancy, sometimes with cramping, is the usual precursor of a miscarriage. With as much bed rest as possible, the pregnancy may continue to full term. This is called a "threatened miscarriage." Should the bleeding continue and increase in intensity, with the cramps turning into contractions, the condition becomes an "inevitable miscarriage" (or inevitable abortion). The fetus is dead, and the process cannot be interrupted.

When the placenta and sac with the fetus are expelled together, the miscarriage is "complete." If the placenta or part of the membranes remain within the uterus, it is known as an "incomplete miscarriage." Your physician must remove whatever remains, or a serious infection may develop. Under anesthesia, the cervix is dilated, and the uterine cavity curetted ("D&C"). Occasionally a fetus will die, but a miscarriage does not occur. This is called a "missed miscarriage." When this happens, the fetus and supporting structures must be removed—if early, by a D&C; otherwise, by induced labor.

Although the causes for most miscarriages are not known, those that are known include an abnormal fetus (the majority of cases), abuse of drugs (including excessive use of alcohol, tobacco, and caffeine-containing beverages), hormonal imbalance, inadequate nutrition, severe emotional stress, and, very rarely, a fall or other injury.

The majority of subsequent pregnancies are normal. Check with your physician to determine if you have any problem that can be corrected. Your doctor will counsel you when to resume intercourse (usually three or four weeks after the miscarriage), and when to plan your next pregnancy (generally after you have had two normal menstrual periods). Do not incriminate yourself or your spouse, but make the appropriate changes in your lifestyles.

Ectopic pregnancy

The term *ectopic* means "not in the normal place," and in pregnancy refers to a fertilized ovum developing outside the uterus or womb, most frequently in the oviduct. For details, see page 1099.

Hypertensive disorders of pregnancy

Toxemias, seen in 5 to 10 percent of all pregnancies, are serious illnesses occurring during the latter part of pregnancy. Symptoms include a rise in blood pressure; an increase in body fluids, with sudden gain in weight and swelling of the tissues of the face and fingers (edema); and the presence of protein in the urine. This condition is known as preeclampsia. With good professional care, mild preeclampsia can be kept under control. This includes rest in bed, a nutritious diet, and plenty of water. The ailment disappears following pregnancy.

Without adequate care, the mother may develop severe preeclampsia, in which she suffers headache, disturbance of vision, severe vomiting, and pain in the stomach. Occasionally

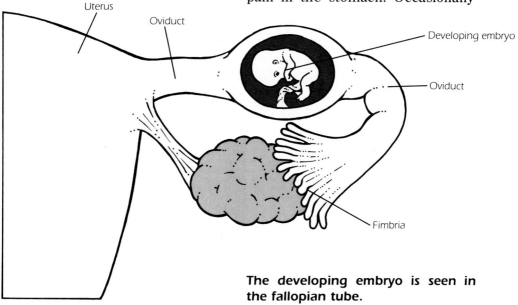

Uterus

Oviduct

Developing embryo

Oviduct

Fimbria

The developing embryo is seen in the fallopian tube.

convulsions may develop, in which case the condition is called **eclampsia.** Should this happen, your physician might decide to terminate the pregnancy by inducing labor or performing a Caesarean section.

The possibility of toxemia and its more serious forms is just one of the many reasons why your physician prefers to observe your pregnancy throughout the nine-month period, rather than seeing you just before delivery.

Umbilical cord problems

Abnormalities of the cord capable of impeding blood flow include loops around the neck; knotting, due to ac-

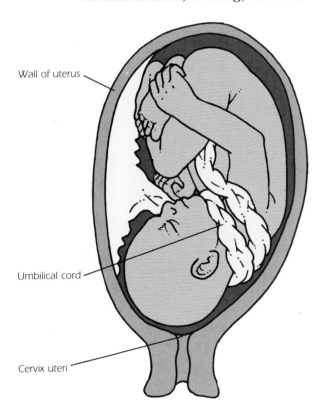

Wall of uterus

Umbilical cord

Cervix uteri

Umbilical cord wrapped around an infant's neck.

tive fetal movements; torsion—the cord becoming twisted; and stricture or narrowing of the cord, usually associated with stillborns.

In approximately one out of four fetuses the umbilical cord is coiled around the neck one or more times, but generally this does no harm. It is an uncommon cause of fetal death. When, at the time of delivery, the cord is felt encircling the neck, it should be pulled over the head. If this is not possible, it should be clamped and cut, and the baby delivered promptly. In twin pregnancies, the possibility of the cords becoming entangled is considerable. The cords may be entwined around one another, or around the neck of a twin.

Placental tumors

In a rare situation the cells of the placenta grow excessively at the expense of the fetus. The most common growth is called a **hydatidiform mole.** For a detailed discussion of this and placental tumors, see page 1103.

Placenta previa and abruptio

In **placenta previa,** the placenta is attached near the cervix or completely covers its opening. In these positions it is poorly attached and can easily break away. Difficulties usually arise during the latter half of the pregnancy, when sporadic bleeding occurs, with the possibility of premature delivery. Ultrasound studies may reveal the extent of the problem. Bed rest and the avoidance of intercourse may delay delivery. Should the bleeding be severe, transfusions are essential to protect the baby from permanent brain damage. When the placenta completely covers the cervical opening, a Cesarean section is the only safe way to deliver the baby.

In **placenta abruptio,** the placenta is normally attached, but because of hypertension, advanced anemia, a severe blow (as in an accident), or an extremely short umbilical cord, the organ suddenly becomes detached from the wall of the uterus. Depending on the extent of the detachment, bleeding may be slight to severe. If severe, pain associated with profuse bleeding will result in shock, with the likely death of both the fetus and the mother. The condition is a medical emergency.

1. *Archives of General Psychiatry,* August 1974, p. 164.

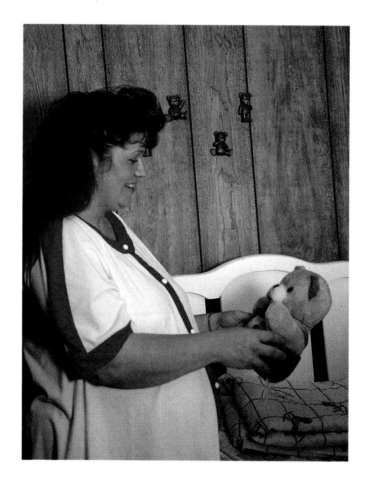

CHAPTER 4

Childbirth

In previous centuries a high percentage of mothers lost their lives at childbirth. "Childbed fever," then a tragic illness due to contamination of the mother during examination before delivery, resulted in a high mortality rate of mothers, and often of their infants.

Fortunately, the progress of medicine has changed this situation. Even as recently as 1930, sixty mothers died for every 10,000 children born alive in the United States. Today, that ratio has been reduced to about one maternal death per 10,000 live births.

There are a number of reasons why the risk of childbirth has been reduced to that of a relatively minor illness. Today, the prenatal care given to an expectant mother throughout the entire period of her pregnancy permits the physician to deal with preventable delivery problems ahead of time. He is able to evaluate the health needs of the mother-to-be and make dietary and other recommendations as might be indicated.

A variety of prenatal training programs are now available to expectant mothers that allow them to cooperate more effectively with the delivery process. They can do exercises that will help them to strengthen their abdominal and pelvic muscles, and they can practice rhythmic breathing that will help them to relax at appropriate times. Such programs are sometimes spoken of as "natural methods of childbirth." Preparations are also made and instruction is given as to how the baby might be breast-fed following birth.

Other improvements in the delivery system include advanced diagnostic techniques that allow the physician to deliver an otherwise difficult birth by means of a Caesarean section. Whereas in the past the majority of women gave birth at home, today the vast majority of women in the United States (about 99 percent) and many other countries go to a hospital or similar facility to give birth. These facilities are specially staffed and equipped to handle emergencies immediately, thus saving many lives of both mothers and children. And, of course, sterile conditions can more readily be maintained in a medical facility.

Signs of impending delivery

If you are an expectant mother, your uterine muscles will contract irregularly throughout much of the period of your pregnancy, but as the time for delivery approaches, these contractions will become stronger and more rhythmic, and they will occur at shorter intervals. As the time for delivery approaches, a mucous plug—a mass of mucus tinged with blood—will be expelled from the vagina. This is a perfectly normal occurrence called **"the show."** It indicates that the cervix of your uterus has begun to dilate (stretch) to make way for the passage of your baby's head.

Either at this time or a little later, a trickle or sudden gush of clear fluid will issue from the vagina. This indicates that the membranes surrounding your baby have broken, allowing part of the amniotic fluid to escape. This event is commonly called the "breaking of the **bag of waters.**" It also indicates that the time has arrived for you, the mother, to go to the hospital or an outpatient facility, or to call your physician if you have arranged to have your delivery at home. It is best not to eat solid food after labor begins, but you may drink plenty of water. In the hospital you will usually be given an enema to prevent the discharge of feces as the baby passes through the birth canal. Generally the hair in the pubic area will be shaved to help prevent contamination by germs and to make it easier to apply disinfectant solutions to the area.

The three stages of labor

Labor is initiated by the softening of the cervix and the beginning of regular contractions. For a first baby this may last up to twenty-four hours. Women who have already borne babies may have a labor period as short as an hour or two, though generally it will last for several hours. Labor is divided into three stages.

First stage

During the first stage of labor, the cervix and the tissues of the vagina will stretch sufficiently to form the birth canal. This is accomplished by the contractions of the uterus, which force the baby's head down through the cervix. These contractions come regularly, beginning with intervals of fifteen to thirty minutes and gradually shortening till they occur every one or two minutes. The contractions also become progressively stronger till they last for thirty seconds or more. Most women experience the greatest discomfort from contractions. If the bag of waters has not already broken, the doctor may hasten the process of dilation by rupturing the mem-

399

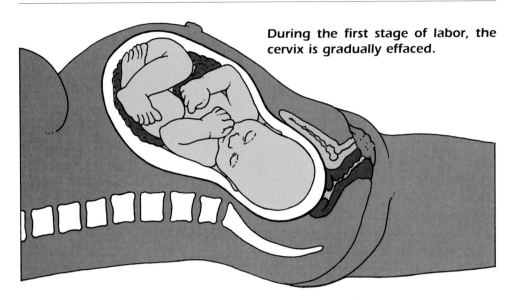

During the first stage of labor, the cervix is gradually effaced.

branes. The first stage ends when the cervix is completely effaced and dilated.

Second stage

The second stage is the actual expulsion of the child. The contractions of the uterus are now joined by those of the abdominal muscles and are accompanied by a strong urge to push. However, you should push only when you are urged to do so by your physician. The head is usually delivered first, followed by the shoulders. The rest of the body follows quickly. This stage normally takes from several minutes to an hour, depending on whether this is your first baby. The second stage ends when the baby is born.

Third stage

The third stage, the expulsion of the placenta (afterbirth) and the other membranes surrounding the infant, usually occurs in five to fifteen

During the second stage of labor, the baby is expelled through the birth canal.

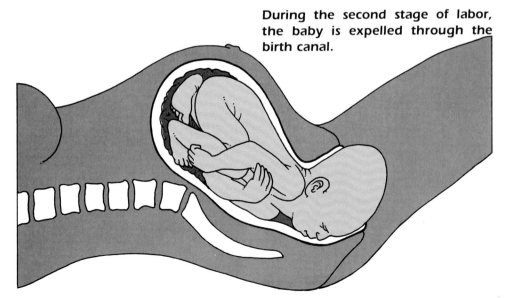

minutes. There is usually very little discomfort. As the uterus continues to contract, the placenta with its accompanying membranes separates from its attachments to the uterine wall. The physician or nurse may manipulate the uterus through the abdominal wall to ensure that it contracts firmly, thus minimizing the loss of blood.

After the birth

Immediately after birth, the infant is placed on the mother's abdomen. If it fails to breathe spontaneously, it is gently rubbed on the back, and a rubber syringe is used to clear its mouth and nostrils of mucus. The cord is usually clamped and cut before the afterbirth is delivered. (For information about gonorrheal infection, see page 1080.)

The physician then examines the infant to determine if there are any abnormalities. Premature infants must be kept warm and placed in an incubator as soon as possible (see "Problems of delivery" below).

Problems of delivery

Ideally, the baby will be delivered with no complications, either for itself or for the mother. However, a number of complications can arise. Some are relatively minor, while others may threaten the life of the baby or the mother, or both.

False labor

Mothers who have had children previously sometimes develop rhythmic contractions of the uterus that do not result in dilation of the cervix. Physical activities such as walking and bending usually cause them to cease. If you have any questions, call your physician.

Premature birth

Normally forty weeks will elapse between the day of conception and the day of childbirth. A baby born before the thirty-seventh week is termed a premature baby or "preemie." Since it is not always possible to determine the precise time of conception, it is generally assumed that any baby much smaller than the average newborn or weighing less than 5.5 pounds (2,500 grams) is probably premature. Premature infants account for some 7 percent of all live births in the United States. The smaller the infant at birth, the higher the risk of its dying. Thus the mortality rate of premature babies is 17 percent, as contrasted to less than 1 percent for full-term infants.

Although often no cause for a premature birth can be found, conditions that may contribute to such births include hypertensive disorders of pregnancy (preeclampsia and eclampsia), placental problems (placenta previa), high blood pressure, diabetes, chronic infections, vaginal bleeding, rupture of the bag of waters, poor nutrition, numerous pregnancies in quick succession, cigarette smoking, a mother who is less than twenty years of age, living at a high altitude, a blow to the abdo-

401

men, intense emotional upset, and, often, having twins and triplets.

What you can do. Should you have indications of a premature birth, call your physician immediately or go to a hospital emergency room.

What your physician can do. Following an examination, your doctor may attempt to stop the labor with a drug that prevents uterine contractions, or he may decide to allow the labor to continue. If he allows the baby to be born, it will require care in a specially equipped nursery.

Premature rupture of the membranes

Rupture of the membranes at term normally initiates labor. When this occurs several weeks before the expected time of delivery, you should notify your physician immediately. Occasionally, if the tear is small, the membrane may repair itself, and the fetus may be carried to term. However, any breaking of the membrane usually indicates that a premature birth is about to take place.

Episiotomy

An episiotomy is an incision made through the outer opening of the vagina to enlarge the birth canal. The procedure is done under a local anesthetic. Your physician will perform an episiotomy when he feels that the descending head may tear the vagina and surrounding tissues or when labor is premature or when forceps are to be used. Tears are more difficult to repair and often leave a weakened pelvic support. Following the

delivery of the placenta, the doctor will close the incision with stitches. The area may remain tender for some time.

Forceps

Obstetrical forceps have saved thousands of infant lives that otherwise would have been lost. They consist of two open blades that can be jointed together. One blade at a time is inserted into the birth canal and placed beside the infant's head. The blades are then locked together (like the two parts of scissors), and the infant is drawn out by gently pulling on its head.

Since forceps increase the risk of injury to both mother and infant, they are only used when normal processes fail: when labor is not progressing properly (especially in premature labor), when the position of the head must be rotated, or when the baby shows signs of distress (asphyxia).

Caesarean section

A Caesarean section is an operation by which the baby is delivered surgically. An incision is made through the mother's abdominal wall and the lower portion of the uterus, and the baby is withdrawn through the opening. The placenta and membranes are also removed, and the incisions are closed with stitches. A general anesthetic or, preferably, a regional nerve-block anesthetic (epidural) is required for the procedure. A Caesarean is done as an emergency measure if during labor the fetus shows signs of distress, usually asphyxia, or the baby cannot be delivered due to maternal exhaustion (preferred to forceps), or the birth canal is found to be too small.

Because of improved techniques, many more Caesareans are performed today than in the past. It is often the preferred method of delivery because of a maternal condition that might make a normal delivery too hazardous, because the birth canal is unsuited for a vaginal delivery, because of possible difficulties arising from an unusual position of the fetus (breech, crosswise), or even because of an unusually large baby. Vaginal birth (a normal delivery) is often possible in a pregnancy following a Caesarean.

Hemorrhage following delivery

The placenta detaches itself from the uterus shortly after delivery. The muscles of the uterus now contract, and in so doing, control the loss of blood from the now torn vessels. Should a portion of the placenta fail to separate **(retained placenta),** the uterus is not able to contract completely, and hemorrhage results. Manual removal of the placenta will resolve the problem. At other times, due to fatigue (following a prolonged labor) or to overstretching of the uterine muscle (from carrying twins), the muscle is unable to contract sufficiently. Medications are available to stimulate the uterine muscle and staunch the bleeding. Bleeding from vaginal tears must be surgically repaired.

Abnormal presentations

The most common position of an infant at birth is with its head pointed downward in the birth canal and with its face directed toward its mother's back. The delivery is more difficult when the face is directed forward. However, the head may rotate spontaneously, or the physician may be able to rotate it. In a breech presentation the baby's buttocks are directed

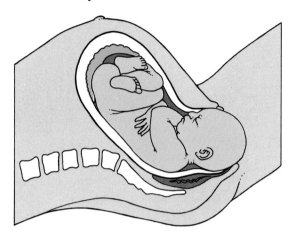

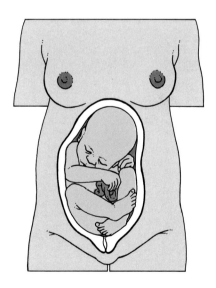

Abnormal presentations make the delivery more difficult. Above, the face is directed forward (occipital posterior); below, the buttocks are directed downward (breech).

403

downward. Occasionally the infant's shoulders or back may lie across the birth canal. Your physician will determine whether a vaginal delivery or a Caesarean section is the safest choice.

Multiple births

Twins are born in approximately one out of ninety births. If a single egg (ovum) is fertilized and soon thereafter splits, forming two developing embryos, identical twins will be born. When two or more eggs are produced at the same time and both are fertilized, the result is fraternal twins or multiple births (triplets, quadruplets, quintuplets). The tendency to have twins seems to run in

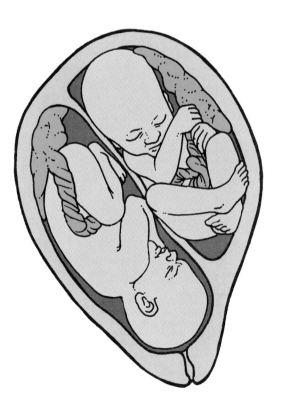

families. Multiple births are rare but have become more common due to the use of certain fertility medications. Delivery of twins or multiple babies is more difficult, and Caesarean sections are more commonly employed.

Respiratory distress syndrome (hyaline membrane disease)

A condition called **respiratory distress syndrome** is the most common cause of death among premature infants. The problem results from a lack of the chemical substance *surfactant* in the air sacs of the infant's lungs. The lungs expand initially but collapse on expiration, and the baby is in danger of suffocating. Surfactant normally prevents the collapse of the air sacs (alveoli). Infants suffering from this disorder require trained personnel for their care in nurseries that are specially equipped.

Birth injuries

Often the change in the shape of a newborn child's head is more apparent than real because some of the tissues of the scalp are swollen as a result of the birth process. The alterations in the head's shape, the bruises, and the swellings usually disappear within a few hours.

Today serious injuries do not occur as often as formerly. This is due in large part to the more frequent use of the Caesarean operation. Now physicians prefer to deliver a child surgically rather than to per-

Fraternal twins with individual placentas.

404

mit birth by the natural route when the examination, before labor begins, indicates that the child's head is too large in relation to the size of the mother's pelvis to permit an easy delivery.

Changes in the newborn's body

Immediately after birth, several major changes occur in the infant's body so that it can live independently from its mother.

The lungs

The baby's lungs expand, allowing it to obtain oxygen directly from the air rather than through the placenta and umbilical cord. Prior to birth, only a small portion of the blood pumped by the fetal heart passed through the lungs, which had not as yet expanded. Instead, because of a special opening in the heart, most of the blood bypassed the lungs. With the first expansion of the lungs, the pressures within the various chambers of the heart change. These pressure changes close the special opening so that the blood is no longer bypassed, but perfuses the infant's lungs.

The skull

Newborn babies frequently have misshapen heads. This is perfectly normal, and is not to be confused with injury to the head that was discussed earlier. The many bones that make up the skull of the fetus are not fused, allowing considerable molding of the baby's head at the time it passes through the birth canal. At times the bones may partially overlap. A few days after birth, the baby's head resumes its normal shape, and over time the bones will fuse together.

Two large areas in the midline of the skull are only covered with a thin membrane (the **fontanelles**) and are easily felt after birth. The larger one is in front and measures about an inch (2.5 cm) across, while the smaller one is in the back. The smaller one closes in about two months, and the larger one in about a year.

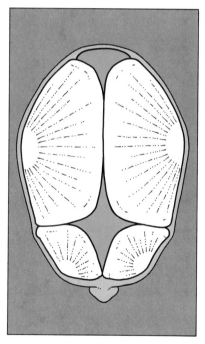

The skull of a newborn infant (as seen from above), with two membranous areas—the larger in front and the smaller behind (anterior and posterior fontanelles).

CHAPTER 5

The newborn

With the newborn's first breath and the severance of the umbilical cord a few minutes later, a new, independent life is launched. But the independence is only relative, for the infant is completely dependent on his parents for the necessities of life, and for the care and protection that will allow him to grow and mature to full adulthood. In this chapter we will discuss the care of an infant through about the first year.

Immediate needs at birth

Doctors and nurses must take several precautions with a newborn baby to prevent health problems. Some of these must be cared for immediately after birth, while the baby is still in the delivery room. Others can wait a few days or weeks.

Gonorrheal infection

Immediately after birth a preparation of either silver nitrate or penicillin ointment is put in the infant's eyes to prevent gonorrheal infection, which could cause blindness. Penicillin is generally used in the United States, but silver nitrate is cheaper and just as effective and is still widely used in other parts of the world. In many countries, including the United States, this procedure is required by law.

Phenylketonuria ("PKU")

Phenylketonuria, or "PKU" for short, is an inherited disorder in which one of the essential amino acids, phenylalanine, is not properly metabolized. This condition, due to a deficiency of a liver enzyme, occurs in 1 in every 15,000 children and, if undetected, causes gradual mental retardation. Many states now have mandatory laws requiring every newborn baby to be tested. A diet low in phenylalanine prevents this abnormal development. Infants with this disorder cannot be breast-fed. For details, see page 1047.

Circumcision

The decision of whether to have a boy baby circumcised should be made by the parents in consultation with their physician. Circumcision is a simple procedure by which the foreskin of the penis is surgically removed, usually during the first week of life. For details, see page 1085.

Vaccinations

Vaccinations (immunizations) stimulate the body's natural defense mechanisms to build up immunity to particular organisms. As a result of the vaccination, the body forms antibodies so that when the infectious agent invades the body, it is recognized, and the body's police forces immediately dispose of it. Generally a vaccination affords protection for life.

Since certain conditions require the exclusion of one or more vaccines, you should ask your physician which vaccines should be administered to your child, in what order, and at what age. A good time is usually when an infant is two months old. Vaccines are not given when an infant is sick, though a mild sniffle should not impede their administration.

Many vaccines can be given in combination. **DTP** and **TOPV** are usually the first to be given. **DTP** immunizes against diphtheria, tetanus, and pertussis (whooping cough).

The letters **TOPV** stand for trivalent oral polio vaccine, which protects against poliomyelitis (infantile paralysis). **MMR** stands for measles, mumps, and rubella (German measles). The last named is very important for girls to receive before they are old enough to become pregnant (see pages 377, 727).

Vaccination carries a certain risk, but the risk of not being vaccinated is many times greater. Occasionally, parents who are opposed to vaccination refuse to allow their children to be immunized, and sometimes these children get by. The fact that they escape a particular disease is probably due to the fact that the people around them have been immunized, making it difficult for the infection to get started. But tragedy often results when a virulent strain of organism arises and the unprotected individual is exposed.

Vaccinations do produce some undesirable side effects, such as pain at the site of injection, low-grade fever, and an occasional rash. However, these will soon pass away. You should immediately report to your physician any more serious reactions such as high fever or an allergic response.

When the baby goes home

Although the parents' involvement with their newborn begins at birth, until the infant leaves the hospital, others have the primary responsibility for its care. The parents' real responsibility begins when the nurse brings their baby from the nursery

and hands it to them, and they take their newborn home.

The mother's role

The mother harbors the greatest concern over how to care for her newborn child, especially when it is her first baby. This is a new experience for her. Though she may have been around babies before and even helped to care for them, she finds the total responsibility of caring for her own almost overwhelming. "If only the baby could talk," she wishes, "and tell me what he needs and what he wants, it would be so much easier."

While the newborn cannot talk, he has many ways of communicating his needs. Babies have a different cry when hungry than when sleepy, and a still different cry when they feel uncomfortable, lonely, or in pain. Sometimes a baby will cry to exercise his developing lungs. The mother can also communicate her feelings to her baby, especially by the tone of her voice, by how tense or relaxed she is, and by the way she handles her child.

Careful observation of your infant and his reactions will provide you with the information essential to respond appropriately to your baby's real needs. If he sleeps peacefully, eats contentedly, and gains weight regularly, and if his skin is warm with normal color, you can rest assured that everything is going well.

While a baby won't break like a doll, you should handle your newborn with care. An infant's nervous system is not very stable, so you should lift him slowly and gently, avoiding noises and sudden movements. Do not lift him by the arms, because they are not yet strong enough to support his weight. When carrying him, support his head and back. Since he cannot change his position, you should do this for him at regular intervals. Some babies sleep quietly, while others make peculiar noises in their sleep.

The father's role

The goal of both parents is to provide a loving home in which their child can grow up to be a healthy, well-adjusted adult. This is best accomplished if the father is also involved in satisfying the needs of the newborn, the infant, the child, and the young adult. Many fathers attend prenatal classes with their wives, stay with them during childbirth, and as time permits, help with the many activities required in raising a child. A few fathers feel that they are too busy to be bothered with their children. Such "one-parent homes" pose problems for the wife and mother, and are often a serious handicap to the child as he matures and reaches adolescence.

Characteristics of the newborn

The life of a fetus in its mother's womb is virtually effortless. Oxygen and nutrients are provided via the umbilical cord, and gaseous and chemical wastes are removed by the same means. Within the womb, the temperature is maintained at very close levels, and injury from outside forces occurs rarely, if ever. But after delivery, and after that first momentous breath, things change rapidly. In a few minutes the newborn is on its own, other than for the support it must receive from the adults who surround it.

The newborn's heart now circulates his blood through his own lungs, carrying oxygen from the lungs to the tissues and transporting the carbon dioxide back from the tissues to be exhaled into the air. A newborn breathes about forty times each minute, which is almost three times as fast as an adult. A healthy, full-term baby can suck vigorously and has the ability to digest and absorb the nutrients present in his mother's milk.

The nervous system

While the newborn's brain and nervous system are still developing rapidly, many senses are already present soon after birth. Sight is incomplete, but newborns can follow a bright light, and studies reveal that they like to look at a human face. Loud noises will startle an infant, while low-pitched, soothing sounds will relax him. Both the sense of smell and taste seem to be present to some degree at birth, the latter more strongly developed than the former. Newborns suck more vigorously when offered something sweet, but will attempt to reject anything bitter.

While a newborn can regulate its body temperature to some degree, you should take care not to expose the baby to extremes of heat or cold. Do not allow it to become too warm or chilled.

A newborn baby can feel pain at birth, and this sense becomes more acute with each passing day. Before the eighth day of life, circumcision can generally be performed on a baby boy without an anesthetic, but not thereafter.

Temperament

Newborn babies usually have distinct temperaments. Some seem placid and respond to attention slowly but enjoy being handled and caressed. Others are overactive, hard to control, and want to be independent. Parents should realize that they themselves have contributed these traits to their children, and they should work understandingly toward encouraging the traits they like and modifying those they feel are undesirable.

Just as no two babies look alike, so no two babies act precisely the same. However, it is typical for a newborn to spend sixteen to seventeen hours a day sleeping. This sleep is roughly divided into equal amounts of regular and irregular (non-REM and REM) sleep (see page 54). Periods of sound sleep, with few if any body movements, will be interspersed with periods of irregular sleep, with twitching of the body and moving of the limbs. At times the infant will be drowsy and at other times alert.

While rigid schedules may not be the best, reasonable times for feeding and sleeping will give the infant's built-in rhythms the best chance for guiding his activities of growth and development. If given a chance, inborn biological clocks regulate an infant's cycles of eating, sleeping, elimination, and wakefulness. Each baby soon develops a schedule of his own if environmental sounds and activities do not interfere. The seventeen hours of sleep are typically divided into periods lasting forty-five to fifty minutes. During its waking hours the infant is usually quiet, active, or crying.

Crying

Crying is probably the most important way a newborn has to communicate its wants. However, it is also a way that the baby obtains exercise. Parents, and especially mothers, should know that the average newborn cries two hours a day during the first month, and this crying is not a reflection on parenting skills.

Crying frequently indicates an infant's needs—hunger, pain, or cold. Or it may exhibit fear or dislike—when it is suddenly moved or when it is abruptly deprived of the breast or a pacifier. Crying may range anywhere from a whimper to a loud cry with kicking and thrashing of arms. Every cry does not imply a need for food and should not be met with a bottle of milk or juice. A restless, crying infant may be quieted by rocking, by soft rhythmic singing, by wrapping it snugly in a blanket, by placing its feet in warm water, or by giving it a slightly sweetened pacifier.

Caring for the newborn

Breast-feeding

The breast milk of mammals is species specific. That is, the milk of a cow is ideally suited for a calf, and the milk of a horse is specifically designed for its foal. The same is true of the human. There is no better food for a newborn than the milk from its own mother. Any other milk, whether from another animal or from a plant source, is a substitute food and should be recognized as such. Mothers should be encouraged to nurse their babies if at all possible.

During the twentieth century, there has been a steady decrease in the number of mothers who nurse their infants, and this tendency is worldwide. Fortunately, in Western countries (including the United States), a growing trend is for mothers to once again breast-feed their infants. Yet in spite of this

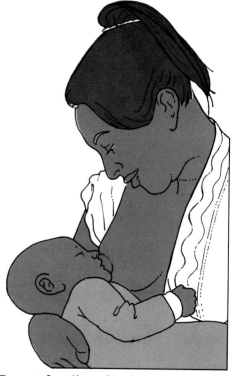

Breast-feeding is the most satisfactory way of feeding an infant.

trend, only about one in every three infants is nursed at the breast, and all too often the period of nursing is for only a few months.

Breast milk contains the specific nutrients in just the right amounts required for the growing child from immediately after birth until he is old enough to eat off the table. The nutrient content of milk is not constant, but continually changes to meet the growth needs of the infant. For example, as the infant's growth rate declines, the concentration of protein in the mother's milk decreases. The mother's breast has been "programmed" to produce just what her baby needs at each stage of growth.

Breast milk does not have to be warmed. It is sterile, readily available, and cheap. It is the ultimate "convenience food." Besides being better nourished, breast-fed infants have less diarrhea, fewer allergies (asthma, hay fever) and infections (colds, coughs, pneumonia, polio, scarlet fever), less tooth decay, and, later in life, less obesity and atherosclerosis. No other food can give the newborn a better start in life.

Breast-feeding an infant brings mother and child into an intimate relationship that appears beneficial to both. Sucking satisfies the infant and stimulates lactation in the mother, which, in turn, is controlled by her hormones. Many nursing mothers obtain a deep personal satisfaction from the experience. And a happy mother tends to produce a more generous supply of milk, and she usually has a healthier, more contented baby.

Some mothers who desire to breast-feed their infants either have insufficient milk or cannot provide milk for their babies. For these, formulas are a lifesaver. Formulas also provide a means for raising millions of children whose mothers do not wish to nurse their babies.

Artificial feeding

While formula is not as desirable as mother's milk, formula-fed infants, especially if they are held and fondled while nursing, grow to be healthy adults. The *sterile* formula has made this possible. Many commercial formulas can be obtained in either liquid or powder form. Infants who are allergic to animal milks can be fed excellent plant milks, usually made from the soybean. These should be prepared in accordance with the manufacturer's instructions.

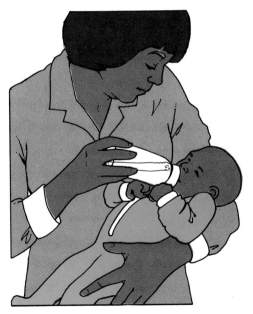

When formula-feeding, hold the infant in the same position as for breast-feeding.

Prepared infant formulas are becoming available around the world, and can also be obtained through various government and private agencies. However, a method for preparing a simple formula from evaporated milk is included here for those situations in which a prepared formula is unavailable. Whole milk contains two times more water than evaporated milk.

Mix in the following proportions: 2 ounces of evaporated milk, 3 ounces of water (1-1/2 ounces water when using whole boiled milk), and 1 teaspoon of corn syrup. This will give 5 ounces of milk with 20 calories per ounce of food energy. Sugar is added because mother's milk contains twice as much sugar as cow's milk.

How much should you feed your baby? Begin by estimating the total calories your baby needs for a day. (Keep in mind that underweight infants may need additional calories, so check with your physician if your baby is underweight.) During the first four months, the average baby needs 2 to 3 ounces of milk per day for each pound of body weight. Thus,

An evaporated-milk formula							
Milk		**Karo**		**Water**		**Total**		**Calories**
oz or ml		tspn or ml		oz or ml		oz or ml		1 oz or 30 ml
2	60	1	5	3	90	5	155	20

Calories and ounces or milliliters (ml) of formula needed per day				
Age of infant **months**	**Calories needed** **per lb**	**per kg**	**Formula** **oz/lb**	**ml/kg**
1-4	55	120	2.75	180
5-8	50	110	2.5	165
9-12	40	88	2.0	130

Formula needed per day, number of feedings, and amount per feeding								
Weight **of infant**		**Formula**		**Total** **volume**		**Feeding**	**Amount of** **feeding**	
lbs	kg	oz/lb	ml/kg	oz	ml	per day	oz	ml
7	3.2	2.75	180	17.0	575	6-7	2.6	66
10	4.5	2.75	180	27.5	850	6-7	4.6	142
15	7.0	2.50	165	37.5	1175	4-5	9.4	294
20	9.0	2.00	130	40.0	1170	3-4	13.3	390

a 10-pound baby would need between 20 and 30 ounces daily. For the next four months, the baby needs only 2.5 ounces per pound per day, and thereafter, 2 ounces of milk per pound per day should be enough since the infant is beginning to eat other foods.

How often should you feed your baby? It should have six to seven feedings per day during the first month, four to five between the second and sixth months, and in most cases three feedings per day after that. To determine the size of each feeding, divide the total amount of formula your baby will need in one day by the number of feedings it will have. If you make up all your baby's milk for the day at one time, you should sterilize (boil) it, pour it into separate sterilized bottles with nipples for each feeding, and keep it in the refrigerator. As your child grows older, you can use bottles and nipples that have been thoroughly cleaned in soap and water. The table on page 412 will give you a summary of directions.

The majority of infants do not need more than 32 ounces of formula per day. When your baby seems to demand more than this, you should probably begin adding solid foods to his diet. Some babies don't know when to stop feeding, and stuffing them until they are obese is not wise. By gradually adding cereals, vegetables, and fruits to your baby's diet, you will provide the calories he needs to make up for those he no longer gets from the formula.

After five or six months, you can begin reducing the amount of karo or sugar you've been adding to your baby's formula. Do it gradually, decreasing the sugar added to the total formula for the day by one teaspoonful (15 grams) every two weeks until you've eliminated sugar altogether. At this point, you can put your baby on boiled whole milk if you wish.

If you use cow's milk, it should be whole milk. Avoid skimmed milk and low-fat milk. The two major proteins in both human and cow's milk are lactalalbumin and casein. The amount of lactalalbumin is the same in both milks, but cow's milk contains more than four times as much casein. If cow's milk is diluted, the amount of lactalalbumin is decreased, and the infant will not grow normally.

The extra protein in cow's milk, together with the extra vitamins and minerals required by rapidly growing animals (but not by human babies—see page 80), must be eliminated by the infant's kidneys. This requires additional water. A breast-fed infant does not need extra water, but a bottle-fed baby does. A formula-fed baby should be encouraged to drink water (slightly sweetened) between regular feedings.

The hole in the bottle's nipple should be just large enough to allow a drop of milk to ooze out and drop off when it is shaken gently. When giving your baby a bottle of milk, hold the baby as though you were nursing him. It is best not to force him to empty every bottle. If he is contented and growing well, he is getting sufficient food. Babies differ in their precise food requirements. For further details on feeding growing children, see pages 130, 131.

Whether your baby is breast-fed or bottle-fed, halfway through and at the end of each feeding, you should burp him. Face him toward your back, place him upright with his head above your shoulder, and rub or pat him gently on his back. Then place him on his right side or on his tummy.

The method by which a baby obtains milk from his mother's breast differs from that required to drink from a bottle. A bottle requires far less muscular action from the muscles of the mouth and those used for chewing. That is why dentists recommend that bottle feeding should be terminated by the time a child is eighteen months old.

Changing the feeding schedule

Babies differ as to the number of feedings they require per day. The midnight feeding is usually the first to be eliminated, after four to six weeks. The next to be dropped is the 10:00 p.m. feeding, when the infant is three to six months old. Generally by the sixth month, a baby will be on three regular feedings a day.

Weaning

Weaning from the breast should be done gradually, over several weeks, with a bottle replacing the breast. If the child is older (some mothers breast-feed their child till it is two or three years old), the baby can take its milk directly from a cup, making the bottle unnecessary. Many children who have not used a bottle for months may suddenly re-

vert and crave a bottle. There is no harm in this, for they will again give it up. A child should not be allowed to have a bottle in its mouth while sleeping as it tends to encourage tooth decay.

Modifying the baby's diet

Since human milk is designed specifically for infants, a breast-fed baby does not require solid foods for at least six months, maybe even longer. Formula-fed infants, on the other hand, have a substitute food, so even though it is from another mammal, the addition of solid foods is a safeguard against deficiency. However, it is unwise to force solid foods at too early an age. Foods other than milk should be in addition to the regular breast-feeding or the bottle.

There is no definite time when solid foods should be started, nor is there any special order for introducing the various foods (cereals, fruits, vegetables). Neither is there any advantage, other than convenience, to the baby foods available in the market over those prepared at home. Home foods should not be seasoned to the adult taste, nor should the parent necessarily enjoy a preprepared infant food, as these are generally not salted or seasoned. The infant's kidneys are not designed to handle the excessive salt intake of the average adult. Home-prepared foods should be thoroughly mashed or pulverized in a blender.

Give your baby very small amounts of food at a time. If he rejects the food, try it again later. Do not rush the process. Your baby will find some foods more acceptable than others, but in time, he will learn to enjoy a wide variety of foods.

Cereals are generally introduced at about four months, pureed fruits and vegetables at four to five months, and egg yolk and, if desired, boiled eggs and cottage cheese at about five to six months. Fruit juices may be started at six months. Cereals should be given one at a time—a small amount of a single cereal, thoroughly cooked. Observe the child's response, especially any adverse reaction. Rice is a good starting cereal since a few infants are allergic to wheat. Whole grain cereals are nutritionally superior to refined cereals (see page 87). Brown rice, finely ground whole-wheat flour (prepared as a cereal), oats, whole cornmeal, and other cereals can be used.

To reduce the possibility of allergies, fruits are usually given cooked until about the age of eight months. Ripe bananas appear to be well tolerated raw. Puréed vegetables may be started after cereals have been accepted. A well-baked or boiled potato is an excellent vegetable. By about eight months of age, chopped foods can be tried. By the time he is one, the average child should be eating from the table.

At six months most babies will hold a piece of dry bread or crust in their hands and enjoy sucking on it. They should be allowed to feed themselves as soon as they wish to.

Foods that might be harmful if inhaled (because of the possibility of choking), such as popcorn and nuts, should not be given to an infant or even to a young child. Small children usually enjoy drinking from a cup once they have learned that it provides them something enjoyable.

The baby's bath

Infants and children enjoy being bathed. Be sure the room is warm. Fill a basin or a small tub with warm (not hot) water. The basin should be large enough that you can place your baby in it comfortably. When he is small, you should support his head with one arm. Use mild soap, and thoroughly rinse the soap off before drying him. If his skin tends to be dry, you may wish to use an oil or lotion. Otherwise, dust his skin with a little powder.

Beware of leaving your baby alone when he is old enough to sit up in the tub by himself. Many children have drowned in the bathtub because they were not watched.

Diapers

You should regularly change your baby's diapers to avoid the possibility of a "diaper rash." A baby's skin is tender and can easily be injured, especially if he develops diarrhea. When changing his diaper, clean between all the folds of skin so that no irritating material is left.

415

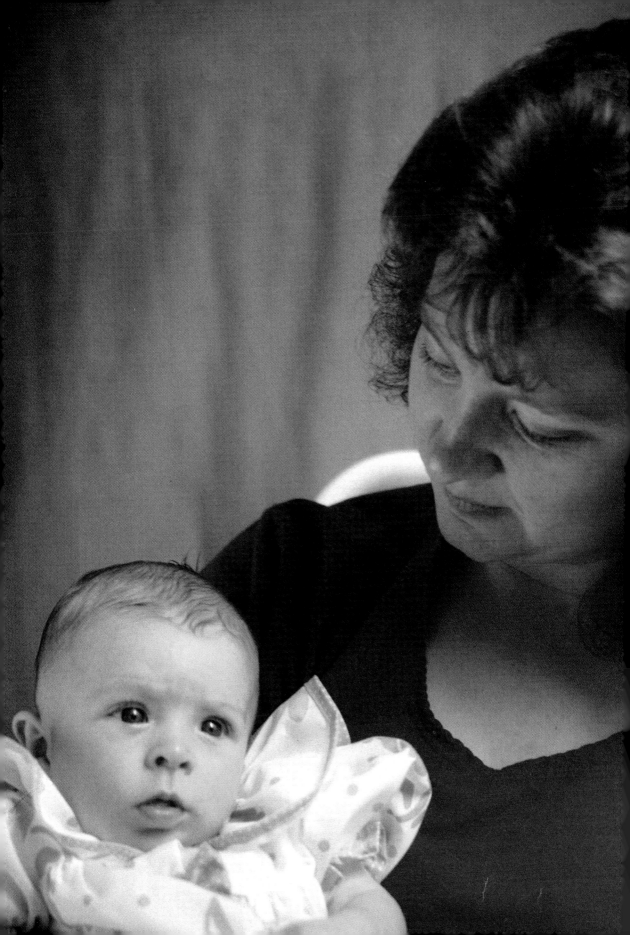

CHAPTER 6

Special problems of the newborn

Newborn babies have special problems that are unique to their stage of life. These problems are complicated by the fact that the baby is not able to tell anyone the symptoms he is experiencing, or even that something is wrong. Yet there are ways that parents and doctors can, in most instances, recognize an infant's needs.

General problems of infancy

Excessive crying

It is perfectly normal for a baby to spend some time each day crying. As mentioned in the previous chapter, normal, healthy babies will cry an average of two hours a day during the first six months of life, and during the teething period they tend to cry even more than that. Other common causes of crying include colic, illness, pain, too much or too little food or water, or a need for more love and attention. If your baby's crying does not seem to be from one of these causes, you may have an "excessive-crying baby." You may wish to check with your doctor. Even though the baby cries, have a regular schedule for his sleeping. Place him where it is quiet and the light is subdued.

As mentioned earlier, babies' temperaments differ. Fussy babies may be more difficult to console and may be quicker to cry from touch, gas pains, or noise. Studies have shown that very fussy babies may cry more than twice as long as do normal infants. Often crying is the greatest during the evening between five and midnight. This "fussy crying" begins two to three weeks after birth and may not end until the baby is three months old. Do not consider yourself a failure if you have a very fussy baby. First try the suggestions for handling a normal crying baby (see

417

page 410). If these do not work, here are some additional suggestions that some mothers have found very helpful.

- Teach your infant to console himself when put to bed. Continual rocking may actually keep a baby from going into a deep plane of sleep because the baby awakens as soon as the motion stops. Put your baby down the way he is to be for the whole night.
- If your baby cries when he is put down, let him cry for fifteen to twenty minutes and console him another fifteen or twenty minutes. Then lay him down to sleep.
- Should he cry again—and he probably will—wait a little longer before picking him up or patting him on the back, etc. After you have again consoled him, put him down again and leave him to sleep.
- Lengthen the intervals before you respond to his crying. He will gradually learn to go to sleep on his own.

Diarrhea

Diarrhea—loose, excessive bowel movements—may be caused by overfeeding, a too-concentrated formula, or, in more severe cases, by an infection or food allergy. If you have given your baby a new article of diet recently, try discontinuing it for a few days. Because a person who has diarrhea excretes more water than normal, you should watch for dehydration. In severe cases, consult your physician. For details regarding diarrhea, see pages 424, 877.

Drooling

In drooling, saliva escapes between the lips rather than being swallowed. A reasonable amount of drooling is normal for an infant. Excessive drooling occurs in the very young infant in those rare cases in which the passageway of the esophagus is not open. An increase in drooling occurs reflexively in response to pain in the mouth, as when the infant's teeth are erupting.

Fever

Body temperature is determined with a thermometer (see page 573). A rectal thermometer should be used to take the temperature of any child under the age of three. We typically associate a rise in body temperature above the normal (98.6°F, 37°C) with illness. However, one's temperature may rise for other reasons. A newborn infant may develop a high temperature merely because his surroundings are too warm. His temperature-regulating mechanism has not yet stabilized, and his temperature may exceed 98.6°F if the nursery is too hot (90°F or 32°C), or if he is dressed too warmly. The infant is sensitive to the loss of water within his body, and his temperature will rise because of dehydration.

Fever is an elevation of the body temperature above the normal range resulting from a disease state. Fever alone does not indicate what kind of illness the baby has. The symptoms present with the fever indicate the problem. A newborn may develop a fever within the first few hours after birth as a result of injury to the brain sustained during childbirth. Serious infections are accompanied by fever—infections such as pneumonia, meningitis, and septicemia. Seek the advice of your physician to determine the underlying cause. Very high fever can be reduced by means of cold applications (see page 598).

Jaundice

About 60 percent of normal babies display jaundice about the second or third day after birth. An excess of bile pigments in the blood causes the skin and the whites of the eyes to develop a yellowish or greenish-yellow color, called jaundice. As they wear out, red blood cells release their hemoglobin—the protein pigment that carries oxygen and carbon dioxide. The hemoglobin, in turn, breaks down to release bilirubin, a substance which full-term babies with a *mature liver* can readily handle. This condition should fade after five or six days.

The *immature livers* of premature infants are unable to break down bilirubin, so its concentration rises. If the levels of this pigment rise too high, the neurons in certain areas of the brain will be damaged. However, exposing such an infant to sunlight or a sunlamp changes the bilirubin molecule to substances that are soluble in water and are easily eliminated by the kidneys, thus doing no harm to the brain.

A more serious form of jaundice is seen at birth and persists longer than a week. This occurs in such conditions as hemolytic disease of the newborn (Rh disease) or some congenital defect of the liver or of the bile passages (see page 816). Consult your physician if your baby's jaundice persists longer than a week after birth.

Teething

Most babies experience a certain amount of discomfort when their teeth are breaking through their gums. The baby becomes irritable, cries more than usual, and may reject some of his feedings. Allowing the baby to bite on a blunt object or massaging the sore spot on his gums with your cloth-covered finger may temporarily ease the discomfort. Make sure that the baby receives abundant fluid even though he refuses some of his regular feedings. If he clutches at an ear and is running a fever, see your physician, as he may have an ear infection.

Thumb-sucking

Thumb-sucking often begins during infancy and reaches its height

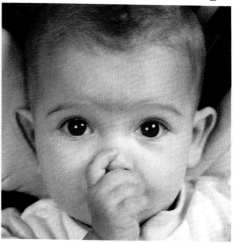

Thumb-sucking often begins during infancy.

419

between one and two years of age. Sucking seems to help an infant feel secure. Most children give up the habit before the age of three. The problem is best handled with an indirect approach: checking on the adequacy of the little ones's diet, keeping the child pleasantly active, and showing him sincere affection.

Rarely, if ever, are mouths or thumbs distorted by thumb-sucking. However, the teeth may become misaligned if the habit continues past the third year. Consult your dentist if your child has difficulty giving up his thumb-sucking.

Scolding the child generally makes the condition worse. Foul-tasting materials are available at the pharmacy that can be applied to the finger. Also, it may help to have the child wear gloves.

Spitting up (regurgitation) and vomiting

Spitting up is common in all babies during the first four to six months of life. Handling the baby more gently and burping him consistently while nursing may help to reduce the frequency and amount. If your baby is growing normally and holding his weight, you need not be concerned about whether he is retaining enough food to maintain health.

See your physician if your baby's weight gain is slow, or if the regurgitation is extensive (**reflux esophagitis,** see page 851), with choking, coughing, and possible aspiration of stomach content into the trachea with wheezing (and possibly pneumonia).

If food is being forcefully expelled (projectile vomiting) and is persistent, there may be an obstruction at the outlet of the stomach or in the upper small intestine. This condition, called **pyloric stenosis**, should be evaluated by your physician (for a detailed discussion, see page 856).

Other causes of vomiting by babies include intolerance to cow's-milk formulas (see "lactose intolerance," pages 454, 858), systemic infections, sepsis, and dehydration. Vomiting may result in dehydration, and dehydration, in turn, causes more vomiting (see pages 455, 561).

Umbilical hernia

Some infants develop a protrusion of soft tissue at the umbilicus (belly-button). Before birth, the umbilical cord, carrying blood from the placenta to the fetus, passed through its abdominal wall. After birth, the umbilical cord was severed, and its stump healed to form the umbilicus.

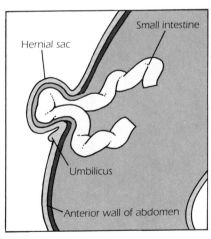

An umbilical hernia. A portion of the small intestine pushes through the weakened abdominal wall near the umbilicus.

To strengthen this soft spot, the connective tissues slowly grow together and reinforce the abdominal wall in the middle.

Sometimes the tissues of the umbilicus protrude when the child cries lustily or strains. The diameter of the hernia may vary from 1/2 inch to 2 inches (1 to 5 cm). By far the larger number of these hernias disappear spontaneously by one year of age. Only in those cases in which the hernia persists beyond three years of age, causes symptoms, or becomes progressively larger should a surgical repair be considered. For further details regarding umbilical hernias, see page 862.

Two infectious diseases of infancy

The diseases in this section and those that follow are mentioned for the convenience of the reader. The details of many of these disorders are found elsewhere under the general discussion of these conditions. Of the many infections and contagious diseases that may afflict an infant, two important ones are mentioned in this section.

Whooping cough (pertussis)

Whooping cough is an acute infectious disease that is easily transmitted from person to person, and even a young infant is susceptible. About half the cases occur in children less than two years of age. The bacteria are sprayed into the air when an infectious person sneezes or coughs. The disease, which is caused by a germ (*Bordetella pertussis*), involves the nose, throat, and upper air passageways. The characteristic spasmodic cough ends with a loud, forced inspiration of air—the "whoop." At the time of the whoop, the child may gag and vomit. In mild cases there may be no whooping or vomiting.

Thanks to immunization (DTP), the disease is relatively rare in the United States today. However, when a baby that is less than a year old gets whooping cough, the condition is most serious and carries a high mortality rate. One of the serious complications is pneumonia, causing over 90 percent of the deaths in children less than three years of age.

The first stage of pertussis begins a week or two after exposure. For about the first two weeks the symptoms are essentially the same as for an ordinary cold, except that the cough becomes persistent and is especially troublesome at night. After the second week the cough is spasmodic and the typical "whoop" is heard. The mucus in the air passageways is thick, tenacious, and difficult to dislodge, and breathing may be difficult during a coughing spell. The whooping stage lasts from three to six weeks, but often continues as a less troublesome cough for several months.

Prevention. Because the disease carries such a high risk, especially for infants and young children, immunization or shots with pertussis vaccine (DTP) should be given at about two months of age.

Treatment. If your child contracts whooping cough, your physician will determine whether he needs to be sent to a hospital or can be cared for at home. An antibiotic (erythromycin) given before the whooping stage begins may prevent its appearance. Many infants and young children should be hospitalized so that the nose and upper air passageways can be cleared of the sticky mucus with suction. Oxygen may also be helpful. The vomiting may cause loss of water and food. Plenty of fluids will correct the dehydration, and the child should be encouraged to eat wholesome food.

Congenital rubella (congenital German measles)

Congenital rubella is a disease of prenatal life and early infancy that occurs when an expectant mother develops rubella (German measles) during her pregnancy. The rubella virus is easily transferred from the mother's blood to that of the fetus. German measles is relatively harmless when it occurs in an older child, or in an adult other than during pregnancy. But the effect on the fetus can be tragic. It often causes death, or, if the child survives, it may interfere with normal development.

Two serious problems are related to the newborn that has congenital German measles. When the mother develops rubella during the first three months of pregnancy, there is a strong probability that the baby may develop congenital heart disease, low birth weight, hepatitis of early infancy, cataracts and other defects of the eyes, hearing loss, mental retardation, or malfunction of the endocrine organs. The prospect is so serious that the mother who has had German measles should discuss the implications with her physician.

The second concern is that the infant born with congenital rubella harbors the virus in his tissues for several months after birth. That is, the infant has a chronic form of the disease and can act as a carrier. During this period, susceptible persons having contact with the infant may develop the disease.

Two skin problems

Many skin diseases affecting infants, children, and adults are discussed elsewhere (see page 971). Two that commonly affect infants are briefly described here.

Atopic dermatitis (eczema)

Atopic dermatitis consists of an inflammatory reaction in the skin—itching, burning, and redness. It seems to especially affect individuals with an inherited hypersensitivity of the skin.

In the infant that contracts this problem, the skin of the face, scalp, and outer surfaces of the arms and legs are particularly affected. There is reddening, blistering, oozing, and crusting. And, unfortunately, there is no cure. The goal of treatment is to relieve the discomfort, prevent infection, and reduce the inflammation.

For details of such treatment, see page 971.

Impetigo

Impetigo is an acute infection of the skin. It can occur at any age but is most commonly seen in children. However, it is seldom dangerous, except in infants, on whom it can become widespread, since the infant's tender skin seems to have little resistance. When the streptococcus organism is involved, it may cause disease of the kidney (glomerulonephritis).

Usually the lesions start on the face, around the mouth and nose. Small red blisters break and form pustules that ooze. These develop into "honey-

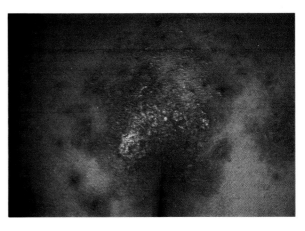

Impetigo is a skin disease. Note the many small blisters.

colored" crusts. The infection spreads along the margins, and is itchy but not painful. For details of treatment and prevention, see page 975.

Respiratory disorders

Bronchiolitis

The bronchioles are the small air passageways that carry the air between the bronchi (large air tubes) and the air sacs (alveoli). The bronchioles are smaller in the infant than they are later in life. Bronchiolitis is a viral infection that fills hospitals with four-to six-month-old infants every winter. The infection starts as a cold. A day or two later the lining of the bronchioles is involved, causing swelling, congestion, and difficult breathing. The infant's condition abruptly becomes worse. There is wheezing, coughing, labored breathing, and cyanosis (blueness of the skin).

In severe cases the infant should be taken to the hospital. There he may require oxygen (in a tent), intravenous fluids, and tube feeding. If no complications develop, the infection normally runs its course in two to three days. It is rarely fatal.

Bronchiolitis may be a precursor to asthma later in life.

Respiratory distress syndrome (RDS)

In this condition the newborn has difficulty breathing, sometimes even taking his first breath. The difficulty is due to a lack of the chemical substance **surfactant**, which normally coats the inner surface of the air cells. Surfactant helps the air sacs to expand and prevents them from collapsing when air is exhaled. This allows for free passage of oxygen to the blood.

In RDS the walls of the tiny air sacs stick together, thus interfering with

423

the entrance of air and endangering the life of the baby from suffocation. It is most commonly seen in premature infants, but also occurs in abnormally large babies, babies born of diabetic mothers, and babies delivered by Caesarean section. Formerly, only about one in four infants with RDS survived. Today, however, three out of four RDS babies survive because of advances in medical knowledge. Specially equipped intensive care units provide an infant with oxygen, intravenous fluids, artificial respiration if needed, and artificial surfactant. Unfortunately, even with these modern technologies, one out of four RDS babies fails to respond.

Sudden infant death syndrome (SIDS)

This tragic, unexpected, and unexplained infant death occurs when an apparently healthy baby is placed in the crib in the evening and is found dead in the morning. These deaths typically occur quietly during the infant's sleep. SIDS is the leading cause of death in infants between two weeks and one year of age, with the highest incidence occurring between two and four months of age.

Several factors appear to predispose a child to SIDS. More male babies die of SIDS than females, and the condition is more common among premature infants and those with low birth weight than full-term babies of normal weight. It is also more frequent among black children than white children, and it is seen more often in infants born of mothers who smoked during pregnancy than among those who did not. However, the actual cause of SIDS is not known. It is presumed to be some defect in the lungs or in the breathing center of the brain.

Unfortunately, but understandably, most parents with a child that died of SIDS develop a sense of guilt. They feel that somehow they should have paid closer attention to their baby as he slept. Actually, no parental negligence is involved, and there is no known way to prevent this tragic occurrence. Respiratory monitors are available, but have not proved to be of significant value. Grief-stricken parents should be comforted and given understanding support.

Endocrine disturbances

Hypothyroidism (cretinism)

No evidence of an abnormality may be evident at birth, but the condition can be detected by a blood test immediately after birth to see if there is a thyroid deficiency.

If no test is made, a baby with this condition begins to show signs and symptoms within a few weeks. It does not grow as rapidly or symmetrically as it should. Its skin thickens and is cool, dry, wrinkled, and sallow. The infant's cry becomes hoarse, its lips become thick, and the tongue is large and protruding. The face is broad and the facial expression piglike, with a short, upturned nose. The teeth develop late. The feet and hands are puffy. If untreated, the child becomes a cretin—a deformed dwarf. Mentally the infant is feebleminded, dull, apathetic, and feels bad.

The prognosis is better when treatment is started before the age of three months. Treatment consists of administering thyroid hormone, and the response may be spectacular. The infant may resume a normal appearance and activity within a few weeks. Delay in starting treatment has serious consequences.

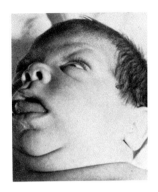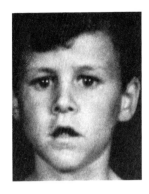

A hypothyroid infant (cretin) before and after treament.

Gastrointestinal disturbances

Many ailments involve the stomach and intestines. However, three that often occur between birth and one year of age are described here. For other disorders, see page 845.

Infant colic

Colic has been on record for hundreds of years, and is seen in all races and social classes. It appears to be less common in cultures where the infant is strapped closely to the mother. It occurs with equal frequency in both sexes, is just as common in breast-fed as in bottle-fed infants, and the firstborn is no more likely to have the disorder than younger brothers or sisters. The cause is not really known.

Colic usually develops two to four weeks after birth. Interestingly, in a premature infant its onset is about three weeks after the due date of delivery. The problem is usually over by the time the infant is three or, at the most, four months old, hence the name **"three-month colic."** It

seems more common in fussy babies. The crying is a loud scream that may last for hours, especially during the evening. Parents become distraught.

For suggestions on consoling the infant, see under "excessive crying" earlier in this chapter. The infant should, of course, be burped, kept in a quiet room, and handled gently and lovingly.

Infectious diarrhea (acute infectious gastroenteritis)

This ailment is associated with diarrhea and vomiting, and is accompanied by a mild fever. The major concern is rapid loss of fluid (dehydration) with a mineral (electrolyte) imbalance that occurs within a few hours in severe cases. The younger the infant, the greater the danger.

Most cases of acute infectious gastroenteritis are caused by viruses in infants, and by bacteria in adults. The diarrhea is profuse and watery, and is accompanied with vomiting.

The infant cries with pain, may be lethargic, and loses interest in feeding. Dehydration is evident when the skin is warm and dry, the lips parched, the eyes sunken, and sucking is weak or absent. The soft spot on the head of a young infant will be depressed.

The principal treatment is to restore the fluid lost by vomiting and diarrhea. In a bottle-fed infant, the formula can be replaced for the first day with water to which has been added a teaspoon of sugar or honey and a half teaspoon of salt for each pint of formula. Depending on the severity of the illness, the formula may be replaced on successive days by making it 1/4 strength, 1/2 strength, 3/4 strength, and full strength for days two, three, four, and five. For a breast-fed infant, encourage the drinking of sweetened water (see above). If the baby refuses to drink, see your physician. It is sometimes necessary to hospitalize the infant in order to provide water and salts, first by vein and later by mouth.

Pyloric stenosis

The tendency to develop this disorder appears to be inherited. In pyloric stenosis, the outlet of the stomach is narrowed, and this interferes with the passage of the stomach's contents into the small intestine (duodenum). It occurs on the average in 1 out of every 200 babies and is more common in boys than in girls. The muscle (pyloric sphincter) that controls the opening between the stomach and duodenum is overdeveloped. Symptoms first appear during the second or third week after birth, and usually become progressively worse.

In pyloric stenosis, food is prevented from entering the intestines. The symptoms include vomiting after feeding, with the vomitus literally being ejected from the mouth (projectile vomiting); active contraction waves in the wall of the stomach that are plainly observed in the infant's abdominal wall; constipation; and

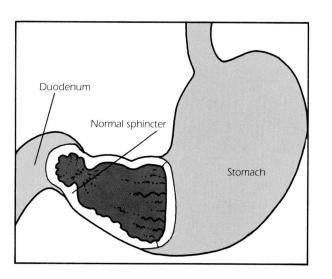

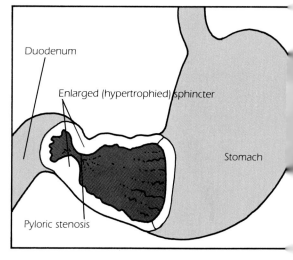

Pyloric stenosis (right). Note the enlarged sphincter muscle.

progressive loss of weight to the point that the baby may weigh less than at birth.

Treatment consists of surgery: the surgeon incises the tissue outside the enlarged muscle (pyloric sphincter). This immediately enlarges the opening from the stomach and permits food to pass through. The infant's feedings are gradually increased for two or three days, after which the baby should make a complete recovery.

Rickets

Rickets is most frequently seen in infants six to eighteen months of age. Incomplete absorption of calcium and phosphorous due to a lack of vitamin D causes the bones to develop poorly near their ends and to be misshapen. The earliest symptoms consist of restlessness, irritability, and sweating of the head. Other causes for rickets are kidney failure and celiac disease. Should you observe any of the above symptoms, consult with your physician. For a more complete discussion of the problem, see page 944.

Hemolytic disease of the newborn (Rh factor disease: erythroblastosis)

Hemolytic disease of the newborn is a serious condition that affects babies born to a mother whose blood contains antibodies that tend to destroy the infant's red blood cells. For a complete discussion of the disorder, see page 775. The problem occurs when the mother's blood type is Rh negative and the blood of the fetus is Rh positive. The mother's antibodies pass to the fetus and destroy its red blood cells.

Giving the mother an injection of "Rh immune globulin" at precisely seventy-two hours after the birth of a child will suppress the production of harmful antibodies and protect any child she may have in the future from Rh factor disease. If this preventive measure was not taken prior to the birth of the present child, the infant's life may be saved by giving it an exchange transfusion, in which the baby's blood is replaced with blood that does not contain the damaging antibodies.

Congenital malformations (deformities)

Of the many types of congenital defects that may occur, only the more common are listed here.

The birth of a child with a congenital defect comes as a shock to the parents. The question naturally arises, "Why did this happen to our child?" The parents feel deeply concerned as to what they might have done wrong. However, frequently these abnormalities are quite unrelated to what the parents did or did not do. Speculation is unproductive. Parents with such a problem would do well to seek the support of an organization composed of parents of defective children. Membership in such an organization serves well as group therapy and helps the parents to emphasize helping the child rather than focusing on their frustration over the child's plight.

Progress in medicine has made it possible to correct, or at least modify, many congenital defects. Procedures once delayed till the child was older can now be done promptly. Infants have been found to tolerate surgical corrections very well.

Following are some of the more common congenital defects, with a reference for finding additional information about each one: **congenital heart disease,** page 797; **spina bi-** **fida,** page 1047; **hydrocephalus,** page 1046; **clubfoot,** page 946; **harelip,** page 845; and **mongolism (Down's syndrome),** page 428.

Congenital glaucoma

In this disorder, faulty development prevents adequate drainage of the fluid formed within the eye. Eighty percent of these cases can be recognized by the time the baby is three months old. The infant is extremely intolerant to light, and the cornea (the clear structure in front of the colored iris) has a hazy or dull appearance. Should you notice either of these conditions, see your physician immediately.

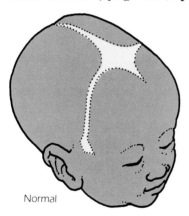
Normal

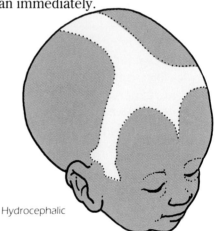
Hydrocephalic

In hydrocephalus, the bones of the skull are pushed apart (right).

Nervous-system disturbances

Cerebral palsy

Cerebral palsy results from an abnormality in the brain that arises sometime during the brain's development. The damage may occur before, during, or soon after birth. Because the site of this damage varies from case to case, so do the specific symptoms. In most cases there is an impairment of the control of the muscles (more commonly in the legs), coupled with spasticity (stiffness), with awkward, jerking movements. Some victims experience involuntary movements such as twisting and twitching. Some have compulsive, impaired speech and a degree of mental deficiency, while others are highly intelligent.

The precise cause is not always known. Possible causes may include an inadequate supply of oxygen due to restricted blood supply (such as during a difficult delivery in which the cord has been compressed or the brain traumatized); prolonged labor; multiple births; and some cases of hemolytic anemia, when high blood levels of bilirubin are present.

Cerebral palsy may be recognized by the newborn's inability to nurse or swallow, decreased general activity, undue stiffness, inability to kick with both legs, and, as the child grows older, inability to crawl, walk, or stand normally.

Treatment should begin without delay, as soon as diagnosis is made. Training programs center around speech training, muscle reeducation, the use of braces, special tutoring in school, and vocational guidance. Many cerebral-palsy victims are capable of living quite normal lives. Physical therapy may be necessary to prevent deformities and ensure joint mobility. Medications are sometimes used to reduce spasticity.

Down's syndrome (mongolism)

Down's syndrome is a congenital condition. The symptoms include mental retardation (a mean intelligence quotient of about 50); stunted growth; a small skull; coarse, scanty hair; a flat face; an upward slope to the eyes; a depressed nose bridge; a thick tongue; short, thick hands and feet; and a laxity of the ligaments (often double-jointed). Many Down's children have abnormalities of the heart, intestines, and teeth (malocclusion and missing teeth).

Down's syndrome is usually associated with a defect of the chromosomes (trisomy 21). The chromosomes designated as pair 21 produce three individual chromosomes rather than the usual two. The condition may be transmitted by either parent. Women over thirty-five are more likely to transmit this abnormality.

Because the condition is congenital, no cure exists. The goals are to train such children to do as much as their limits permit and to shelter them from life's competitions. Some are responsive, pleasant, and loving. Some are best cared for by relatives, whereas others fare better when placed in an institution.

A procedure called **amniocentesis** can be performed by which it can be known before birth whether a baby will be born with Down's syndrome. Amniocentesis is generally performed between the fourteenth and sixteenth weeks for women whose fetuses are most likely to suffer from Down's—those over thirty-five and those with a family history of Down's syndrome. If the procedure indicates Down's syndrome, the woman and her husband should discuss the implications with her physician.

CHAPTER 7

Growth and development

From the moment of conception to birth and on to adulthood, each person's cells, tissues, and organs grow and develop steadily until he or she reaches full maturity. Not only do the person's physical components form, but his personality also unfolds. This growth, which encompasses all of a person's characteristics, does not occur symmetrically, but rather, by spurts. Certain organ systems may grow at a faster rate at one time, while other systems will accelerate their growth at a later time.

During the first six or seven years of life the nervous and lymphatic systems develop rapidly, so that the brain of a seven-year-old has almost reached adult size! As adolescence approaches, the sex organs, which grew but little during the earlier years, now undergo rapid development. On the other hand, the lymphatic system, with its large mass of lymphoid tissues (thymus, adenoids, tonsils), not only stops growing at this time, but actually regresses. The thymus atrophies, and the tonsils and adenoids shrink.

Thus, the body's organ systems follow their individual patterns of development, with some progressing at a faster rate than others. Also, there are certain differences between males and females. Even within the same sex, some individuals develop at a faster rate than others.

The pattern of growth and development

While nutritional, environmental, and emotional factors play an important role, the **basic pattern** of an individual's growth and development is determined largely by the combination of chromosomes and genes at the time of his conception. Whether the person will be tall, stocky, or of athletic build is a matter of heredity. The hormones produced by the endocrine glands play an important part in all the changes that occur.

Adolescence

Until adolescence, the growth rate for both boys and girls follows the same pattern. But with the onset of adolescence, this plan abruptly changes. Girls generally begin to mature two to three years earlier than do boys, reaching their peak growth spurt during their thirteenth and fourteenth years. Boys have their growth spurt during their fifteenth and sixteenth years.

At the beginning of adolescence, the pituitary gland produces a hormone known as gonadotropin. This hormone stimulates the sex organs, either male or female, to produce androgens in the boy and estrogens in the girl.

Androgens are produced by the testes in the male, and also in the cortex of his adrenal glands. As these hormones circulate throughout his body, they trigger the growth of the long bones. This accounts for the rather sudden increase in height—the typical "growth spurt"—so noticeable in adolescent boys. The androgens also bring about a maturing of the male organs and other changes in body contour, growth of hair on the chin and cheeks, and the lowering of the voice that are so characteristic of the male.

In an adolescent girl, the estrogen hormones are produced by the ovaries. These stimulate the growth of the long bones, increasing the young woman's height, but the stimulation is not as great as that produced by androgens in a male. Thus, the average girl does not grow to be quite as tall as the average boy. Estrogens cause a maturing of the female sex organs and modify the pattern of growth to provide for the feminine features and characteristics, including development of the breasts.

While the rate of growth is changing from month to month and year to year, each individual has his or her own order of progression. The curves in the diagram on p. 432 illustrate the growth of boys and girls from birth to maturity. These curves represent percentiles of growth from five to ninety-five, the average being the fiftieth percentile. Some children will start life in the ninety-fifth percentile, while another might begin at the fifth. After a few weeks, each child will settle into his/her level of growth. It is quite evident that some children are small, while others are large.

The importance of such growth profiles is not so much the particular percentile the child happens to be in, but rather that growth continue steadily upward at a constant rate. For example, if a child has been growing in the seventy-fifth percentile and suddenly drops to the fiftieth or fortieth level, this indicates that something is wrong. Moving to a higher percentile of growth is acceptable as long as it can be maintained. The cause for shifts from one percentile to another should be determined by your physician.

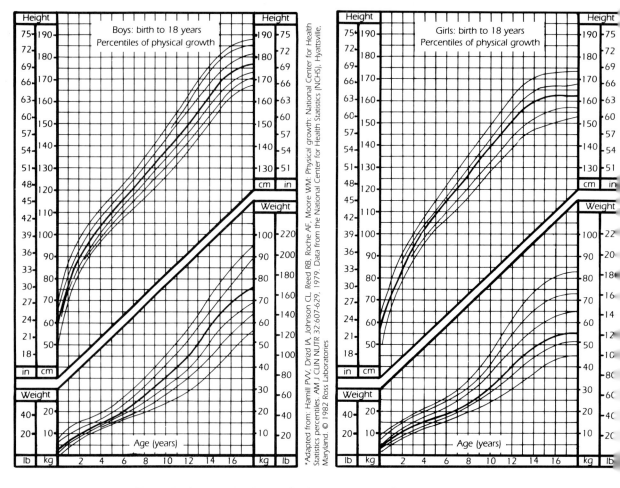

*Adapted from: Hamill P.V.V., Drizd IA, Johnson CL, Reed RB, Roche AF, Moore WM: Physical growth: National Center for Health Statistics percentiles. AM J CLIN NUTR 32:607-629, 1979. Data from the National Center for Health Statistics (NCHS), Hyattsville, Maryland. © 1982 Ross Laboratories

Growth, in percentiles, of girls and boys from birth to maturity.

Changing proportions

Even though the main features of the human body are present during the early part of fetal life, the proportions of the various parts are quite different when compared with those of the adult. Even at birth, an infant is not just a scaled-down version of what it will be a few years later. Its head is usually large, and its arms and legs are relatively small.

The various parts mature at different rates. The large head of the fetus and young infant is necessary because the brain develops relatively early as compared with other organs, whose functions become important a little later. The brain and the other parts of the nervous system must be able to control the movements of the muscles and perform other functions of regulation that are necessary during the early phases of development.

As the chart on page 433 indicates, the relatively large head accounts for about half of the total height of a two-month-old fetus. At birth, the head accounts for one-fourth the infant's length, whereas in the adult, the head accounts for only about one-eighth of the total height. This reduction does not mean, of course, that the head has decreased in size. The head continues to grow throughout fetal life, and, at a slower rate, throughout childhood. But because the head grew faster than other parts of the body during the earlier stages of development, its slower growth later allows the other parts of the body to assume their share of the adult height by the time physical maturity is attained.

A child's face differs from that of an adult. We speak of it as a "baby face." In a child's face, the bridge of the nose divides the face about evenly, with about as much of the head above this point as below. As a child matures, the lower face length-

birth, the greatest amount of growth occurs in the trunk. At one year, the child's large trunk and big head contrast with his short, fat legs, which are often bowed. But after the first year, the legs grow faster than other body parts.

Until the onset of adolescence, the body build of boys and girls remains similar. Some are slender, and some are chubby, but this variation occurs in both boys and girls. But beginning with adolescence, when the growth spurt occurs, the male follows a different pattern than the female.

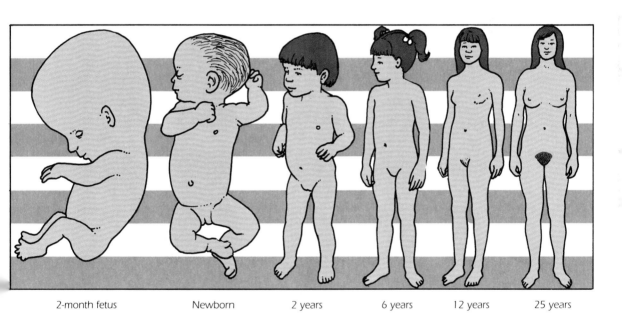

| 2-month fetus | Newborn | 2 years | 6 years | 12 years | 25 years |

The body proportions constantly change from conception to birth, and from birth to maturity.

ens, so that by adulthood, one-third of the face is above the bridge of the nose and about two-thirds are below.

Significant changes also take place in the relative lengths of the trunk and limbs. During the first year after

As mentioned earlier, girls usually reach adolescence two to three years earlier than boys, and this accounts for two interesting observations. First, for a short time in their early teens, girls are often larger and taller

433

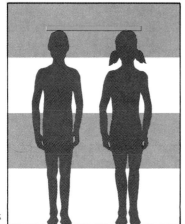

9 years

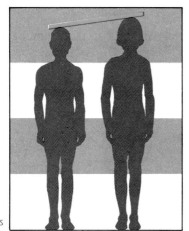

13 years

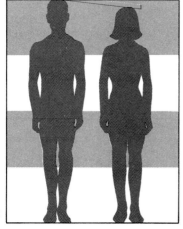

16 years

Girls have their accelerated rate of growth earlier and mature at a younger age than do boys.

than boys of the same age—a phenomenon that causes considerable embarrassment to some adolescent boys! Second, the period during which a boy's legs grow faster than the other parts of his body continues longer. Thus, when both boys and girls have completed their growth spurts, the average boy is taller than the average girl because his legs are longer, but the body is about the same length in both adult men and adult women, as is evident when watching them sit side by side.

Men also tend to have broader shoulders than women. This makes it appear that men have narrower hips than women, but in reality, the hips are about the same size for both.

Variations in the rate of growth

The rate of growth is fastest during the nine months prior to birth. *Rate* of growth means the comparative increase in weight and height, as when either of these measures increases by 50 or 100 percent. The rate of growth is fastest before birth because the starting point is very near zero.

Even after birth, the rate of growth continues to be rapid at first, with the average infant weighing three times as much on his first birthday as when he was born. However, height does not increase at such a rapid rate. The four-year-old is twice as tall as at birth.

While total growth is rapid during the first four years of life, the *rate* of growth actually slows down. The infant grows twice as much during the

434

first year as the second, twice as much the second year as the third, and so on for the next two years. On close examination it is also apparent that infants grow twice as fast during the first month as the second, and twice as fast the first week as the second week. Thus, it is evident that the body's growth rate begins slowing down immediately after birth.

From the fifth to the ninth or tenth years of life, the child grows only a little each year. During this period a slow rate of growth and decreased appetite are perfectly normal. An understanding of this fact has important

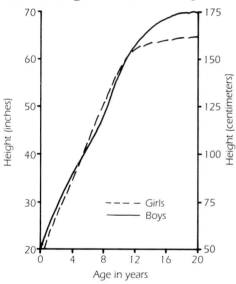

Boys and girls grow at about the same rate until puberty. Girls mature earlier and stop growing sooner, and are therefore usually shorter.

implications. Some parents worry that their children are not eating enough or that they have stopped growing. However, rarely are either of these fears justified. Food intake, in a healthy child, parallels the rate of growth. The faster the body tissues are being formed, the more the child will eat. Giving him extra vitamins and minerals "to make him grow faster" is unwise. Just wait for the adolescent growth spurt.

Someone has calculated that if a child's height continued to increase after birth at the same average rate that it increased before birth, he would be about 23 feet (7 meters) tall by age ten! Parents can be thankful that their children's growth slows down between the ages of five and nine!

We may speculate as to why it takes the human child so long to reach his adult size, while most domestic animals reach their adult size within a matter of months. Actually, the Creator had a purpose in this arrangement. The slower rate of growth and development in humans allows time for the development of personality and character. It gives parents an opportunity to train and direct their children's way of life. Later in life, children can develop their own characters and personalities through their choices and decisions. Because their nervous systems are still completing their development, within reasonable limits, children can become the kinds of people they want to be.

Ultimate size

Many parents would like to predict how tall their children will be when they reach maturity. This wish is often shared by their children! Inasmuch as inherited patterns of growth and development provide for a certain sequence of events, the child's size, at any stage of his

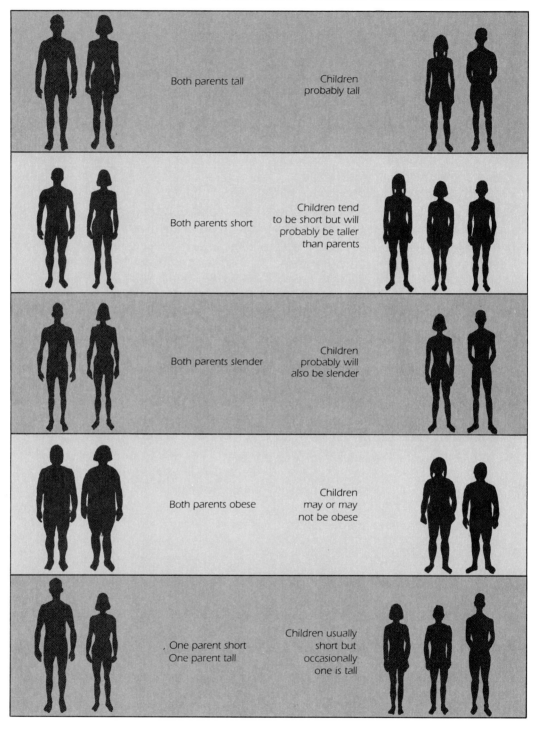

Both parents tall

Children probably tall

Both parents short

Children tend to be short but will probably be taller than parents

Both parents slender

Children probably will also be slender

Both parents obese

Children may or may not be obese

One parent short
One parent tall

Children usually short but occasionally one is tall

The diagrams illustrate how a child tends to inherit the characteristics of the parents.

growth, can be a predictor of his ultimate size. A baby that measures longer than average at birth will very likely become a tall adult. Interestingly, a child's height on his second birthday is generally very close to half of what his adult height will be.

Children must generally live to sixteen or eighteen, and occasionally longer, to reach their full adult height. However, a number of factors may retard the development specified in the hereditary blueprint, including faulty nutrition, severe illnesses, and unfavorable emotional experiences. If these interferences last only a short time, the adolescent growth spurt may compensate for them to a large extent.

Parents often become concerned because their children appear too big or too small for their age. Again, such fears are generally unfounded. Each child passes the various milestones of the journey toward maturity at the rate prescribed by his or her genetic pattern, some speeding through the sequence of events at a faster pace than others. A few perfectly normal children will reach their physical maturity as early as fourteen years of age, while others will not arrive at this stage of development until they are twenty or twenty-one.

The child who matures at a slower pace is just as normal as one who rushes through the sequence. The slow-maturing child will have all the capacities of the one who develops earlier. There is nothing anyone can do to hasten or slow the progress toward maturity. The goal should be to maintain the best health possible,

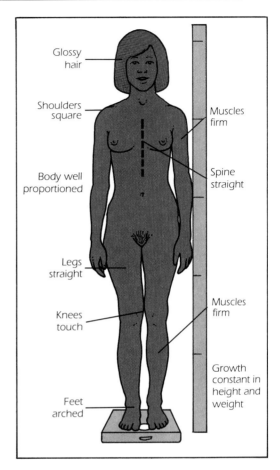

The physical characteristics of a healthy child.

which, in turn, will provide the very best circumstances for the maximum development of the child's entire hereditary potential.

Interestingly, people grow taller today than they did a hundred years ago. Various explanations have been suggested for this increase. The best evidence indicates that children with improved environmental conditions, better nutrition, and freedom from childhood diseases (due to vaccinations) grow a little faster and a little larger than those whose circumstances are not so favorable.

437

Behavioral development

Equally as important as physical growth is the development of a child's pattern of behavior. And just as there are stages in physical development, so there are stages in the ability to think and act.

Children with favorable living conditions and adequate nutrition make automatic, predictable progress in their physical growth and development, and about all parents can do is

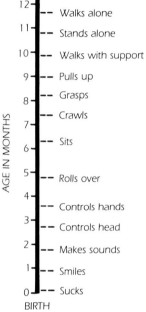

Behavioral development during the first year of life.

to be sure their children's circumstances are as favorable as possible. But with behavioral development, parents carry a far greater responsibility. Their personal influence, their methods of encouragement, and their ways of dealing with unacceptable behavior impact their children for better or for worse.

Actually, physical and behavioral development are more closely related than we sometimes realize. A child's behavior can be modified and controlled only within the limits that his developing nervous system permits. A two-year-old may try to do things that are characteristically easy for a four-year-old, but he is not yet able to do them because the nerve pathways in his brain and other parts of his body are not yet tuned to the four-year-old's more complicated behavior.

Parents make a mistake in trying to encourage or force their children to do things beyond their age. A precocious child does not have a better chance of ultimate success than the child who follows a more leisurely pace in the development of his personality. A child's own zest for activity and progress is the best guide in determining what he is capable of doing.

Normal course of development

As already mentioned, each child has his own pattern of development, and, except perhaps for identical twins, no two children have identical rates of growth. In the outline on the next page, only the more common capabilities of the average child are listed. These have been grouped together at three- to six-month intervals.

During the first three years of life, the body's organ systems are de-

438

Age	Progressive development
At three months	Smiles, holds head erect (with some wobbling), sits when supported, moves arms toward objects, turns from side to back, listens to sounds, eyes follow moving objects, coos and gurgles.
At six months	Rolls over from back to side, holds head, sits steadily when held, plays with hands and clothing, transfers objects from hand to hand, babbles, tries to stand when helped.
At nine months	Sits without support, rolls over from back to stomach, pulls up to standing position, crawls with arms and drags legs, uses thumb to pick up objects, recognizes parents, especially mother, responds to name.
At twelve months	Stands alone (for several moments), walks with help, picks up objects, places one object on top of another, says a few words.
At twenty-four months	Walks well, runs fairly well, jumps short distances, walks up and down stairs, stacks three or more blocks, turns pages in book, identifies pictures in book, listens to stories, tries to draw with pencil, feeds self with spoon, opens doors, tries to dress.
At thirty months	Jumps up from floor, down from chair, can stand on one foot momentarily, hands and fingers work together, stacks blocks very well, wants to do things himself, knows his full name, enjoys books and stories.
At thirty-six months	Runs well, stands on one foot, rides tricycle, can walk up and down stairs with alternate feet, pulls toys with a string, buttons and unbuttons clothes, speaks in short sentences, listens to stories and asks them to be repeated, tries to sing, feeds himself (although messily), extremely curious and active, is often demanding.

veloping rapidly, and with this development, the control of the central nervous system becomes increasingly fine tuned. As the nervous system matures, the child is increasingly able to coordinate the movements of eyes and ears, head and body, hands and feet, so that activities are done intelligently, for a purpose. The child's understanding of the events around him increases rapidly, and he becomes ever more capable of expressing his own desires and preferences.

The critical period of training

Many parents feel that the toddler is too young to train and discipline. As a result, activities that at a later stage would be considered unacceptable are regarded as "cute." This is a serious mistake. Your little ones are quite aware of what you want and do not want. Little children can understand that certain things must be done and certain other things are not permitted—"no-no's"—and you do not need to use harsh physical measures to obtain compliance.

Children can be taught the little courtesies and niceties of behavior at a very young age. Tiny tots can learn to say Please and Thank you. This is especially true if the parents are polite to each other and to their children. Children have tender feelings, just like adults. You do not need to raise your voice in order to gain obedience. Speak to your children as though you were talking to a friend. If your child only obeys when you have made your request two or three times in louder and louder tones, and you have to change your voice to be more threatening, you are not teaching your child obedience. Speak once, clearly, in a matter-of-fact way, and expect compliance.

Consistency is the key. Toddlers do not inherently know what is right and wrong. To them, right and wrong are what Daddy and Mother say is right or wrong. An object or activity that is denied one time and allowed another time confuses the little one. Parents must carefully decide which activities and behaviors are acceptable and which are not, including the things that can be touched or played with.

It is important to understand that without a permanent memory, one cannot make true decisions. Few of us remember events that occurred before we were five or six years old. We have no recollection whether we were made to go to our room or received a spanking for some misbehavior. The first five or six years are a period for conditioning a child in the way he should go. This should be done lovingly, consistently, and firmly. Never deny something you really don't mind your child doing or having, and never allow anything you do not believe he should have or do.

Danger signs to watch for at this time include excessive recourse to tantrums and failure to conform to *reasonable* discipline. When a child understands what should or should not be done, but does not wish to do it, the parent must kindly and lovingly see that he obeys. Waffling on the part of the parents leaves the little mind perplexed and befuddled, without guide or compass. If, as parents, you need counsel, seek help from a professional or from parents who have successfully negotiated these situations.

The preschooler

A three- to six-year-old child is generally slender, graceful, lithe, active, and talkative. His primary concern is himself. Self-centeredness is a typical characteristic. He has become interested in the differences between boys and girls and asks questions about where babies come from and about other intimate matters. He is now less dependent on his mother and takes pride in doing things unassisted. He has good coordination and usually has good control of his organs of elimination, both day and night.

The preschool child uses language well, imitating the sentence structure and the pronunciation of words that he hears in the home. He can carry a tune and loves songs and rhythms. He still likes stories and pictures, and he enjoys looking at books, which he handles well without tearing the pages.

The preschooler also does well at eating and drinking. He eats what the family eats and seldom spills his food or drink. He wants to be part of the group at mealtime. He is fascinated by picnics and other variations in the pattern of eating. His growth rate is rather slow, and his actual consumption of food appears to be small.

At play, the preschooler is often dramatic and acts out the life scenes that he sees around him. He plays cooperatively with others of his age, but if such playmates are not available, he finds pleasure in the make-believe world of his toys, his toy animals, and pets.

The parents of a preschool child should be alert for such signs as persistent bed-wetting, excessive tantrums, overdependence on the mother, inability to take care of simple personal needs, or late development of language ability. However, keep in mind that perfectly normal children may progress at rates different from those suggested in this discussion. Parents should be tolerant of variations so long as these do not indicate a radical departure from the usual sequence of events. It is important that parents play with their children as companions in these early years, and at all times exert a steady, gentle, guiding influence.

The school-age child

A child starts losing his deciduous teeth when he is about six, and this continues to somewhere between eleven and fifteen years of age, when he comes to his adolescent growth spurt.

The school-age child is in a period of slow but continuous growth. Steady growth in height and weight is an indication that he is progressing normally. However, look for a hidden health problem, such as poor nutrition, lack of sleep, insufficient physical exercise, or overwhelming emotional stress, if he goes longer than three months without gaining any weight.

In most cases, a child's health is good throughout this period. His immunity to illness should have improved, and thus he should have fewer colds, earaches, and infections.

This is the time to develop good muscular coordination, so encourage activities that require motor skills and muscular exertion. Unfortunately, in today's developed societies, children are allowed to spend long hours sitting or lying in front of a television set, which seriously handicaps them in later years.

Normally a child of this age does well in school and should be encouraged to read books, acquire hobbies, and become curious regarding the world of nature. Parents should become interested in what their children are doing in school. If your child is doing poorly, find out the reason. The problem may be simply irregularities in sleeping (staying up too late) or eating (too much sugar), insufficient interest in his studies, associating with the wrong friends, or becoming involved in drugs. On the other hand, the problem may be due to a physical handicap such as poor vision or poor hearing. Whatever the problem, try to identify it and correct it.

Some children demand independence. They want to do "their own thing." Do not weaken in exercising your parental control over home affairs and over the necessary guidance your child needs at this age. Children actually respect their parents for being firm, as long as they feel that their parents are reasonable. The earlier years of careful, consistent conditioning in the ways the child should behave will now pay big dividends.

This is the age when a child establishes the foundations of his ethical and moral values for the future. He is a keen observer of his parents and of his teachers, as well as of those his own age. When he detects that his parents are sincere, consistent, and impartial in their loyalty to the ideals they profess, he is favorably impressed and inclined to follow their example. But if he observes that they profess one thing and practice something different, he becomes confused in his development of ideals and begins to think of what he can get out of life, rather than what he can contribute to the good of others.

Parents should be alert to the telltale signs of difficulty in a child of school age. If he does poorly at his schoolwork; if he has symptoms of illness, either real or imagined; if he becomes involved in lying or stealing or other antisocial behavior—any such indications of trouble should prompt them to consult a person who has both training and experience in handling the problems of childhood.

CHAPTER 8

Common childhood problems and complaints

Parents are often frustrated to know how to deal with their children's peculiarities. One of the heartening things about rearing children is that very few problems are peculiar to one child. If you are at your wit's end to know how to cope with tantrums, bed-wetting, or a child's refusal to eat, rest assured that other parents have walked these paths and crossed these bridges ahead of you.

The major cause of death among children in the United States today is accidents. However, in the adult population the killer diseases are those that are brought on by long-term unhealthful habits of life. Often the unhealthful lifestyle commences in early childhood. Atherosclerosis, with resulting coronary heart disease and stroke, and cancer, high blood pressure, diabetes, and chronic kidney failure appear to have their origins in the way children learn to eat and live.

Parents carry a great responsibility for the health of their children, not only while they are small, but throughout their entire adult life. The principles of a healthy lifestyle are simple: good food and right eating habits; plenty of physical exercise; adequate rest and sleep; respect for the human body through the avoidance of tobacco, alcohol, caffeine-containing beverages, and drugs; and a wholesome mental and emotional attitude in a loving, supportive environment.

To a great extent, the health that is enjoyed by an adult depends on his faithful adherence to these principles during childhood, for it is in childhood that the habit patterns of life are established. And the robust child, even as a child, will do better at home, at school, and in life.

Childhood problems

Problems related to eating

In this discussion we will focus on the problems encountered in the eating habits of children, rather than on what constitutes sound nutrition, which is discussed elsewhere (see pages 83, 237). A good diet means reducing to a minimum the consumption of refined foods. These foods include refined sugar, refined fats and oils, refined cereals, and products made largely from them. Each meal should include a small variety of simple, unrefined foods. The diet for an entire day should include a larger variety, and, of course, a wide variety should be included in any one season, according to what the season provides. Cereal grains and their products, together with fruits, vegetables, nuts, and generally selected animal products make up the ideal diet.

Meals should be regularly spaced, and no food should be eaten between meals. Snack foods tend to be high in sugar and fat. When these foods are eaten at irregular times, the child comes to the meal with his appetite blunted for simple, nutritious food. Because he is not hungry, he will not eat enough to last him till the next meal. Two hours later he complains of being hungry and is allowed another snack. In this way a most unfortunate habit is established.

If food is available only at regular mealtimes, the child will soon learn to eat enough to meet his needs. However, do not try to force a child to eat more than he desires. Do not force him to clean his plate, especially by offering dessert as a reward. This only encourages overeating, which contributes to overweight. Do not try to make a child eat hurriedly. Give him *small* servings. Second and third helpings are better than being wasteful with food.

This does not mean that parents should ignore the fact that their children leave food on their plates. When the child serves himself, warn him not to take too much. If he overloads his plate anyway—and most children do, at first—let him eat what he wants. When he indicates that he's had enough, excuse him from the table, but put away his plate with the food just as he left it. At the next meal, tell him that he must finish his leftovers before he can have anything else. Generally you will need to do this only once or twice before the child learns his lesson—and the lesson is an important one.

If *you* overestimate your child's appetite and put too much food on his plate, let him leave the table as soon as he lets you know that he is full; then discard the leftovers.

Remember that children are not adults. Their handling of knives and forks will be clumsy. Show them good manners by your own example. Say Please and Thank you for all foods passed to you. This will make mealtime a pleasant occasion, and this is most important. A happy spirit at the table binds a family together. Ancient kings had court jesters who kept the king and his guests enjoying themselves while they ate. Only when absolutely essential should a child be rebuked or punished during a meal.

Some children dislike certain foods. Parents should remember that they, too, have likes and dislikes about food. There is no need to force a child to eat food he does not like, nor is there any need to make an issue over his preferences. Here is a simple technique that works very well—a rule of the home for both children and adults: Every member of the family will eat a little bit of *all* the main foods provided at each meal. A little may be a mere half teaspoonful at first. The important thing is to make no exceptions to the rule. In this way, over a period of years, most children and adults learn to enjoy the very foods they once disliked! Of course, both children and adults should be given larger servings of the foods they do like.

Often children are allowed to eat fruit or drink fruit juices between meals, on the supposition that fruit somehow is not a food. This is a great mistake. Fruit contains nutrients that require just as much digestion as vegetables and cereals. Eating fruit or drinking fruit juice at odd times interferes with the digestion of the previous meal and disturbs the appetite for the next meal.

When preparing lunches for children to take to school, design the foods so that they can be eaten in the time allotted. Foods that are hard to chew or that take a long time to eat cause children to feel embarrassed in front of their friends. Make your children's lunches attractive so they will have pleasure in eating them.

Toilet training

Young children should be encouraged, but not forced, to use the pottie. There is no need to make the bathroom a battleground. Bowel training can easily be accomplished if it is begun at about eighteen months. Begin by giving your child plenty of fluids (water, juices) and foods rich in fiber (fruits, vegetables, legumes, whole grains). This will prevent the stool from being hard and painful to pass. Bladder training should begin at a slightly older age, keeping in mind, of course, that some children learn earlier than others. Place the child on the pottie for about five minutes immediately after each meal. Give him something special to play with at such times.

Parents should be deliberately casual in their attitude toward these body functions. Appearing repulsed by the odors or calling the child naughty—to say nothing of punishment—sets the stage for emotional problems. Encouragement will make the child want to learn toilet habits and will make training easier.

Bed-wetting (enuresis)

Bed-wetting occurs somewhat more commonly among boys than among girls. Some children develop the ability to remain dry all night at an earlier age than others. One study indicates that by the age of eight, 7 percent of children still wet the bed. A few do not gain full control until about the age of twelve.

The child who wets the bed does

not do so intentionally and should not be punished for it. Sympathy and understanding go much farther toward helping the child to overcome this problem than do reprimands and punishment. Brothers and sisters who have gained control should not be allowed to ridicule a sibling who is still struggling. This only tends to precipitate emotional problems.

It is not known whether bed-wetting is a physical or psychological problem. Some children sleep so soundly that the brain does not over-rule the local reflexes for emptying the bladder. In others, the capacity of the bladder does not increase as fast as does the general growth of the body. It is estimated that in 20 percent of bed-wetting children, there is an actual hindrance to the free flow of urine somewhere between the bladder and the outside. This hindrance does not prevent the emptying of the bladder when the child is awake, but disturbs the controls sufficiently to cause bed-wetting at night. These hindrances may consist of a stricture (narrowing) or folds in the lining membrane of the urethra.

Bed-wetting does not indicate that a child has emotional problems, for many bed-wetters show up among perfectly stable children. More plausible is the view that bed-wetting demonstrates a delay in the development of the nervous controls that regulate the emptying of the bladder, at least in some children. Here are some simple methods that may help your child to control bed-wetting:

- Have the child develop the ability to hold his urine longer and longer during his waking hours. Put a chart in his room to record how long he held his urine, and a container to measure the volume of the urine he passed. Give him a reward for increasing the duration and quantity of urine he holds between times.
- Encourage your child to drink plenty of water during the afternoon, and then to gradually decrease the amount toward evening.
- Praise your child whenever he has a dry night.
- Have the child urinate just before going to bed. Wake him up and take him to the toilet an hour later and again before you go to bed. Set an alarm and take him to the toilet a couple of hours after you retire. Gradually increase the time between trips to the bathroom to the point that the child is only going once a night. In due time, he will start waking up on his own.

Most children respond well to these methods. While they take a bit of the parents' time, they are probably less work, especially for the mother, than washing sheets every day.

Electronic devices seem to work for some children, especially those over eight years of age. A bed-wetting electronic device consists of a metal pad that is placed underneath the child's sheet. Whenever the metal gets wet, it establishes a low-voltage electrical contact (battery operated), which, in turn, sets off an alarm. The alarm goes off anytime the child begins to void, waking him up to finish the process in the bathroom.

If nothing seems to work, have your child examined by a urologist. He will correct any physical defects that may be contributing to the problem. He may also recommend a medication that helps some children. Encourage your child to do his best, and assure him that he will outgrow the problem in due time, which is nearly always the case.

You should suspect an infection, diabetes, or an emotional problem if your child has been dry and suddenly starts wetting again. Consult your physician if this happens.

Constipation

In constipation, bowel movements occur less frequently than usual, and the fecal matter is so dry that its passage is uncomfortable. Keep in mind, though, that the frequency of bowel movements varies a great deal from person to person, even among those in good health.

A common cause of constipation in children is a lack of sufficient bulk in the diet, such as is provided by whole grains, fruits, and vegetables. Another common cause is failure to drink enough water. Psychological factors, such as too great an emphasis on toilet training, may cause a child to resist the normal urges that signal his need for a bowel movement. Sometimes a child deliberately ignores the desire to go to the toilet because it interferes with his play. In a small percentage of cases, a small anal opening or a pain-producing break in the membrane that lines the anal canal may interfere with the passage of the stool.

Occasionally, in a case of neglected constipation, the mass of fecal material within the rectum becomes so hard and dry that more fluid bowel contents from the upper part of the bowel find their way around the hard mass and cause the child to soil his clothing. This condition can even be mistaken for diarrhea.

If your child becomes too constipated to have a bowel movement at all, you will need to help him get rid of the hard mass. Prepared chemical enemas are available at any pharmacy, or you may wish to use a small (2 to 4 oz or 60 to 120 ml) retention enema consisting of mineral oil, tap water, or water with a teaspoonful of salt to the pint. (See page 574 for details on how to use an enema.)

However, avoid repeated use of enemas to treat chronic constipation. It is much better to diagnose the underlying cause and correct that. One of the first things to do is to increase the amount of water your child drinks each day. Try increasing the amount of fruits in his diet, especially prunes, apricots, and figs. Also encourage him to eat foods that are high in fiber: whole wheat, oatmeal, and green leafy vegetables. If the condition persists, discuss the problem with your physician.

Bedtime problems

Some children resist going to bed at the designated time. They may cry when left alone in their bed, or they may slip out of bed and find their parents. Children who are allowed to persist in this behavior develop a serious habit that is very difficult to break. Neither punishment, scolding, nor giving in to the child's whims will solve the problem. Consistency is extremely important. Once all your child's needs have been met—going to the pottie, sipping water, saying "good night"—he must learn that bedtime has arrived.

Look for the underlying cause. Among the more common causes of wakefulness in children are long naps taken late in the afternoon, overstimulating play in the evening just before bedtime, and emotional tension in the home. Avoid the cause, whatever it is, and be firm and kind about the child going to bed when bedtime arrives. Place the child in bed in a comfortable position with her favorite doll, his stuffed animal, or blanket. You may leave the bedroom door ajar or a dim night light burning.

Some children are troubled with terrible dreams or **nightmares.** These often follow some intense emotional experience, the viewing of scary movies, or a violent TV program. These night terrors are frequently noted in children between the ages of four and eight, and sometimes they are accompanied by **sleepwalking.** If these dreams occur *frequently*, one to two hours after going to sleep, try waking your child up about a half hour before the usual occurrence several nights in a row. This may cure the problem. When these episodes do occur, give the child love and assurance, and arrange suitable types of entertainment.

Childhood fears

An infant is relatively helpless. He depends on those closest to him for protection and loving care.

Separation anxiety is a problem of little children, beginning at about six months and continuing at least through the first three years. Having learned to depend on his mother for security and comfort, the child becomes terrified when suddenly she is not with him. To avoid this panic, parents should arrange to have one or more other persons become acquainted with the child and share in his care. Then, when the mother must be absent, the child can still feel at ease with a baby sitter that he has already become acquainted with.

Fears of people, animals, and things develop at about three to four years of age. A child of this age or even younger is terrified by manifestations of his parents' anger. In controlling such fears, the example of the parents very largely determines how the child will react, especially the mother, whom he tends to imitate. He observes whether his parents remain calm and confident when strange things happen. A child of this age can understand the explanations his parents make of the things that cause him to be afraid, but these explanations must be repeated over and over again. A loving, sympathetic attitude helps the child develop his ability to cope.

School phobia affects some children when they start school. In this new experience, the child is surrounded with new faces and feels uncertain about what is expected. He has learned to rely on his mother for the guidance and assurance he needs in new experiences, but she is not there. Suddenly he feels alone, even though surrounded by others.

His reaction to school depends greatly on whether he has learned to cope with fear-producing experiences earlier in life. Here, again, the child needs sympathetic understanding and encouragement. Of course, his mother cannot be with him at school. But it may help if a child he knows can accompany him to school. It also helps for him to become personally acquainted with the teacher outside of school. Patience, reassurance, and commendation for what he does well will help him to develop self-assurance.

The hyperactive child (attention deficit disorder, hyperkinetic child)

The term "hyperactive child" refers to several behavior abnormalities that affect children. Sometimes the problem is called **minimal brain dysfunction syndrome,** although many investigators have failed to find any brain damage. It is also called an **attention deficit disorder,** with or without hyperactivity. The major areas are: attention deficit, in which the child has an extremely short attention span, is easily distracted, appears not to listen, and does not complete assignments; impulsive behavior, in which the child does things on an impulse without thinking or planning what he will say or do, is impatient, and cannot complete assigned tasks; and hyperactivity, in which the child is constantly on the move, cannot sit still, cannot stop doing something, and goes from one thing to another. About 3 percent of American children are afflicted with these problems, which occur more often in boys than girls.

The cause of this handicap is presumed to be some unusual circumstance in the child's history. He may have been born prematurely. His mother may have had complications during her pregnancy or at the time of his birth. She may have used alcohol and other drugs during her pregnancy. The child himself may have had an attack of mild encephalitis, considered at the time as only the flu. Most of these children have a family history of hyperactivity (hyperkinesis).

In such cases, there may or may not be structural change in the brain. Usually the child's electroencephalogram (brain-wave tracing) is perfectly normal, or shows only slight variations from normal. At one time hyperactive children were thought to be allergic to certain food dyes, especially those of red color, but this theory has not proved to be valid.

Active children should not be confused with *hyperactive* children. Many normal children have a high level of activity. Often children with learning disabilities are assumed to be hyperactive.

No magic cure exists for these problems. The proper handling of a hyperactive child involves cooperation between parents, teachers, and physicians. The parents need to establish and maintain a home atmosphere in which the child feels comfortable, and yet in which he is not treated as different or abnormal. Limits must be set, and parents must stand together on these restrictions, or the child will learn to play one against the other. The teacher's role

449

is also difficult. In metropolitan areas, some schools provide special classes for hyperactive children that are conducted by teachers with special training.

Various treatments have been tried. Many of these children can be helped with stimulants, but the dosage requires careful adjustment by someone experienced in handling this disorder.

Large numbers of these children have learning disorders and psychological problems in addition to an attention deficit disorder. A team approach involving parents, physicians, educators, and psychologists is needed to help them learn to function in society and feel good about themselves.

A few hyperactive children appear to be helped by diet, but this is hard to prove and probably represents a small percentage of these children. Popular fads that are aired on TV talk shows are rarely successful, and often are presented by those who have had little experience in dealing with hyperactivity.

Without treatment, 40 to 50 percent of these children end up on the streets, in juvenile hall, on drugs, or in jail. Often they are unable to hold jobs. This is a serious problem. With all the pregnant teenagers and broken homes, the number of children with this disorder is increasing rapidly.

Tantrums

Temper tantrums are quite common in children during certain periods of development, notably at about two-and-a-half years of age, and again at about six. A tantrum is an uninhibited expression of rage that is triggered by frustration or by the child's inability to do certain things he would like to do. Parents should patiently and tactfully help their children find better ways of reacting.

A child uses tantrums to get his own way when he is deprived of what he wants. When a reasonable request has been made, the parent must insist on compliance, tantrum or no tantrum. The child must learn that throwing a tantrum does not pay. The best way to do this is to deprive him of that for which he threw the tantrum. Should he have a tantrum when playing with other children, he should be isolated in his room until he has calmed down. Giving in to a child's demands will just reinforce his angry behavior.

Poor eyesight

Vision is involved in almost everything a person does, especially in learning. A child with poor eyesight is handicapped in school. Many such children have been considered feebleminded, when poor vision was the real problem. About one child out of every twenty has a vision problem. Early detection, especially before the child starts school, is very important. For particular problems related to the eyes, see page 1128. You may request a "Home Eye Test for Preschoolers," from the National Society to Prevent Blindness, 79 Madison Avenue, New York, New York 10016.

Hearing problems

Children with hearing problems will show faulty development in other areas, and will especially experience learning difficulties in school. For some of the problems encountered, see under "congenital deafness," pages 469, 1153. Consult your physician if you suspect that your child has a hearing disability.

Speech defects

Speech is the most effective way in which humans communicate. Speech is a highly complex activity involving the speech area of the brain, where ideas are organized and words are selected to express those ideas; the nerves that activate the speech organs; the larynx, where sound is produced; and the modification of the sounds by the larynx, palate, tongue, cheeks, lips, and breathing muscles. A defect or malfunction in any of these areas will cause problems with speech.

Speech problems seen in children may result from several causes: a disorder of **expression,** where the child has normal comprehension; a disorder of **comprehension,** where expression is normal; and a disorder of **articulation,** where speech sounds are not correctly formed. Should you be concerned about any of these problems with your child, talk to your physician or consult a speech therapist.

Stuttering

Stuttering and stammering are synonymous terms referring to a form of speech difficulty in which the flow of speech is interrupted by pauses and the repetition of sounds and syllables. Facial grimaces will often accompany the effort to enunciate the desired word.

Stuttering typically appears in children sometime between the ages of two and ten. It affects about 1 percent of all school-age children, and is six times more common in boys than in girls. Usually, the fault is not with the organs of speech but is a symptom of some emotional disturbance, such as the child's feeling that his personal security or well-being are threatened.

A child's stuttering may be exaggerated by such circumstances as starting to school too soon, being pushed to carry schoolwork scholastically beyond his present stage of development, feeling insecure in personal relations at home, or being resentful of an older brother or sister's domination.

A child learns to speak by imitating the voices he hears. A mother should talk to her baby while bathing, dressing, and feeding him. The parents of a young child should encourage him to express himself, and never laugh at or ridicule these efforts. The greater assurance parents can give a child, the more readily he will develop the calm attitude that will make a smooth flow of speech possible. Spend time with your child in congenial companionship.

If at all possible, a child who stutters should be placed under the professional care of a speech therapist. Teaching the child how to relax is generally very helpful (see under "progressive relaxation," page 601).

Rhythmic movements

Some children exhibit rhythmic movements such as body rocking, head banging, and head rolling. Occasionally such movements as body rocking carry through into young adulthood, usually being manifested at times of emotional stress. For the most part, these rhythmic movements are harmless and occur in normal children. Those who develop such behavior patterns use them especially when they feel self-conscious or tired. One pediatrician suggested, partly in jest, that if mothers would spend more time rocking their babies, children would not resort to rocking themselves.

Accidents

Accidents stand at the head of the list—and way out in front—as a cause of death among children. Millions of accidents also happen each year which do not result in death. Children are particularly susceptible to accidents because of their lack of experience, their great curiosity, and their abundant energy. Responsible parents begin early in their children's lives to coach them on the importance of being alert to dangers and showing them how to take proper precautions. For additional information on accidents of the home, see pages 537-539; 544-547.

Burns

Burns may seriously endanger the life of a child. With infants and toddlers, the immersion scald burn, usually caused by overturned containers of hot liquid, is common and may be fatal. Flame burns from ignited clothing are most common among preschoolers. Burns affecting school-age boys are usually of the trash-fire type. For the care and treatment of burns, see under "burns," pages 537-540.

Poisonings

Children are especially susceptible to poisonings because they are curious, and because they imitate what they see the other members of the family do. Eighty percent of poisonings occurring in childhood take place between the ages of one and four. The precautions that parents should take to prevent childhood poisonings are discussed under "poisons," page 519.

Common complaints of children

A child's constant complaint about a particular problem should alert the parents to the possibility of an illness. The more common complaints are presented below.

Itching

Itching may result from a local problem, or may it be an indication of a systemic disease (see page 626). Itching of the skin may be caused by lice (page 982), scabies (page 981), eczema (page 678), and, in the rectal area, by pinworms (page 754).

Welts and wheals (hives)

Firm, raised spots that appear on the skin very suddenly and itch intensely are probably an allergic reaction (see page 989).

Sneezing, with itching of the eyes and nose

This problem is typical of hay fever or allergic rhinitis. (See page 910 for additional information.)

Wheezing (with difficult breathing)

This problem is generally caused by asthma. (See page 920 for additional information.)

Cough

A number of things can cause a child to cough, some of which are unimportant, but others can be very serious. Coughing is nature's response to some condition that interferes with the passage of air to and from the lungs.

Such simple things as choking or inhaling an irritating substance may cause a child to cough. Infection of the air passages (bronchitis) causes the membranes lining the passages to secrete an excess of mucus, and coughing helps to bring this mucus to the back of the throat so that it can be spat out. Severe coughing occurs in cases of whooping cough (pertussis). Coughing also accompanies influenza, late stages of the common cold, pneumonia, the early phases of measles, and asthma.

In managing a cough, the underlying problem should be treated. However, immediate relief may be obtained by using a humidifier, which moistens and warms the air. A makeshift way to bring warm moisture in is to keep a kettle of water boiling on a stove (see page 594). Also, simple cough syrups are available at any pharmacy. Should the cough persist, see your physician.

Earache

The most common cause of earache in a child is middle-ear infection (otitis media). For this and other causes of childhood earache, see page 1148.

Fever

The normal or average temperature of the body is 98.6°F (37°C). Fever is an elevation of the body temperature above this normal level because of illness. Vigorous physical activity in a hot environment will also raise the body temperature, but such a rise is not called a "fever." Fever commonly accompanies infections caused by germs such as the staphylococcus, streptococcus, and pneuomococcus, and is one of the symptoms of the contagious diseases of childhood. It sometimes occurs after a child has been vaccinated or when he has been given a medication. Fever is even seen in some healthy children in whom no specific illness can be discovered.

For instructions on taking a child's temperature, see page 573; to lower a fever, see pages 596, 598 ; for information on the role fever plays in disease, see page 703.

Growing pains

About 15 percent of children will complain at some time or another of pain in their limbs, especially at night, most commonly in the thigh, the calf, and the back of the knee. The pain may be in a muscle or in and around a joint. These attacks may last up to an hour, and may occur as often as once a day or as infrequently as once or twice a month. The child usually outgrows these episodes within a few weeks or months, but they may recur.

Such symptoms are typical of rheumatic fever and juvenile rheumatoid arthritis, so the child should be examined by a physician. If no disease is found, the child should be treated with supportive measures such as heat and massage to the affected areas (see pages 599, 601).

Headaches

Children get headaches, as do adults, and these complaints deserve due attention. They may accompany an infection in the nasal sinus (sinusitis) or in the middle ear (otitis media). A child with poor vision, or one who needs glasses to correct refractive errors, may develop headaches because of persistent contraction of the muscles of the neck and face from his efforts to see clearly. Migraine headaches may start in late childhood (see page 1051). A head injury (see page 1035) or brain tumor (see page 1046) may also cause headaches.

Nosebleed

Noseblood is a frequent childhood problem. It often occurs spontaneously, but may simply be the result of the child picking his nose. For controlling a nosebleed, see page 907.

"Stitch in the side"

Many children experience discomfort in one side or the other, just under the ribs, when they exercise vigorously. This problem is sometimes called "stitch in the side." A child soon learns that this pain disappears when he rests. The pain is probably due to a spasm of some of the muscles involved in breathing.

"Bellyache"

Bellyache is usually the result of vigorous, wavelike (peristaltic) contractions of the intestines. The most common cause is constipation (see page 877). Often it is nothing more than an indication of the child's urgent need to go to the toilet.

Recurrent abdominal pain

Observe carefully the circumstances under which recurrent abdominal pain occurs. It may be due to some disturbance of the digestive organs, such as the child's diet or habits of bowel elimination, or it may be due to the child's inability to digest lactose, the sugar naturally present in milk. The digestion of this sugar requires a special enzyme, lactase. Some children (and some adults) lose the ability to produce this enzyme, and after drinking milk, they experience abdominal pain, gas, bloating, and diarrhea. This is called **lactose intolerance.**

You can get an initial idea of whether this is your child's problem by having him abstain from milk and milk products for a few days. Most persons so affected can tolerate small amounts of milk, and have no problems with cultured milk or yogurt (which have lost their lactose). If the pain seems unrelated to the above factors, see your physician.

Acute abdominal pain

An acute abdominal pain begins suddenly, is intense, and can occur during infancy, childhood, or adulthood. In infancy it is often due to the telescoping of the intestines (intussusception), appendicitis, or infection of the urinary organs.

Numerous conditions may cause acute abdominal pain during childhood, including gastroenteritis, acute ileitis, constipation with fecal impaction, gastritis, intestinal obstruction, appendicitis, peptic ulcer, pancreatitis, hepatitis, kidney stones, pneumonia, and even a black-widow-spider bite. See the general index for the page number of each condition.

Skin rash

Skin rash may result from a number of childhood diseases, as well as from contact with certain plants and chemicals, and from the taking of certain drugs (drug sensitivity). The characteristics, location, and duration of the rash will vary from one type of illness to another. For possible clues as to the cause, see under "skin rash," pages 723, 972.

Sore throat

A sore throat is an inflammation of the pharynx so that swallowing becomes painful. Sore throat is typically associated with the common cold, or with some other infection of the breathing organs. It may be caused by a virus (as in the common cold), or the streptococcus germs (strep throat). The latter can pose serious problems in children (see page 913).

For a simple treatment for an ordinary sore throat, see page 593. Should the sore throat persist or be associated with fever and other symptoms, see your physician.

Stiff neck

A stiff, painful neck may be due to several conditions. Tenderness and swelling of the lymph nodes in the front and sides of the neck may indicate an infection in the mouth, throat, or ear (see pages 913, 1148). If your child has a fever and is acutely ill, a stiff neck could be due to meningitis (see page 1043). A wryneck (see page 964) may become a chronic problem.

Vomiting

Vomiting is the automatic and forceful discharge of the contents of the stomach through the mouth. The condition may simply be due to an upset stomach, or it may be caused by a more serious problem.

Among the causes of vomiting are motion sickness, certain poisons, a number of illnesses with fever, a head injury, a tumor of the brain, meningitis, infections of the intestine, intestinal obstruction, and appendicitis.

Children may become dehydrated by the constant loss of fluid through vomiting (even more rapidly when associated with diarrhea). If the fluid cannot be replaced by drinking (sipping small amounts every few minutes), or by means of a retention enema, fluids should be given by vein. Call your physician and follow his directions.

455

CHAPTER 9

Common diseases and disorders of childhood

Many of the diseases and disorders common to children are also common to infants and even to adults. Should a disease have been described elsewhere, a reference where detailed information is available on that particular disease will be given here for your convenience. However, certain details are given here regarding some of the diseases to aid parents in recognizing problems and caring for their children.

Heart and vascular diseases

Congenital heart disease

Defects of the heart and blood vessels are fairly common, but thanks to advances in heart surgery, many can be saved to live happy, healthy lives, which only a few years ago would have died. In live-born babies, about one out of every thousand has some structural heart defect.

Depending on the nature of the defect, the symptoms will vary. Some of the more common evidences of a heart problem include: **cyanosis,** or a dusky color of the skin; **delayed growth,** seen during infancy and early childhood; **shortness of breath,** especially when active; and **resting frequently** while at play.

Generally, many of the disorders are discovered during the first examination following delivery. However, other methods are available. Among these are X-rays of the chest, electrocardiography (EKG), echocardiography (ultrasound), and cardiac catheterization.

Depending on the defect, your physician will advise as to what should be done. For a more detailed discussion, see page 797.

Rheumatic heart disease

Rheumatic heart disease is a serious complication of rheumatic fever (see page 473), and the damage done persists throughout life and may not become obvious until years later. For further discussion, see page 795.

Infective endocarditis

This disorder consists of an infection of the lining of the heart and is caused by several types of germs, which are carried in the bloodstream from an infection somewhere else in the body. Children who have a history of congenital heart disease or rheumatic heart disease are more susceptible. For details, see page 795.

Hypertension

Generally, high blood pressure has been considered a disease of the adult. However this is not the case. Children should be periodically examined to determine the level of their blood pressure. If the pressure becomes elevated, they should be under the care of a physician. For additional information, see page 785.

Arteriosclerosis and atherosclerosis

These disorders appear to have their origin early in life. The diet of the westerner—high in fat, especially saturated (animal) fat, and low in dietary fiber—along with lack of exercise, appears to contribute to the development of atherosclerosis. Physical inactivity is no longer a problem only of adults. Children are also affected by the mechanized society of the Western world, where less and less demand is made for muscular exertion. For a discussion of the causes and the methods of preventing the problem, see pages 777, 779.

Anemia

Anemia is not uncommon among children. Evidences of its presence consist of pallor, weakness, rapid breathing, and shortness of breath on exertion. Weakness and shortness of breath stem from a reduced supply of oxygen. The fast breathing and rapid heartbeat represent the body's effort to compensate by providing more oxygen by pumping blood more rapidly. For further details, see page 813. Should you suspect your child has anemia, see your physician.

Respiratory diseases

Bronchiolitis

Bronchiolitis is a virus infection that starts as a cold.

A day or two later, the lining of the bronchioles is involved, causing swelling, congestion, and difficult breathing. The condition of the infant abruptly becomes worse, with wheezing, coughing, labored breathing, and cyanosis (blueness of the skin). For further information see page 422.

The common cold

The common cold affects persons of all ages, from about six months right through adulthood. But it occurs most frequently in early childhood, up to about seven years of age. During these years, the average child has from three to six colds per year. A person's susceptibility to colds depends somewhat on his general health or physical fitness, which appears to increase resistance to disease, and on the number of contacts with others who have colds. This is especially true if the contact is in a closed area where persons with colds are sneezing, coughing, and contaminating objects that they handle. For details regarding this disease and suggestions as to treatment, see page 909.

Influenza

Influenza is a very common, troublesome illness that affects children as well as adults. It is caused by any one of several viruses. The disease strikes suddenly with headache, pain in the muscles, chills, and associated fever usually lasting two or three days. These symptoms then subside, with the disease next targeting the air passages and lungs, causing a cough and feelings of weakness, which may last for a week or more.

In younger children, such complications as convulsions, vomiting, diarrhea, and otitis media (middle ear infection) may develop. Among other such hazards are relapse, sinusitis, and pneumonia. For details, see page 725.

Bronchial asthma

Asthma affects people of all ages. In infants it often follows a common cold, influenza, or some other viral infection, such as bronchiolitis (see above). Fortunately its severity decreases as the child grows older. In others, manifestations of allergy may develop, such as hay fever. This disorder has been discussed in detail (see page 920).

Available medications provide relief, but there is no specific cure. An important point that parents should remember is that they should administer the bronchodilators (medications that cause the air passages to open up or dilate) *early*, when the infant starts to wheeze, rather than waiting until it is gasping and needs emergency-room treatment.

Croup

Croup is a complication of a mild attack of the common cold, in which a child (usually six months to three years of age) awakens during the night with a "barking" cough and severe difficulty drawing air into his lungs. This contrasts with asthma, in which the difficulty is in exhaling. The child may appear well during the day except for his persistent cold. Cool night air may precipitate an attack.

The treatment in uncomplicated cases of croup is to place the child in an environment of warm, humid air. This can be provided in a number of ways: the steam from a hot shower in a warm bathroom; a steaming kettle or a boiling pan of water in a kitchen, or a commercial steam inhalator placed close to the bed with the doors and windows of the room closed.

If the croup is complicated with a fever, heavy breathing, and cyanosis (blueness of the skin), see your physician immediately, as the child may need to be taken to the hospital for oxygen in a tent or by a face mask. Occasionally there may be swelling of the air passage above the larynx, called **acute epiglottitis.** This may demand the passage of a tube or a surgical opening through the neck (tracheotomy) to provide the child oxygen. Antibiotics may be required for secondary infections.

Pneumonia

Pneumonia is an inflammation of the tissues of the lung and is due most commonly to a viral or bacterial infection (more rarely to a fungus). The inflamed tissues pour out mucus, fluid, and lost cells, which fill the air passageways, making breathing difficult. The infection, when patchy and widespread, is known as **bronchopneumonia.** It may follow a common cold and is a complication of chickenpox, measles, and whooping cough. If the infection affects one or more lobes of the lung, it is called **lobar pneumonia.**

The symptoms include a rising temperature; coughing; wheezing; heavy, rapid breathing, with or without cyanosis (blueness of the skin, indicating shortage of oxygen); and chest pain.

For the treatment and further discussion of these disorders, see page 923.

Digestive disorders

Diseases of the mouth and pharynx

Many of the diseases that affect the mouth and pharynx of adults may also occur in children, particularly two: herpangina and primary herpes simplex.

Herpangina, an acute, infectious disease caused by a group of viruses (coxsackieviruses), affects children between one and seven years of age. The illness begins with a sudden high fever, loss of appetite, sore throat, and sometimes vomiting. The back of the throat appears red and soon develops many small vesicles, which form discrete ulcers. Recovery occurs in about ten days. The treatment is symptomatic—plenty of fluids and an easily digested diet.

Primary herpes simplex refers to the first time the herpes simplex virus causes an infection. This virus is responsible for the common "cold sore" appearing on the lip of an individual. The initial infection causes generalized symptoms (see pages 846, 979). In the mouth, the lesions resemble those of herpangina, but are restricted to the mouth and gums. The lymph nodes in the neck are generally swollen and tender. The infection tends to abate in about two weeks. The treatment is symptomatic.

459

Peptic ulcer

While peptic ulcers are usually considered a disease of adults, they do occur in children. The risk of a child having an ulcer is increased if a parent has a peptic ulcer, or if the child drinks coffee and soft drinks (those containing caffeine) and takes aspirin.

The symptoms are abdominal pain and blood vomited or lost in the stool. In younger children, the timing of the pain is not always related to mealtime. In children over ten years of age, the symptoms resemble those of adults.

For a more detailed discussion of the causes, symptoms, and treatment, see page 855.

Infectious diarrhea (acute infectious gastroenteritis)

A major cause of diarrhea in children throughout the world is the rotavirus, the single most common agent of diarrhea in infants less than two years of age that requires medical attention. Outbreaks are most prevalent during the cooler months in temperate climates, but elsewhere they may occur at any time of year. It is a very important cause of acute gastroenteritis in day-care centers. Death from dehydration is a major cause of mortality in developing areas of the world but rare in developed countries.

Symptoms. Diarrhea may vary from mildly loose stools to violent purges, accompanied with cramping and abdominal pain, fever, and blood-tinged stools. *Important:* See your physician immediately if your child is listless or excessively thirsty, con-tinues vomiting, fails to urinate, or if the diarrhea is profuse.

Treatment. It is extremely important to give the child fluids to prevent dehydration. Oral rehydration solutions are available in most countries and through the World Health Organization. These preparations prevent the loss of salt, potassium, and water until the bowel can recover.

Do not give fruit or fruit juices until the diarrhea subsides. The sorbitol (a type of sugar) in fruit increases the diarrhea. A *nonfiber* diet during the acute phase is important (rice, noodles, mashed potatoes, white bread lightly toasted, *strained* carrots, and squash). If a commercially available broth or clear soup is given, remember to dilute it with water, as it contains too much salt for small children.

If your child fails to show signs of improvement, see your physician or take the child to an emergency room. Intravenous fluids may be necessary.

Prevention. The virus is spread by contact with contaminated stools and secretions from the mouth. In day-care facilities it is important that care givers, especially those handling infants in diapers, wash their hands frequently. Ideally, food preparers should not do diapering during an outbreak. Family members must wash their hands constantly.

Ulcerative colitis

Ulcerative colitis is a chronic, persistent ailment in which the lining membrane of the large intestine (colon) is inflamed. In severe cases the patient has multiple bowel movements a day, abdominal cramps, fever, anemia, weight loss, and signs of malnutrition. While generally seen in adults, it is also seen in children, mainly above the age of ten. For a full discussion of the causes and treatment, see page 865.

Appendicitis

Appendicitis is an acute inflammation of the appendix, a slender, blind tube attached to the first portion of the large intestine. In children, appendicitis occurs mainly in those between four and twelve years of age. The principal symptoms are pain, usually beginning in the vicinity of the umbilicus and gradually shifting to the lower right area of the abdomen. The child may vomit and run a low fever. Pressure on the right lower abdomen causes increased pain. The treatment is surgical removal. For a full discussion of the disorder, see page 863.

Hernias

A hernia is a protrusion of one of the body's internal structures through a weak place in the wall that encloses it. The common hernia occurring in infancy is the umbilical hernia, protruding through the abdominal wall at the site of the umbilicus. In childhood, the common hernia is an inguinal hernia, in which the weak place is in the lower abdominal wall in the region of the groin. A loop of intestine pushes outward and downward, forming a soft bulge. The bulge may disappear when the child lies down. The hernia may sometimes extend into the scrotum of a boy. For a complete discussion as to causes and treatment, see page 862.

Hepatitis

Hepatitis, an inflammation of the liver, is seen in children as well as adults. The infection is caused by either hepatitis A virus, usually seen in children, or hepatitis B virus, more often occurring in adolescents. In children, the illness is usually mild, with a duration of a few weeks. The symptoms begin suddenly with fever, loss of appetite, vomiting, and discomfort in the upper abdomen. The urine soon becomes dark, and the liver enlarges. The whites of the eyes and the skin turn yellow (jaundiced). For details as to treatment, see page 869.

Cystic fibrosis

This serious disease of hereditary origin begins in infancy and continues through childhood and as long as the patient survives—an average of fifteen to twenty years. Cystic fibrosis is possibly the most common lethal genetic disease among children in the United States. Its cause is not known. It typically affects the glands that produce secretions in the pancreas, the respiratory organs, and the skin.

When the pancreas is involved, it does not produce its usual quota of digestive enzymes, and malnutrition results. In skin involvement, the child is susceptible to heat exhaustion because of excessive activity of the sweat glands and resulting salt depletion. In the lungs the glands lining the air passages do not function normally (for discussion, see page 922).

461

The treatment consists of attempting to relieve the symptoms, as there is no specific cure. Pancreatic enzymes that are deficient are taken by mouth. When the skin is involved, a liberal use of salt is included in the food eaten. Respiratory problems result in infections, which are best controlled by appropriate antibiotic therapy.

Skin disorders

The disorders listed below are discussed in detail either under "disorders of the skin" or under "infectious diseases." Brief mention is made of each one in order to aid in its recognition. For the details regarding the disorder, the reference page is provided for your convenience.

Eczema (atopic dermatitis)

Atopic dermatitis consists of an inflammatory reaction in the skin, with itching, burning, and redness. It occurs in persons who have inherited hypersensitive skin, and frequently appears in infants, children, and young adults. (See the illustration on the next page.)

The disorder varies in intensity from time to time. There is intense itching, with blistering, oozing, and later, crusting. In children it usually affects the skin on the surface of the arms and legs. Scratching further aggravates the situation. The problems get less severe as one gets older.

A number of factors can provoke or intensify the dermatitis. For additional details, see page 871.

Freckles

Freckles are merely spots of skin in which more than the usual amount of normal pigment has been deposited. They are harmless and cause no distress, except to the appearance. They are more common in blondes and redheads, are more prominent in areas exposed to excessive sunlight, and tend to fade in winter. Freckles can be made less conspicuous by the use of a "cover-up" stick or cream. Certain lotions and creams cause the skin to peel and the freckles to be less obvious. However, these should be used only on the advice of your physician.

Birthmark (hemangioma, vascular nevus)

The ordinary birthmark of reddish or purplish color is composed of a mass or network of tiny blood vessels in the skin. In severe cases, the skin may be thickened, or the area may show one or more "blood blisters" or appear as a tumor mass. The unsightliness is the chief disadvantage. The majority of hemangiomas lighten and disappear by age seven, even if untreated. If the birthmark is large or increases in size, see your physician.

Home remedies should not be used. As with freckles, a "cover-up" stick or cream may make the birthmark less conspicuous. Should the lesion be large or cause emotional distress to the child, consult with your physician or a dermatologist regarding its removal.

462

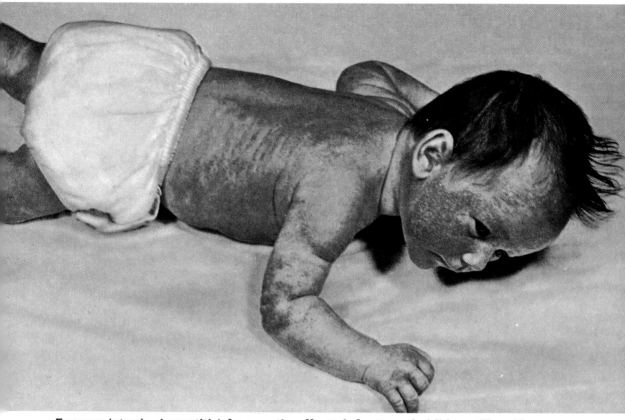

Eczema (atopic dermatitis) frequently affects infants and children. The skin is red, itches, and burns.

Moles

Moles are benign growths of pigment-producing cells and are usually present at birth or may appear early in life. In time, they may grow larger. The vast majority of moles cause no trouble, but occasionally one may become cancerous. Should a mole suddenly change in size, shape, or color, immediately see your physician. Also see page 994.

Warts (verrucae)

Warts are small, benign tumors of the skin caused by a virus invading the skin cells. Common warts

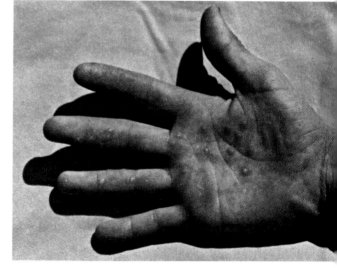

In children, warts often occur on the palm of the hand.

463

frequently occur in children, singly or in groups, especially on the fingers and hands. Given time, most warts will disappear. For a more complete discussion of the various types of warts and their treatment, see page 980.

Ringworm (tinea)

Ringworm is caused, not by a worm, but by a group of fungi that attack the skin of various parts of the body. The name "ringworm" derives from the fact that the lesions tend to heal at their centers and spread in a widening ring. Infections are especially common among children, as they spread from person to person or from animals (as pets) to persons. They can be spread by contaminated towels, combs, and showers. Ringworm infections may occur in the scalp, on the body, and in the groin. Athlete's foot (tinea pedis) is considered one type of ringworm. For a discussion of the various types of the disease and their treatment, see page 978.

Louse infestations (pediculosis)

Children who are infected with body lice and head lice tend to scratch, causing secondary bacterial infections to develop that aggravate the situation. For the manner of spread and methods of treatments, see page 982.

Scabies (the itch)

Children are not infrequently infected by the itch mite, which burrows into the skin, where it lays its eggs. This causes intense itching,

and the Latin word from which *scabies* is derived means "scratching." Because of scratching, the skin may become infected. For further discussion, see page 981.

Poison ivy and poison oak (allergic dermatitis)

Approximately 75 percent of the population react to contact with poison ivy or poison oak. Sensitivity usually develops following a previous exposure. These plants are widespread in the United States, and children are highly susceptible as they romp and play in areas where these plants grow. The first signs may be

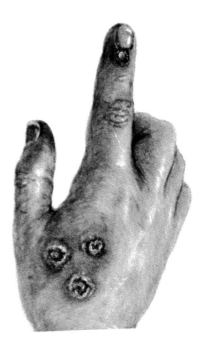

Ringworm (tinea) infection. The lesions are red and ringlike.

the puffiness of the eyes and face. Exposed areas of the skin become red; blisters form and later break and ooze. For details as to treatment and prevention, see page 973.

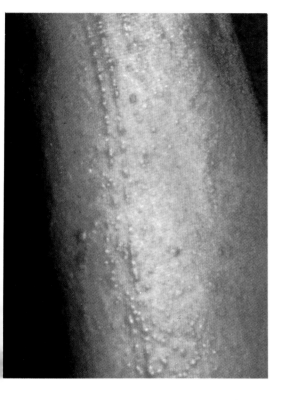

Ichthyosis (fish-skin disease, xeroderma)

Ichthyosis is a thickening of the outer layer of the skin (epidermis), which becomes dry, rough, and scaly, giving it a fish-scale appearance. Cracks form, and the surface tends to peel. The face, hands, and feet are rarely affected. There are several types of the disorder. For further discussion and treatment, see page 988.

Impetigo

Impetigo, one of the more common skin infections of children, is an acute and highly contagious disease, usually caused by staphylococcus bacteria. The lesions, which itch, generally develop on the face and spread readily by scratching. Small red blisters break and fuse, forming pustules, which ooze. Golden yellow crusts form in one or two days. For details as to treatment, see page 975.

Skin reaction to poison ivy or poison oak. The skin is red, blisters, and oozes.

Urinary tract infections

Such infections are extremely common in girls. Failure to keep the superficial areas of the perineum and the vulva clean increases the risk of infections. Pinworms, causing intense itching and scratching, further increase the possibility of getting an infection.

Symptoms of urinary tract infection in a child consist of fever, increased frequency of urination, a sudden onset of bed-wetting, discomfort on passing urine, and inability to delay the passage of urine once the desire develops. In a preschool child, the additional symptoms of abdominal pain, vomiting, and strong-smelling urine may be present. Such infections should be promptly treated lest they produce serious complications. For details of the different infections, see pages 1068-1081.

465

Female reproductive organ disorders

A girl's reproductive organs do not function as do those of a woman, but they are subject to infections and injury. Should a girl show a discharge or bleeding, she should be examined by a physician.

Vulvovaginitis

This disorder is an inflammation of the skin covering the folds (vulva) that surround the opening of the vagina. The affected area is red, sore, and itchy. There may or may not be discharge, which can be foul smelling. Because the opening of the urethra (from the bladder) is close by, a girl may also have a burning sensation at the time of urination.

The irritation develops quite commonly from an infection, the germs being carried from the opening of the rectum to the vulva. Following a bowel movement, girls should be taught to wipe backward or away from the genital area. Soiled underclothing may have the same effect. Contaminated fingers from a girl's nose or mouth may carry the infection. Pinworm infection, because of the intense itching followed by scratching, may also be responsible. Little girls who play in a sandbox may unwittingly introduce sand between the labia and thus develop an infection. The problem may also arise from a skin allergy, with sensitivity to detergents, soaps, and certain fabrics.

See your physician to rule out any serious disorder. Usually good hygiene will cure the infection. Daily bathing and frequent changing of underclothes will help. Protective creams may be applied. Your physician may order an anti-infective.

Injuries to the genitalia

Injuries to the genital area of a girl's body consist either of straddle-type injuries or penetrating injuries. Unless the straddle-type injury is so severe as to cause damage to the pelvic bones, it is not as hazardous as the penetrating type of injury. A simple examination following a penetrating injury often does not indicate the extent of the damage. Even in the case of a deep penetration, there may be very little bleeding. Therefore, in all penetrating injuries of this area, a physician should make a thorough examination, for the child's life may be in danger because of the possibility of an infection in the pelvic cavity.

Vaginal bleeding

Vaginal bleeding in girls younger than ten or eleven may be due to the presence of a foreign body (piece of a toy, any small object) in the vagina. Often these are inserted out of innocent curiosity. Plastic materials may not be detected by an X-ray. Such bleeding should be checked by a physician.

Very infrequently, menstrual bleeding occurs prematurely in a girl of a young age. It may be due to hormones produced by a tumor or some problem with other endocrine glands. Injury to the organs or attempted rape may also cause bleed-ing from the vagina. These conditions should be examined by a physician. For other disorders, see page 1101.

Nervous system disorders

Head and brain injuries

Injuries to the head and brain during the years of childhood happen most often between the ages of four and nine. They most frequently result from traffic accidents, with injuries from falls coming second. Although head injuries involving the face cause suffering and possible disfigurement, the greatest danger to future health—and even to life itself—comes from injury to the brain. See page 1035.

Sydenham's chorea (Saint Vitus' dance)

Most children who develop chorea have had a recent attack of rheumatic fever. In fact, the disorder is considered a late manifestation of rheumatic fever. See page 474.

Reye's syndrome

This disease generally follows a viral infection and affects the brain and some of the abdominal organs, especially the liver. The disease occurs chiefly in children and adolescents. The symptoms are nausea, vomiting, and a change in the child's mental status, which may progress from lethargy to seizures and unconsciousness. There is no specific remedy, so the treatment is symptomatic. Survivors recover in a few days. **Do not give aspirin or other salicy-**lates to persons with chickenpox or influenza. If you suspect your child has this disorder, see your physician immediately. For additional information, see page 732.

Brain abscess

An abscess of the brain is a localized infectious process with destruction of tissue. A cavity in the brain is formed and fills with pus. The infection is usually carried from some other part of the body, although it may result from a penetrating head wound or a fracture of the skull. Children with infective endocarditis are especially prone to develop this disorder. For further discussion of symptoms and treatment, see page 1043.

Meningitis

Meningitis consists of an acute inflammation of the meninges (coverings of the brain and spinal cord). The infection may be caused by viruses, bacteria, fungi, or yeasts. The causative organisms are usually brought to the meninges from an infection elsewhere in the body, such as from the middle ear, the tonsils, the lungs, or the valves of the heart. Meningococcal meningitis is a particularly serious form of the disease, which affects children. Meningitis is always a serious illness. For a more complete discussion of this disease, see page 1043.

Encephalitis

About half of the cases of encephalitis occur in children. In infants, the symptoms of encephalitis are not distinctive and may consist of only a sudden onset of fever, which, frequently, is accompanied by convulsions. In older children, the symptoms are headache, fever, drowsiness, possible convulsions, rigidity of the neck, vomiting, and supersensitivity to light. See page 1044.

Cancer of the brain

Cancer is the second most common cause of death among children under fifteen, accidents being the first. Leukemia (cancer of the blood) is the most common, followed by cancer of the brain. See page 1046.

Down's syndrome (mongolism)

This inherited condition of mental retardation is usually identified at the time of birth, and a full description is found in the chapter "Special problems of the newborn," page 428.

Cerebral palsy (Little's disease)

Cerebral palsy is often recognized during infancy, so it has been described in detail in the chapter "Special problems of the newborn." See page 427.

Eye disorders

Infections

Infections involving the eyelids and membranes of the eye are common in children. The germs are carried to the eye by carelessness in hygiene. A child's fingers are easily contaminated, and these are used to rub the eyes.

Conjunctivitis is an inflammation of the "white of the eye" and the lining of the eyelids. A severe, acute form is called "pinkeye," a highly contagious disease easily transmitted by fingers, soiled towels, or handkerchiefs. The disease may also be due to an allergic reaction, as in hay fever (see page 1132).

Blepharitis, commonly seen in children, is an inflammation of the margins of the eyelids (see page 1130). A **sty,** a miniature boil, develops in a hair follicle (eyelash) or in one of the gland openings contained in the eyelids. For a full discussion, see page 1130.

Refractive errors

Parents should be aware that about 10 percent of children age seven and older can have their vision improved by wearing glasses. Farsightedness often shows up in children who experience headaches and have difficulty reading. It is better for children to be treated at an early age, and it is suggested that all children age four should have their eyes examined. For a more detailed consideration of these and other problems, see page 1136.

Congenital glaucoma

See under "special problems of the newborn," page 1135.

Cross-eye and walleye (squint, strabismus)

Treatment of these disorders should be started at the earliest possible age. Even during infancy is not too soon.

The brain tends to use only one eye, ignoring the other. As a result, the eye that is not used gradually loses its usefulness, and it is very difficult, if not impossible, to restore such vision once it has been lost. For further details, see page 1140.

Ear, nose, and throat disorders

Congenital deafness

Children born deaf are often considered feebleminded. Parents should be alert to any unusual behavior of their child, especially if he fails to respond. See page 1153.

Acute suppurative otitis media

Recurrent infections are common under two years of age. In children of this age, the shorter, straighter shape of the eustachian tube (auditory canal) makes it easier for germs to get into the middle ear cavity. Another reason for recurrent infections is the underdeveloped immunity of small children.

Consider the following if your child has recurrent infections, or an infection fails to clear up:

- The child may have an allergy, which causes increased nasal mucus, and may be susceptible to colds and respiratory infections.
- Check with your physician as to whether the organism is resistant to the prescribed antibiotic.
- Ask your physician about the need

of a tympanogram, which enables him to determine if the eardrum is free to move.

If your child appears to have hearing loss after a cold, see your physician immediately, as fluid may have accumulated behind the eardrum. A hearing loss may delay speech development.

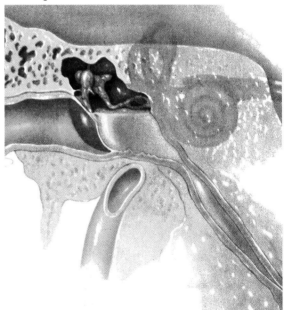

Inflammation of the middle ear. Note pus in the middle chamber.

For a further discussion of middle ear infections, see page 1149.

Otitis media with effusion

This type of inflammation is not caused by infection but by congestion or obstruction of the auditory tube, and is seen more frequently in younger than in older children. Typical symptoms are fullness in the ear, some hearing loss, and a mild, dull earache. For details, see page 1149.

Tonsillitis and adenoiditis

The tonsils and adenoids are composed of lymphoid tissue. The right and left tonsils are located on either side of the pharynx (throat), while the adenoids lie between the openings of the right and left auditory canals in the back part of the nose. The audi-

tory canals extend between the back of the nose and the middle ear cavities. On occasion, the lymphoid tissue of the adenoids enlarge so as to interfere with the passage of air into and out of the middle ears.

Inflammation of the tonsils, called tonsillitis, causes intense soreness of the throat, difficulty in swallowing, and high fever with aching back and limbs. Swelling of the adenoids and obstruction of the auditory canals may cause loss of hearing and infections in the middle ears. These conditions, quite common in younger children, are often outgrown as they get older. Should you observe any of these problems, see your physician, because untreated, they may cause serious complications. For a full discussion, see pages 829, 908, 913.

Allergic disorders

Allergic disorders are those in which the body responds to the presence of some aggravating agent called an allergen. Since individuals react differently in their responses to allergens, some are said to be more allergic than others. For a more detailed discussion of allergies, see page 672. Some of the more common allergies that affect children are outlined below.

Asthma

Asthma consists of periodic attacks of coughing, wheezing, and difficult breathing. The problem lies in exhaling, with the sufferer struggling to force the air out of his lungs. About 25 percent of all asthmatics develop the

disorder before the age of five. About half these children outgrow asthma as they become adults. For a more inclusive discussion of causes, symptoms, and treatment, see page 920.

Contact dermatitis

This condition consists of an irritation of the skin, caused by either a direct contact with some irritating chemical substance or an allergic reaction to a substance to which the individual is sensitive. For details about these disorders, see page 972.

Hay fever (allergic rhinitis)

Hay fever is an inflammation of the membranes lining the nasal cavities due to sensitivity to one or more allergens. These allergens include a wide variety of substances, including plant pollens, animal and human dander, and house and plant dust. The reaction of the membranes causes itching, runny nose, sneezing, and red, watery eyes. A dry cough may be present, but there is usually no wheezing. For suggestions as to treatment and prevention, see page 910.

Urticaria (hives)

Hives—red, itchy areas of the skin—develop firm, elevated wheals, often with a white spot in the center. They usually fade away in minutes. A single hive is usually due to an insect sting. Multiple hives can be due to an allergic response to certain foods, pollens, house dust, feathers, molds, and drugs. Certain forms of hives are very serious, namely, **angioneurotic edema** and **anaphylactic shock.** For further discussion, see page 989.

Sensitivity to drugs

Many types of drugs may cause an allergic reaction in sensitive persons. The antibiotic penicillin and the analgesic aspirin are common examples. A skin rash and hives are the two most likely allergic reactions. Should your child show an unusual response to a medication, notify your physician. For further details, see page 679.

Sensitivity to foods

Many people believe they are allergic to certain foods, when actually they are not. Those who are allergic consistently show specific symptoms. Occasionally it is easy to iden-

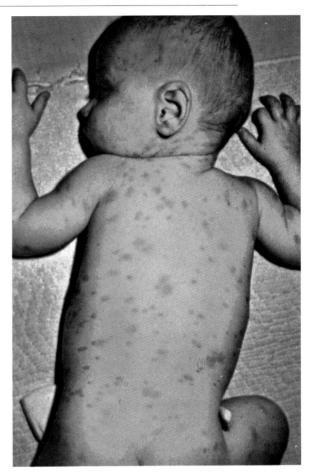

Hives or urticaria. The lesions are red, raised, and itchy.

tify some of the foods to which a child is sensitive, but generally it is a long and difficult process. For a discussion of the subject, see pages 677, 877.

Serum sickness

Serum sickness was first described when an allergic reaction was triggered by the injection of a serum of animal origin (usually a horse). The adverse response may be immediate or delayed. There is fever, enlargement of lymph nodes, skin eruptions, pain in the joints, nausea, and abdominal pain. Several

471

drugs can cause serum sickness, among the more common being penicillin, streptomycin, and sulfonamides. Should these symptoms develop following the administration of a medication, see your physician immediately. For further discussion, see page 679.

Infectious diseases

Thanks to immunizations, many of the so-called childhood diseases no longer pose serious problems. These diseases can affect infants to adults, but are seen more commonly in children.

Several common diseases of children give a rash, including chickenpox, measles, German measles, erythema infectiosum, roseola, and enterovirus.

Chickenpox

Chickenpox, a highly contagious viral disease, usually occurs in children under nine years of age. There is generally a mild fever, chilliness, aching in the back and limbs, and vomiting. The rash starts as small red spots, becomes bumps, then blisters and breaks, forming scabs, starting on the face and spreading to the chest and back. Recovery is in about two weeks. For care of the child, see page 723.

Measles (rubeola, "hard measles")

Measles is doubtless the most serious contagious viral disease of childhood. It is spread by invisible discharges from the nose and mouth, and develops in about two weeks from exposure. It starts with a runny nose; mild fever; hoarse, dry cough; pain in the chest; and redness of the eyes, with sensitivity to light. The fever steadily rises to reach 105°F (40.5°C). Pink spots appear after the third day, first behind the ears, on the neck, scalp, and forehead, then on the trunk and limbs. The spots run together, forming blotches. White spots are seen on the lining of the mouth. The child appears gravely ill but usually makes an abrupt recovery.

The disease can be prevented by a vaccination given during infancy or early childhood. For details of the disease and its treatment, see page 726.

German measles (rubella)

German measles, a mild, infectious viral disease, starts with symptoms of a common cold, along with a sore throat and cough. A fever may develop, and the child feels ill and has a headache with muscle pains. Lymph nodes may be enlarged behind the ears and sides of the neck. On the second day, a faint reddish blotchy rash usually appears on the face and neck, quickly spreading to the trunk and limbs. It lasts about two days.

Children should be routinely vaccinated for measles, along with other vaccinations. The disease may do serious damage to the fetus of a pregnant woman who has not been vaccinated, so any girl who has not developed the disease should be vaccinated at age ten (even though vaccinated in infancy). For further discussion of the disease, see page 727.

Erythema infectiosum (fifth disease)

This is a mildly contagious viral (parvovirus) disease of childhood (occasionally passed on to adults) with a suddenly appearing rash. The intense, fiery red rash is first seen on the face, giving a "slapped cheek" appearance with pallor around the lips. This is followed in one to four days with a lacelike rash on the arms, moving down to the trunk and thighs. The rash fluctuates in intensity with sunlight and heat.

Outbreaks occur in school-age children, usually in the winter and spring. The incubation period is from four to fourteen days, and the disease lasts one to three weeks. The contagious period is not more than a few days after the rash appears. The treatment is symptomatic.

Roseola infantum (exanthema subitum)

This is an acute viral disease affecting infants and young children (six months to three years of age) and is associated with spiking high fever (102-105°F) that lasts three to five days and ends abruptly (crisis). When the temperature becomes normal, a skin rash (red spots), which lasts for two to three days, appears mainly on the trunk, arms, and legs. Generally there are few other symp-

toms. Sometimes the symptoms may be only a fever and a convulsion. There is no specific treatment. Cool sponges, sponge baths, or an alcohol rub may be used to lower the high temperatures. Activity should be restricted until the temperature returns to normal. Recovery is usually complete.

Enterovirus

This is a very large group of viruses. Infection caused by many varieties may begin as a cold, with vomiting, diarrhea, and a faint rash on the abdomen. The coxsackieviruses may cause small ulcers in the mouth and blisters on the palms and soles. For treatment of the infections, see under "diarrhea," pages 460, 878.

Rheumatic fever

Rheumatic fever, an inflammatory disease that follows a throat infection caused by **streptococcus** bacteria (group A), may involve many systems of the body. It occurs most frequently in children five to fifteen years of age, but adults are also susceptible, especially those under thirty. It has been said that rheumatic fever "bites the heart and licks the joints." This is more true of children than adults, although the pattern in children may be changing.

The typical clinical sequence is (1) an acute infection by streptococcal bacteria (strep throat, tonsillitis, scarlet fever) with recovery usually in a week; (2) a period of three days to three weeks during which the patient appears to have recuperated; (3) a gradual reappearance of acute symptoms: fatigue, fever, joint pains, and a red rash. This phase of the illness may last a few weeks to more than a year; and (4) the possible chronic results of damage inflicted on the heart and brain.

The joints affected are usually the larger joints of the extremities: ankles, knees, elbows, and wrists. They are tender, swollen, red, hot, and painful. Not all joints are affected at the same time, the infection moving from one to another. Generally within a month the inflammation of the joints disappears without permanent damage.

Involvement of the heart is the most serious complication of the disease, with the occurrence of pericarditis, myocarditis, and, most often, endocarditis. The heart valves are damaged, with the damage persisting for the remainder of life (see "rheumatic heart disease," page 795).

An occasional complication is the development of chorea (Sydenham's), often many months after the original infection. The presence of chorea is evidenced by uncontrolled, purposeless movements and emotional instability. There may be slurring of speech. This condition, however, clears completely.

Without treatment, attacks of rheumatic fever tend to recur from time to time, and each time the possibility lurks of introducing or aggravating the serious complications of the disease.

Treatment. Your child must be under the care of a physician. Immediate care usually requires bed rest, especially with involvement of the heart and joints. For the streptococcal infection, antibiotic therapy (penicillin, erythromycin) is given. Anti-inflammatory agents (aspirin, steroids) aid healing in the heart and joints. Your physician will decide whether a long-term preventive program (using anti-infectives) is advisable.

Whooping cough (pertussis)

Whooping cough, an acute infectious disease caused by a germ (*Bordetella pertussis*), involves the nose, throat, and other air passageways. There is a characteristic spasmodic cough that ends with a loud, forced inspiration—the whoop. At the time of the whoop, the child may gag and vomit. (In mild cases there may be no whoop or vomiting.) For additional information see page 420.

Other diseases

Cancer in children

Accidents cause more deaths of children than any other single factor, but accidents are not a disease. Cancer kills more children than any other disease. Leukemia heads the list, accounting for 30 percent of cancers. Cancers of the central nervous system come next, with 19 percent. Lymphomas and others make up the remainder. The types of cancers are the same in children and adults (see page 680).

Rickets

Rickets is most frequently seen in infants six to eighteen months of age. For a full discussion, see page 944.

Insulin-dependent diabetes (type I, juvenile-onset)

This type of diabetes is more serious and requires more precise medical supervision than diabetes that develops in adults. It requires careful attention to the daily routine of food intake, insulin administration, physical activity, and steady encouragement to stay with the program. The American Diabetic Association and other agencies support camps for diabetic youngsters, where they can associate with others with like problems and receive counsel and guidance. See pages 1013-1018.

Tooth decay (dental caries)

Tooth decay, a serious childhood disorder, causes the destruction and loss of the baby, as well as the permanent, teeth. The loss of the baby (deciduous) teeth has important consequences. For a detailed discussion as to causes, consequences, and treatment, see page 891.

Periodontal disease

Periodontal disease involves the soft tissues that surround the teeth (gums). For a detailed discussion of the problem, see page 895.

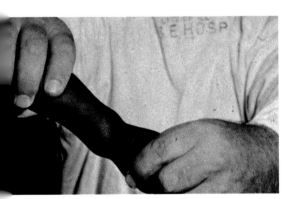

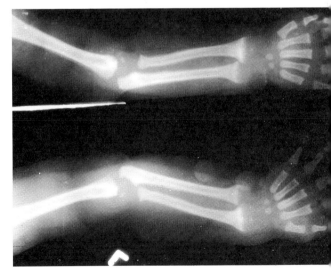

Note the enlargment of the wrists in a child with rickets.

475

CHAPTER 10

The adolescent

Adolescence is the period when a child is being transformed into an adult. Nature provides a good analogy of this change. A caterpillar, a chrysalis, and a butterfly or moth are three distinct stages in the life of a single organism. Similarly, the child, adolescent, and adult are different stages in the life of a single individual. Parents must realize that they are no longer dealing with a child, nor are they yet dealing with an adult, but with a unique individual, nevertheless, who is changing physically, mentally, and emotionally.

Adolescence begins in girls about two years earlier than it does in boys, and in the United States the average age is eleven for girls and thirteen for boys, though the time varies. Adolescence will last only a short time in some cases, while in others it will be longer. In any case, whether it is early or late, short or long, adolescence brings physical changes that make boys into men and girls into women. These changes are largely controlled by hereditary factors operating through the endocrine glands.

As a girl blossoms into young womanhood, she gives attention to developing feminine traits, and she begins to cherish the self-image of a young woman rather than that of a girl. As her sexual drives emerge, her mind focuses on romance. Since most girls mature at an earlier age than boys, boys of the same age will still be indifferent to romance. Thus the boys will be tempted to think the girls are "silly," and the girls will think the boys are "dumb." This transition time often brings confusion into the family and the classroom. Old friendships may break up and new ones form.

Intellectual and emotional changes are also taking place during adolescence, but these are not as automatically controlled as are the physical changes. The quality of the intellectual and emotional changes depends, to a large degree, on the young person's previous experiences and influences during childhood, together with that "something" on the inside that sparks in young people a desire to make those choices most opportune for their advancement. During this period the responsibility for life's choices shifts from the parents to the adolescent.

Shift of responsibility

Although it is too early at the beginning of adolescence for the young person to know precisely what his or her ultimate life goals will be or what the future holds, preferences are emerging. During these years a young person will make major decisions that will shape the course of his or her later life.

Often these decisions have profound, sometimes irreversible, consequences, yet it seems that life is built backward. A person's future is handed to him in his teens, yet during this time of life he has neither the knowledge nor the wisdom that comes from experience to guide and temper his choices and decisions. A youth is entrusted with the care, not only of his physical body, but also with the development of his character and personality. Fortunately, if the teenager's background has prepared him for this time, he will seek the counsel of parents, teachers, and friends.

Character formation

To fulfill any goal, especially when it requires long-term planning and implementation, the adolescent, like anyone else, must have the stamina to stay with the course that he and his counselors have mapped out. This very requirement helps to develop in the emerging adult the traits of personality and character that, along with his education and training, will make his life successful,

honorable, and happy. As they are repeated, these traits become established in the young person's pattern of living. A teenager who insists on being honest and dependable quickly earns the respect of others, and this helps him in his progress toward success.

Plan for success

Unfortunately, some teenagers squander their adolescence without realizing the importance of the opportunities that beckon them at this time of their lives. Thus they loose valuable time in preparing for success. They also fall into habits of carelessness that must be unlearned at a later time if they are to make real progress. This is especially true in homes where compliant parents give in to the demands of their adolescent children. Many parents give their teenagers the material things (cars, pleasure equipment, clothes, money) that the parents themselves had to acquire with a lifetime of hard work.

Any parent who says, "I don't want my child to have to work as hard as I did to make it in life" is doing his child a terrible disservice, for a teenager whose life imposes no responsibilities or hard work is likely to drift into patterns of living that will destroy his health and character. Careless in study, indulgent in artificial pleasures (alcohol, tobacco, and abusive drugs), demanding a continuous round of entertainment, uninhibited in releasing the emerging sexual drives—such an adolescent is on an ocean whose irresistible currents carry him to a rockbound shore.

The foundation for a successful transition from childhood to adulthood is laid during childhood and preadolescence. These are the years when the loving relationship between child and parent must be developed, thus making it possible for the adult to successfully navigate the adolescent through the storms of life.

It is imperative that young people always have before them a definite goal toward which they can direct their efforts. The goal may change, but with each change, new plans will emerge, together with appropriate efforts toward achieving the goal. This will give focus to a young person's life and provide stability during an unstable period. With perseverance on the part of the youth and continuing encouragement and support on the part of his parents, success in life is assured.

Physical development

Profound changes are taking place in the structures and functions of an adolescent's body. The rate of growth, which has been steadily decreasing since birth, now speeds up (see page 434). Some adolescents grow steadily for two or more years, while others reach their adult height in less than one year. Height usually increases by 25 percent during this time. A boy who is four to five feet tall when rapid growth begins may be six feet or more when it is over, and his body weight may double. If he weighed ninety pounds at age twelve, he may weigh 180 pounds when he is seventeen. The growth of girls is also spectacular.

While the age when this growth spurt will begin is different in different children, in both boys and girls, once it starts, it follows the same sequence. Puberty is affected by a number of factors. Heredity is one. The adolescent's growth pattern will very likely be similar to that of his or her parents. If a girl's mother entered puberty at a late age, the girl is likely to start late also. If a boy's father matured early, the boy will very likely do the same. Children who are sick and undernourished tend to begin puberty at an older age, while those who are overnourished (obese) begin earlier.

Although the rate of growth is relatively slow until adolescence, it does continue year by year. This partially explains why boys, who grow an extra two years before entering puberty, end up taller than girls. Children who mature early tend to be tall, while those maturing late are often short. Obese children and those from high socioeconomic groups are generally taller than those of normal weight and who come from more deprived backgrounds.

The various parts of the body also change during adolescence. A man develops more muscle and bone than a woman. His shoulders broaden, and his hands grow rapidly. A woman's hips will enlarge, and the ratio of fat to the rest of her body changes. About 25 percent of an adult woman's body will be fat, compared to only about 15 percent in a man. The fat is also distributed differently. In a woman, fatty tissue tends to grow in the hips, breasts, and upper back. Thus there is a clear difference in the contours of a mature male and a mature female.

Growth patterns in adolescents

The chart below shows summarizes the observable charac-

clumsy. He may knock things over and stumble over his own feet. As he becomes stronger, a boy's face will lengthen, and his nose and chin become more prominent. Hair will grow on his face, and he will begin to shave. In response to the stimulus of his male hormones, pimples will break out on his face as the ducts of his overactive skin glands become plugged and infected. Fortunately, these pimples generally disappear with time.

Tufts of hair begin growing over

Male characteristics Ages 12 to 18	Female characteristics Ages 10 to 16
Sex organs: penis, testicles, scrotum	Sex organs: breasts, nipples
Hair: pubic, underarm, face	Hair: pubic, underarm
Emergence of apocrine sweat glands	Emergence of apocrine sweat glands
Voice deepens	Menstruation begins

teristics of sexual development in boys and girls. You should consult your physician if any of these characteristics fail to develop by the time your daughter is sixteen or your son is eighteen.

The beginnings of manhood

Because a boy's body proportions change rapidly during the teen years, he will probably feel awkward and

the pubis and under the arms of the adolescent boy, and smaller hairs will appear on his arms and legs. His voice box (larynx), located on the midline in the front part of his neck, will enlarge and becomes prominent, and his voice will deepen. These changes are brought about by the male hormone testosterone that is produced by the testicles.

The testicles, or testes, also produce the male sex cells called

sperm. Sperm are not produced by the testes until adolescence, but once their production has commenced, they are manufactured in enormous numbers throughout the male's active life. In the course of a man's lifetime, only a few of his sperm ever unite with female sex cells (ova) to start a new life, so most of his sperm are never used.

After they are formed, the sperm are stored in the tubules of the **epididymis**—an almond-sized organ attached to each testicle. The epididymis also produces a fluid called **semen** in which the sperm are suspended. As an adolescent matures, the stored semen containing sperm is expelled every few days through the urethra, which lies within the penis. These seminal emissions occur during sleep, and are known as "night loss" or "wet dreams." While they are harmless, they do cause some inconvenience by soiling the bedclothes. When a young man becomes a husband, the discharge of semen (ejaculation) normally and appropriately occurs at the time of sexual intercourse.

The penis (see page 1084) ordinarily hangs limply downward. The urethra traverses its entire length, connecting the bladder with the outside. Another duct, the **vas deferens,** carries the semen and sperm from the epididymis to the base of the bladder, where it unites with the urethra (see page 1084). Emotions associated with sex cause the tissues surrounding the urethra to become engorged with blood, which in turn causes the penis to enlarge, elongate, and stand erect. This is called an **erection.**

As an adolescent boy matures, he will experience occasional erections and seminal emissions. Once the semen is discharged, the penis normally returns to its relaxed condition. Erection permits a husband and wife to engage in sexual intercourse.

The beginnings of womanhood

Throughout childhood a girl's physical appearance is almost the same as that of a boy. Her hips are no broader, and her shoulders no smaller than his. The strength of her muscles is about the same, and her chest is relatively flat, just like a boy's.

However, with the advent of adolescence, a girl takes on a more feminine appearance. Her breasts enlarge, her hips become wider, and the various angles of her body are rounded out by delicate layers of fat beneath the skin. Her lower face also lengthens, and she no longer looks like a child. Her figure takes on the characteristic female curves, in contrast to the angular figure of a man.

Girls, like boys, go through an awkward period, but it is usually less troublesome. They also suffer from pimples because of the generous production of hormones. A girl's ovaries, although not visible, also enlarge and produce the female hormones called the **estrogens.** These hormones are partly responsible for stimulating growth at the time of adolescence, along with the broadening hips, the developing breasts, and the production of hair under the arms and in the pubic area.

The ovaries also produce the female sex cells, or ova. The right and left ovaries take turns in forming an ovum each month (except during pregnancy) until a woman is about fifty years old, after which no more ova are produced and pregnancy is no longer possible. This is in contrast with the male sex cells, or sperm, which are produced constantly and in lavish numbers throughout a man's life.

In order for conception to occur—the start of a new life—a sperm must enter an ovum. This should not occur until a husband joins his wife in sexual intercourse. Until an ovum is fertilized by a sperm, the ovum that a woman's body produces each month travels through the oviduct into the uterus and perishes as it passes out through the vagina (see page 1087).

The uterus, another of the female reproductive organs, begins to function at the time of adolescence (for details, see page 1087). The lining membrane, or mucosa, of this organ undergoes monthly changes, becoming thick and vascular, only to break apart and be lost from the vagina over a period of about four days. This monthly loss of tissue and blood is known as **menstruation** and is one of the signs that a girl is becoming a woman.

The mucosa of the uterus becomes thick and lush at the time the ovum is passing down the oviduct. If the ovum is fertilized with a sperm, the mucosal cells accept the ovum, which attaches itself to the uterine wall and develops for the next nine months into a new human being. An unfertilized ovum is swept out with the menses.

In order to prevent the loss of too much blood at the time of menstruation, the uterus becomes quite firm—so firm that it may cause a certain amount of pain, commonly called **menstrual cramps.** An adolescent girl should be informed in advance that she will menstruate so that she can be prepared to wear a sanitary napkin or tampon during her period. Girls differ in the degree of discomfort (cramps, tension) felt during these monthly cycles, in the length of the menstrual period, and in its precise timing.

For convenience, the events of the monthly cycle are reckoned from the first day of menstruation. The usual time between the first day of menstruation one month and the first day of menstruation the next month is twenty-eight days, in which case the ovum escapes from the ovary on the thirteenth or fourteenth day.

In some women, the menstrual month is either longer or shorter than twenty-eight days, in which case the ovum leaves the ovary correspondingly earlier or later than the thirteenth or fourteenth day of the menstrual month. For example, when the interval between menstruations is thirty-one days, the ovum will escape from the ovary on about the fifteenth or sixteenth day.

The ovum remains available for conception (union with a sperm) for only about twenty-four hours after being expelled from the ovary. If it is not fertilized, it simply passes through the remaining portion of the oviduct into the uterus and perishes.

481

Sexual interaction

As the reproductive organs of a boy or girl begin to function, he or she develops new interests in matters of sex and experiences new sensations in the sex organs. This is part of the natural preparation for eventually becoming a husband or wife.

An adolescent boy becomes interested in girls in a new way. Conversation with an attractive girl does something to him that he never experienced before. He admires her not only for her personality but for her beauty and her femininity. He begins to notice her figure, and there wells up in his thoughts an interest in her distinctly different from that directed toward boys of his age. This attraction will eventually lead to his desire to "go out" with a particular girl (to date her). As this interest continues toward one girl, it will ultimately lead a young man to select her as his wife.

Girls experience similar feelings toward boys. They admire their angular faces, broad shoulders, and deeper voices, and they become interested in boys in ways that are different from their interest in girls. In time their attention will focus on a particular young man. Part of a young woman's unique adolescent development is the ability to attract a young man to want to spend time with her. As these feelings focus on one man, and as they spend time with each other, she will eventually select him to be her husband.

Being in the presence of a person of the opposite sex generates sensations in a young person's body, whether boy or girl, that automatically awaken sexual interest. Even when still in his teens, it is normal for a boy to experience a mild erection when he is near a girl or thinking about her. Similar feelings in a girl may cause her to secrete vaginal fluid. The reflexes that prompt these responses are powerful, and without good judgment and self-control, young people sometimes act prematurely and inappropriately in expressing affection for each other.

The Creator in His wisdom arranged our bodies so that the reproductive organs become active a few years before the appropriate age for marriage (early twenties). Sexual interest, which did not exist before adolescence, allows the boy and girl to evaluate the personality and emotional makeup of members of the opposite sex. However, it is important to understand that personality and emotional makeup are constantly changing during the years between adolescence and young adulthood. The girl whom the young man "loves" at seventeen he may despise when he is nineteen. A girl who is "in love" with a boy at sixteen may find that she can't tolerate him at seventeen. These formative years, when personalities are taking shape, allow young people to carefully evaluate members of the opposite sex to see what the mature young man or young woman will really be like.

This is also a time when young people must learn to master their desires rather than allowing their desires to control them. Such self-discipline is beneficial for young people, because it prepares them for

482

the responsibilities and privileges of a stable and happy marriage. It allows time for them to exercise wise moral judgment, to recognize the sacredness of the human body, the importance of intimate relations, and the need to develop their lives in ways that will ensure a lasting and successful marriage.

The external sex organs are so designed as to be very sensitive to stimulation, causing them to respond with a readiness for sexual activity. In the case of a boy, an erection of the penis will occur. In a girl, a similar and comparable response occurs in the tissues at the entrance of the vagina. This is the way it should be for the intimate relationship established by marriage. In both sexes, intercourse normally culminates in orgasm (see below).

Sexual stimulation apart from intercourse

When the sex organs are stimulated by manipulation (usually with the hands) rather than through sexual intercourse with a person of the opposite sex, the sexual reflexes are activated, and in due time a climax will occur. In a boy this climax is accompanied by a release of semen **(ejaculation),** just as in a seminal emission. In both sexes, a tension develops that consumes a great deal of nervous energy. This tension is relieved very suddenly by an explosion of energy that leaves the person relaxed and exhausted. This explosive release of tension is called **orgasm.**

Ejaculation and orgasm that are brought about by manipulation of the sex organs outside of intercourse are essentially the same as those that occur normally when husband and wife reach orgasm through sexual intercourse, but when attained by stimulation apart from intercourse they are spoken of as **masturbation.**

Masturbation may be accomplished by the individual himself or by someone else. Sexual stimulation by another person of the same sex is called **homosexuality.** Anyone who stimulates himself, or who allows himself or herself to be stimulated by another person of the same sex, arouses some of the most powerful emotions known to human beings in a way that was not intended by the Creator. These practices often result in a compelling desire to engage in the practice again. Thus, almost without the person realizing it, a habit is formed that may be very difficult to break.

Experience has shown that certain undesirable consequences tend to accompany masturbation. Very frequent masturbation may use up an excessive amount of nervous energy, leaving the individual weary and listless after an orgasm occurs. This can interfere with study, work, and other normal activities of life.

Masturbation often lowers a person's sense of self-worth. The practice is typically performed in solitude or alone with someone else who has similar interests. It is associated psychologically with fear of discovery and humiliation. Many people who masturbate find that they are robbed of that inner sense of self-worth to square their shoulders and face life without apology or embarrassment.

483

Masturbation may result in the formation of a dominant habit that controls conduct. Once the habit is established, the events of the day seem to circle around the opportunity to masturbate. For many people, the habit, once established, tends to rob them of the ability to remain in command of their own conduct.

Masturbation is a powerful habit, but there is no habit that cannot be brought under control when God's help is solicited. In principle, the secret of avoiding masturbation is to steer away from the circumstances that permit self-manipulation of the external sex organs. The guidelines below may help if you would like to discontinue masturbating.

- Keep busy. The desire to masturbate is greatest when a person has leisure time alone, so keep busy with interesting and profitable pursuits, and spend time around others. This will help you to avoid those situations that encourage the habit.
- Avoid wakefulness in bed. The desire to masturbate is greatest when a person lies awake instead of sleeping. One of the best ways to drop off to sleep is to develop a personal physical fitness program. This will also strengthen your willpower in overcoming the habit. When you awake in the morning, rise quickly from your bed and enter into the responsibilities of the day.

- Avoid sexual suggestions. If you wish to overcome the habit of masturbation, you must not read pornographic literature or listen to stories or conversations that will arouse your sexual desires.
- Choose your friends wisely. Avoid friendships with those whose minds constantly dwell on sexual matters and who constantly talk about sex. Seek the companionship of those who find enjoyment in nonsexual activities, and whose interests and aspirations focus on the responsibilities of life.

The future

It is normal for a child to look forward to the time when he or she will be an adult. With the coming of adolescence, this childhood desire meets its fulfillment. Suddenly, new opportunities, new possibilities, and new capacities develop. Adolescence is a thrilling and gratifying time of life. But the adolescent's arrival at adulthood is not an end in itself. For a youth of this age, the important phases of life are now just beginning.

With the onset of adolescence, youth are entrusted with their future life. If they act wisely, the opportunities for continued progress and success lie open before them. If, on the other hand, they think only of the now, are impetuous, make foolish decisions, and take unwise actions, they may find themselves with lifetime handicaps.

CHAPTER 11

The teenager's problems and illnesses

Teenagers should have good health. Their bodies are young. Few have had any serious illness. Yet the fact remains that many of them suffer from reduced health and diminished energy. Why should this be so? Here are two possible reasons.

The physiological and psychological transition from childhood to adulthood, although a natural process in growth and development, requires major adjustments in the maturing child's way of life. Physical and emotional stresses imposed on the adolescent are handled less easily by some than by others. Complaints of fatigue, headache, and joint pains are not uncommon. As a girl enters womanhood, she begins to menstruate and periodically loses blood. Some may develop anemia. The concerns of growing too little or too much, plus those associated with their changing appearance and how they are accepted by their parents and their peers, all tap the energy re-serves of both boys and girls.

But doubtless the major reason is that teenagers tend to be careless about their health, and do more to break it down than to build it up. They too frequently tend to break away from the regular program of the home. They stay up late, thus not receiving sufficient rest and sleep. They often eat what they want, of foods that are popular but not neces-sarily nutritious. They frequently take up unhealthful habits of smok-ing and drinking, and even worse, drugs. They often engage in premari-tal sex, with its drain on emotional resources. Their pace of living con-tinually exceeds their physical capa-bilities. Their lifestyles make them vulnerable to infections and disease.

Questions teenagers should ask themselves

The reality of aging has not yet caught up with the teenager, and life seems eternal. He doesn't mind trad-

485

ing a little of his energy for what seems like fun. However, there are telltale signs that even a teenager is using his life's resources wastefully, in ways that are likely to shorten his life at the other end. The following questions can help a teenager to assess his lifestyle in light of what twenty to thirty years from now will become a much more compelling issue: How much longer do I have to live?

Do you feel strong and well? If you can fulfill all your responsibilities and do them well, you should feel comfortably fatigued by the end of the day, and after a good night's sleep, awake refreshed in the morning. If you feel listless much of the time, many days having to "drag" yourself to school or work, you should reassess your habits so that you feel good most of the time.

Do you recover quickly from fatigue? Any normal, healthy teenager will get tired from time to time, but a good night's sleep or a short rest will rejuvenate him and restore his energy supply. If you feel tired most of the time and wake up most mornings hating to start the day, ask yourself what changes you might make in your lifestyle so that you have more energy through the day.

Are you making good progress in school? Are your grades excellent, good, or poor? Are you improving or at least maintaining your relative position in class, or are you losing ground? Debilitating health habits are not the only cause of poor grades, but they can be a contributing factor.

Is your skin clear and ruddy, and are your muscles well developed? If you are sallow complexioned and your face is filled with pimples, you are probably not exercising or resting enough. Perhaps you are eating too much of the wrong kind of food. Insufficient exercise will allow your muscles to weaken and dull your skin.

Are you optimistic and cheerful? You should be active and purposeful in what you do, and have a zest for living. If you habitually feel downcast or unusually irritable, check your habits of life.

Are you using any health-destroying substances? Chemicals that give a passing, artificial "high" are all too popular. Unfortunately, these agents enslave the user, destroying him physically, mentally, emotionally, and socially. No intelligent person should ever become involved in their use. If you are using any of them, the sooner you seek professional help, the sooner your life will come together again.

Habits for a long life

During these important teenage years, you are developing a pattern of living that will stay with you throughout the rest of your life. Here are some simple activities, which, if incorporated into your lifestyle, will pay you rich dividends a few years years from now.

Regular exercise. Relatively few young people really get enough exercise. A few get on a ball team. Another few lift weights, jog, or ride a bicycle. But the majority in today's technologically advanced society usually get transported to and from school, and when old enough, own a car. Power tools, power lawn mowers, elevators, and escalators have removed the need to use our muscles. And by the time adulthood is reached, the stage has already been set for the degenerative diseases that are today's major killers.

degeneration and disease.

Sufficient rest and sleep. The normal activities of life and the wear and tear of everyday living cause fatigue. To continue operating efficiently, your body needs periods for rest and recuperation. Sleep is nature's way of restoring your energy (see page 53). During a good

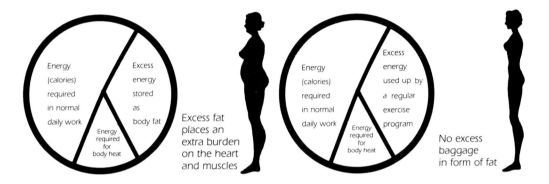

Exercise burns food energy (calories) rather than storing it as fat.

Exercise is an absolute essential for good health (see page 40). The only body system that you control is your voluntary muscles, which attach to your bones. All the other major systems—cardiovascular, respiratory, digestive, and eliminative—are programmed to operate without your intervention. But interestingly, their well-being depends on the use you make of the one system you do control: your voluntary muscles. It is only when you use these muscles, in moderate to vigorous exercise or work, that these other organ systems are called into activity. And this is the only way to strengthen and protect them against

night's sleep, taken at regular intervals, both the physical and nervous components of your body are recharged for the next day's enterprises.

Put yourself on a regular program, with set times for eating, exercising, sleeping, working, and playing. And never mix work and play. The amount of sleep you need may differ from that required for some of your companions. Experience will tell you how many hours you require to awake rested and refreshed. If you study regularly and faithfully, you won't have to stay up late preparing for examinations. A rested mind is a sharper mind (see page 46). Your

487

grades will be better, and your chance of success in life far greater.

A nutritious diet. In the United States, studies have repeatedly shown that the diet of the average teenager is the poorest, nutritionally, of all diets consumed in this country. If you get a major share of your food energy from "fast-food counters," your diet will be high in calories; high in refined cereals; high in refined oils and animal fats; high in refined sugar; high in products made from refined cereals, fats, and sugar; and high in salt. Such a diet is low in complex carbohydrates, low in fiber, low in vitamins, and low in minerals. It encourages the development, at an early age, of coronary heart disease, diabetes, hypertension, obesity, cancer, and chronic kidney failure.

In place of the above diet, use whole grain cereals and products made from them, together with vegetables, fruits, and nuts. Reduce the amount of sugar, refined fats, and oils—and foods made largely from them—that you eat. Eat at regular times, have a good breakfast, and do not eat between meals. And even though you are a growing teenager, do not overeat. It is best to eat only the amount of food required to keep you in your desirable weight range. For details on a good diet, see page 96.

A small group of teenagers, mostly girls, actually suffer from malnutrition, not because they cannot afford enough food, but because they are afraid they might become overweight, even though their present weight is normal or even less than normal. In one form of this problem, **anorexia nervosa,** a girl will actually starve, deliberately denying herself the food she needs. With the other problem, **bulimia,** the individual eats food, only to vomit it up later (see page 239). Both of these practices cause serious problems that require the immediate counsel of your physician.

Mental and emotional balance. Adolescence is a time of change during which a child becomes an adult. As a maturing individual, you are experiencing new thoughts and feelings, which, in turn, produce emotions you never felt before. You can no longer behave as a child, nor can you quite act as an adult. You and your associates find yourselves in situations that are different. As you begin to think new thoughts and your mind ventures into new areas, you find yourself uncertain and emotionally unsure. This leaves you tense and tired.

Unfortunately, the teenage years are often years of turmoil. The constant beat of high-decibel music envelops you wherever you go. Modern audio sound systems blare out from cars, stores, homes, and from portable units carried in your pockets and plugged into your ears. The hours spent by the television, with its emotion-stirring programs, neither rest nor calm your nerves. You travel in the fast lane from dawn to dusk. Many of you come from single-parent homes, or from homes in which division and conflict constantly exist. Other homes have working parents, and often working teenagers too.

That inner calm that mind and

body need does not come from the perpetual round of activities just described. It comes from reading a good book, listening to restful music, a quiet walk in the evening, sitting on a park bench watching the ducks swimming in a pond, or listening to the twittering of birds in the trees. It comes from reading the Scriptures, from meditation, and from prayer. It comes from communion with yourself, with nature, and with God. Nothing else will balance your mind and quiet your emotions so well.

Clean outside and in. You don't need to wear expensive clothes or have your hair done up in some extravagant way to look well groomed. Clean and appropriate clothes give you a dignity and poise that will build your self-worth. Bathe often, look neat and tidy, drink plenty of water, expose yourself to sun and air, keep an orderly room, stay away from tobacco, alcohol, and drugs, be polite and pleasant.

Skin disorders

Eczema (atopic dermatitis), acne. Acne has been spoken of as the "scourge of adolescence." About 80 percent of adolescents experience some degree of acne, which appeares in the early teens and often continues into the twenties. In most cases the problem is nothing more than "troublesome pimples." However, about one teenager in five experiences a condition that is more severe and may leave permanent scars on the skin. See page 982.

Blackheads (comedones). Blackheads frequently develop at

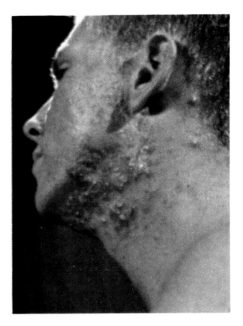

Acne, the "scourge of adolescents."

about the same time and are characteristic of acne (see page 983).

Heart problems

The heart problems affecting adolescents are most frequently **congenital,** that is, deformities of the heart with which a person is born (**congenital heart disease**—see page 797), and damage to the heart resulting from rheumatic fever (**rheumatic heart disease**—see page 795). Today, thanks to modern advances in diagnostic methods and in heart surgery, many heart defects can be recognized even before birth and can be successfully repaired. Rheumatic fever can be satisfactorily treated so that heart damage occurs only infrequently, and those who do suffer damage can have repairs made on their hearts in due time.

489

Sex-organ disorders

Enlargement of the male breast (gynecomastia)

A boy's breasts contain the same fundamental tissue elements as a girl's. However, as a girl reaches womanhood, the newly produced female sex hormones stimulate the growth of her breasts in harmony with the feminine pattern. These hormones are not generally active in a boy's body, but occasionally they do become active, and when this happens, his breast tissue responds in the same way as a girl's. In most cases, only one breast enlarges, and may be uncomfortable and sometimes slightly tender. Boys naturally feel greatly embarrassed when this happens, but they should not be concerned. The condition will disappear in a few months as their endocrine system stabilizes. Occasionally the enlargement may continue for a year or two.

Delayed sexual maturation (male or female)

The exact age of transition from childhood to adulthood varies from person to person over a period of several years. In practically all cases, even though development is a little late, the boy or girl will be just as masculine or just as feminine as those who develop at an earlier age. It is understandable, of course, that the young person will be anxious. You should consult your physician if your boy's testicles have not begun to enlarge by age fourteen or if your girl's breasts have not started to develop by age thirteen or her first menstrual period does not occur by age sixteen.

Irregular menstruation

For a normal young-adult woman, menstruation occurs quite regularly at intervals of about one month, except at times of pregnancy. But for the teenager who has just begun to menstruate, the time of menstruation may occur irregularly and somewhat unpredictably during the first year or two after the first menstruation, or menarche.

Once the regular pattern of menstruation has become established, then a missed period (amenorrhea) should be investigated. In some cases of poor health, a young woman's body will conserve vitality by ceasing menstruation for one or more occasions. There are even cases in which menstruation has halted temporarily because of emotional tensions. Menstruation stops, of course, when a pregnancy occurs.

Menstrual cramps

A certain amount of discomfort—cramps—is normal at the time of menstruation. These painful cramps are caused by the contraction of the strong muscles in the wall of the uterus as it produces the pressure needed to expel the lining of the uterus. This menstrual discomfort is

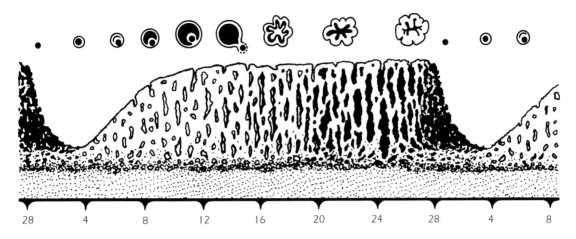

Diagrammatic portrayal of events occurring in the ovary and uterine lining (mucosa) during the menstrual month.

usually not as great after a young woman gives birth to her first child. In the event of extreme discomfort at the time of menstruation, the teenage girl should consult her physician. In the large majority of cases, exercises, such as those suggested in the accompanying diagrams, will do much to relieve the discomfort. These exercises should be taken daily between menstrual periods as well as during menstruation. For further details, see below.

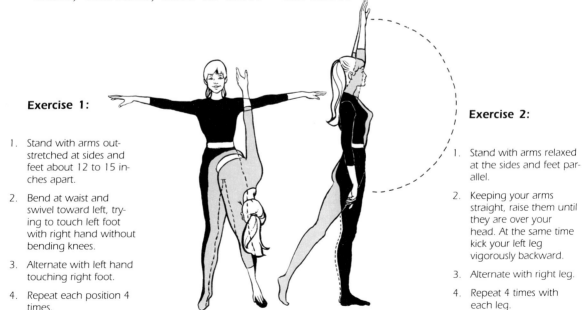

Exercise 1:

1. Stand with arms out-stretched at sides and feet about 12 to 15 inches apart.

2. Bend at waist and swivel toward left, try-ing to touch left foot with right hand without bending knees.

3. Alternate with left hand touching right foot.

4. Repeat each position 4 times.

Exercise 2:

1. Stand with arms relaxed at the sides and feet par-allel.

2. Keeping your arms straight, raise them until they are over your head. At the same time kick your left leg vigorously backward.

3. Alternate with right leg.

4. Repeat 4 times with each leg.

Menstrual cramps are often relieved by simple exercises.

491

Increase in vaginal fluid (leukorrhea)

The interior of the vagina is kept moist by the secretions from small glands located within the lining of the vagina. It is normal for the amount of this secretion to increase as a girl arrives at adolescence.

This is a nuisance, but unless the secretion is foul smelling, or thick and tenacious, it is probably within the limits of normal. Once an adolescent girl begins to menstruate, the amount of this secretion should decline except for a few days about the middle of her menstrual month, at the time the ovary is producing another ovum (female sex cell).

In certain cases, however, inflammations and mild infections develop in the lining of the vagina, causing the discharge of a thick, white secretion that may cause irritation and itching at the external outlet of the vagina. This is more common in older girls and in women than in adolescents. For the treatment of this condition, see your physician. For further details, see page 1108.

Rape

Rape is an unfortunate circumstance in which a girl or woman is assaulted by a male and forced to yield to sexual intercourse against her will. Rape involves a woman in both legal and medical problems. In this book the primary concern is the medical problems—the care and well-being of the girl or woman thus assaulted.

She should report at once to a physician, who can advise her on the handling of the legal complications and who will care for her physically. His professional health care will deal with two possibilities: pregnancy and exposure to venereal disease. He can deal with both of these possibilities much better if he is consulted as soon as possible following the sexual attack.

Anemia

Adolescents, especially girls (though boys to some extent), are particularly susceptible to iron-deficiency anemia. This condition, which results from insufficient iron in the diet, causes an abnormally low level of hemoglobin (the oxygen-carrying pigment) in the red cells of the blood. The average loss of iron by a woman, including that present in the blood lost in her period, is about 2 milligrams per day. The loss of iron in a man is approximately 1 milligram per day. These amounts can easily be supplied by a good diet.

However, during the rapid growth period, an adolescent's body manufactures more blood, and therefore, needs more iron. If the diet at this time is poor, the tissues will not be supplied with sufficient iron, and anemia may develop. An inadequate diet is a problem to both boys and girls, but, because of her monthly loss of blood through menstruation, the adolescent girl is more likely to incur an iron deficiency than the adolescent boy. A nutritious diet will correct the problem. However, your physician will advise as to whether an iron supplement is desirable. For details of iron-deficiency anemia, see page 814.

Hepatitis

Hepatitis occurs in two forms: type A and type B. Type A, a mild form, is typically seen in young children, and often occurs in epidemics. Type B is a serious infection, and more commonly affects teenagers and adults. For details as to its spread, symptoms, and treatment, see page 869.

Lactose intolerance (milk intolerance)

Lactose is the sugar contained in milk, whether human or animal. A special enzyme in the intestine digests or breaks lactose down so that it can be utilized by the body. When this enzyme is missing, the lactose is not absorbed, and abdominal distress occurs. For details about handling this problem, see page 858.

Drug abuse

Drug abuse is a major problem today, especially among teenagers and young adults. The most popular drugs are mind-altering agents, which cause a short-lived feeling of well-being. Their continued use soon makes the person dependent on the drug. Obtaining more of the drug becomes a compelling force in life, and every other interest is subordinated to this one goal. Family, education, health, making a living—all take second place. The addict's craving for the drug is so strong that he will often resort to crime to get the money to purchase the substance.

The question may be asked, If teenagers are aware of the effects of drugs, why do they become involved with them? There are a number of reasons. People of all ages tend not to learn from the experience of others, but want to experiment for themselves, and this tendency is particularly common among teenagers, who are anxious to make their own choices and establish their own identity. Teenagers also do not want their friends to think they are different, and so are subject to peer pressure. The fear of being different and the desire to be a good sport are hard to resist. And, of course, drugs are readily available. Thus teenagers are easily persuaded to "give it a try."

Alcoholic beverages are commonly used by the adults in the homes of most teenagers today. Many smoke, and almost everyone uses beverages that contain caffeine. All of these social habits cause addiction. In the medicine cabinet other addictive agents are found: sleeping pills, tranquilizers, appetite suppressants, and pain-relieving pills. While most of these are not used by the addict, they may serve as a starting point.

The drug pusher may be a classmate or a teenager who has dropped out of school. Whoever he is, the pusher probably obtains his supply of drugs from another teenage pusher, who, in turn, patronizes an adult peddler. The peddler gets his drugs from a smuggler, who brings drugs into the country illegally. Thus, in its travel from the original source to the user, the drug has passed through several hands. There is no easy way to trace the series of transactions, nor is there a way to check on the quality of the product being transferred.

Persons engaged in the handling

of drugs are prone to deceive. Their first motive is to make as much money as possible. They often mix the products they handle with cheaper substances that are not easily recognized. A drug handler, obtaining 10 ounces of heroin, may mix it with 10 ounces of an inert substance, giving him 20 ounces to sell. As it passes from one dealer to another, the substance is further diluted. Sometimes it is diluted with a cheaper drug.

More than this, should a drug handler receive a request for a certain drug that he does not have available, he may sell what he has under the guise of its being what was called for. As a result, the drug user at the end of the chain really does not know what he obtains from his pusher, and he is usually afraid to double-check.

The user of a certain drug becomes accustomed to its effects. He learns how much to take in order to obtain the usual result. Much of the drug that he obtains has been diluted many times. But on occasion the drug he buys has not been diluted to the same extent as before. Thus the user takes an overdose, which may be fatal.

The user also risks the possibility that in the adulteration of the drug as it is passed from one person to another, a substitution was made, not with some harmless substance, but with a drug to which the user is sensitive. As a result, a toxic, if not a fatal, response may occur.

The sensible teenager will see wisdom in not experimenting with drugs—not even once. It is far better to lose a friend who is using drugs than to be trapped in a habit that will destroy your personality, your self-respect, and even life itself.

Perspective on life

Teenagers find themselves facing the real world. They have not yet had time to gain the experience that will provide them the wisdom to make the decisions essential to success and self-reliance. Peer pressure is probably at an all-time high, and it may conflict with the standards already established at home and school. New friendships are being made and broken. Emotional imbalance and mood changes are common.

If you are a teenager reading this book, seek the counsel of someone you trust, whom you sense has the ability to give you good advice about the course you should take. If your parents have fostered a good relationship with you, you can approach them with your problems in a trusting, understanding, matter-of-fact way. Otherwise, seek the counsel of trusted teacher, a family friend, a physician, or a minister.

CHAPTER 12

Problems of later life

At the time of this writing, some 25 million people, or 11 percent of the total population, are sixty-five years of age or older. For the most part, the illnesses that affect persons in the older age group are the same as those occurring among younger adults, but some problems more frequently befall those of advancing age. While one should not anticipate illness because of age, the human body, like any machine, cannot help but show signs of wear and tear from a lifetime of work and activity, even when maintenance has been at its best. Unfortunately, the preservation of health has all too frequently been neglected, resulting in the premature breakdown of body systems.

Each individual, like a chain, breaks at his or her "weakest link." Inherited weaknesses, even though held in abeyance through a lifetime of healthful living, may eventually make their appearance. Unhealthful habits and practices established in youth and left uncorrected now take their toll. Osteoporosis, with its demineralizing and weakening of the bones; atherosclerosis and hardening of the arter-

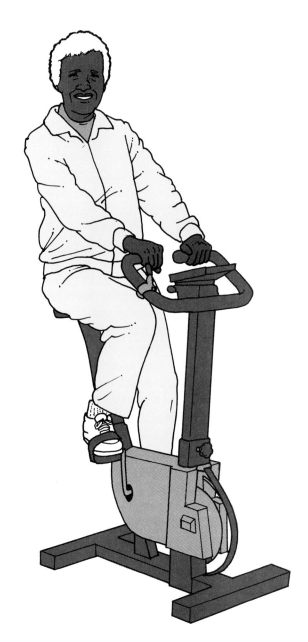

Regular exercise delays aging.

ies; cataracts; and hearing loss are among the problems most commonly seen in older persons.

Some illnesses strike older people harder than those who are younger. The greater severity stems largely from the older person's lower resistance to disease. Acute illnesses often last longer in older people, and in most cases recovery from any illness also takes longer.

An older person may not respond to medication as he did when he was younger. The body's ability to break down and eliminate a medicine may have decreased so that the drug, when taken, may have a greater effect, resulting in overdosage.

Most older people experience more frequent problems associated with their aging, and as a consequence need more professional attention. But fortunately, remedies are available for many of these ailments, and the period of comfortable living can be extended. Older people's tolerance for surgery is remarkably good, even for those in their late seventies and eighties.

The maxim, "You're as old as you feel," carries considerable truth. Mental attitudes profoundly affect our well-being. Those who keep their minds and bodies active and who continue to involve themselves in community activities remain alert and spry. Some are old at sixty, while others are "young" at eighty.

Yet we must all recognize that no one in this world lives forever. The time comes when our bodies no longer perform the tasks they should. The disorders may be physical, mental, or both, and these problems present difficulties to the persons afflicted, as well as to their relatives and others responsible for their care.

In this chapter, only the more common problems of the aged will be mentioned, and, where applicable, page references will be given where additional discussion of a particular problem can be found.

High blood pressure

High blood pressure in the elderly is usually a carry-over from earlier years. Depending on your age and general health, you may be able to alleviate the problem by reducing your salt intake, losing weight, and stopping smoking (smoking tends to enhance atherosclerosis). Also, if you lead a sedentary life, check with your physician about going on an exercise program.

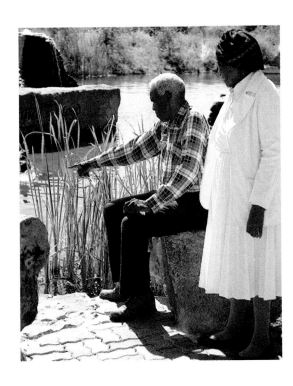

Regardless of your age, you should have your blood pressure under control, because high blood pressure poses the risk of serious complications such as stroke, heart disease, and kidney failure. However, an older person needs to be careful how he *lowers* his blood pressure. By the time a person reaches sixty-five, the supply of blood to certain vital organs—the brain, the heart, and the kidneys—is not as great as in younger years, but an elevated blood pressure forces the blood through these organs anyway, keeping them functioning quite well. Abruptly reducing the blood pressure to these organs may result in an insufficient blood supply and impaired function.

Your physician, in managing your high blood pressure, will attempt to avoid excessive reduction, but at the same time will try to protect you from the complications of stroke, heart disease, or kidney failure. Medications are available, and he will reduce your pressure gradually, observing your response and the extent to which it should be decreased.

Heart problems

If an elevated blood cholesterol level is added to the factors mentioned above—which are factors likely to cause high blood pressure—the chance of your having a **coronary heart attack** is greatly increased.

A program of graduated exercise, adapted to your needs, together with a modified diet (if your cholesterol is high) and steps to reduce any remaining risk factors, will go a long way toward postponing or preventing an attack. In a person with some coronary atherosclerosis, regular exercise encourages the development of tiny, supplementary blood vessels within the heart wall. Thus the sudden closing of one of the coronary artery branches is not as disastrous in older patients as in those who are younger. For this reason, should you have a heart attack, your risk of sudden death is less than if it occurred in your forties and fifties. For details, see page 788.

Heart failure occurs when the muscle of the heart wall has gradually weakened, usually by continuous overload, so that it can no longer pump the volume of blood required by the various tissues of the body. The telltale signs and symptoms include breathlessness on exertion, swelling of the ankles, generalized weakness, and a blue coloration of the lips and the fingernail beds. Appropriate therapy by your physician can strengthen your heart, improve your well-being, and prolong your life. For details, see page 787.

Nutritional problems

Good health depends on eating good food, regardless of your age. Adequate nutrition is vital to provide your body with all the essential elements necessary to replace those depleted by the function and repair of your organs. A good diet promotes the body's defense mechanisms for resisting disease.

Unfortunately, some elderly persons fail to provide an adequate, well-balanced diet for themselves, and carelessness is not the only cause of the problem. Those who live alone may have no motivation to prepare a

497

meal only to eat it alone. Often, because an older person's sense of smell and taste is diminished, his appetite is not as keen as it once was. Loss of teeth makes it difficult for some older people to chew satisfactorily, and unsteady hands further complicate the eating of food. For these reasons, older people need to be especially careful of their diets, particularly if they live alone.

The ingredients of a good diet are simple and are outlined elsewhere (see page 96). Contrary to the opinion of those selling them, studies have shown that supplements such as vitamin pills cannot convert a poor diet into a nutritious one. Do your best to eat simple, nutritious food. If you feel strongly that you should take a supplement, consult your physician.

Constipation

Constipation is a common problem among the elderly. In constipation, the bowel movements are infrequent, small, and often hard and difficult to pass. A number of factors contribute to the disorder, among them a failure to answer the "call of nature," a diet high in refined foods, insufficient water, insufficient exercise, emotional tension, and painful hemorrhoids.

Treatment requires rectifying any of the underlying conditions: establishing a regular time for elimination, eating foods high in fiber (fruits, vegetables, whole grain cereals), drinking plenty of water at regular intervals during the day, and an appropriate amount of exercise. For a full discussion of the condition, see page 877.

Problems of the bones, joints, and muscles

Arthritis is probably the most common problem affecting older people in the bones and joints (see page 954). Unfortunately, no satisfactory way has been found to prevent the problem, nor is there any satisfactory way of restoring the affected structures to their original condition. Judicious use of the affected joint as long as possible will help to retain function. Your physician can advise about the treatments that offer the best approach to your problem, whether it be medication or surgery.

Osteoporosis, a condition in which the bones are weakened due to mineral loss (calcium and phosphorous), and therefore break easily, is commonly seen in the elderly, especially in women. Mineral loss starts when a person, man or woman, begins to cut down on physical activity. In women, the problem is intensified following menopause because of decreased estrogen production. Osteoporosis tends to become progressively more severe.

Supplementation with calcium and other minerals will not cure the problem. A nutritious diet, a good exercise program, and, in women, the judicious use of estrogen will improve the condition. If you suspect that you have osteoporosis, see your physician to determine how advanced it is, and follow his recommendations.

Muscle spasms (leg pains) Muscles have a way of signaling distress when the blood does not supply

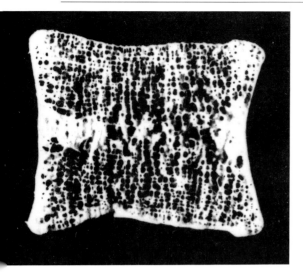

Bone density of normal (A) and osteoporotic (B) vertebrae.

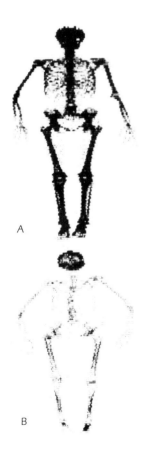

X-rays of normal (A) and osteo-porotic (B) skeleton.

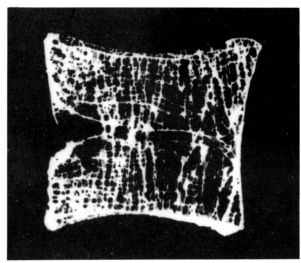

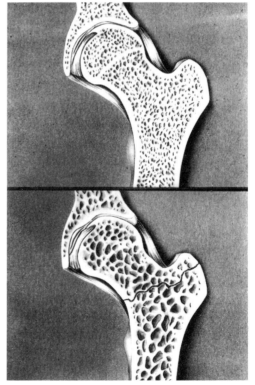

Sections of the upper end of the femur showing normal (A) and re-rified (B) bone density due to osteo-porosis.

them with enough oxygen. The demand is highest when a person is active. In some elderly persons, particularly those who have been sedentary and who have developed atherosclerosis (which reduces the flow of blood through their arteries), oxygen deficiency, with pain in the leg muscles, will occur on walking. The cramping pain will first be noticed on walking briskly or uphill. As the condition progresses, pain may be felt, even with mild, sustained exercise. This pain in active muscles is due to **claudication.**

If you have this problem, the following simple exercise program may help to relieve the condition:

- Walk at a moderate pace until pain develops.
- Rest until it subsides.
- Retrace your steps to the starting point.
- Later in the same day or the next day, try to walk a little farther than the point at which the pain first developed. When the pain occurs, rest and return to your starting point.
- Increase the walking distance slightly each day until you can tolerate a reasonable amount of exercise.
- Continue this daily exercise program until your leg muscles can tolerate exercise without cramping.
- Then continue the daily exercise program indefinitely to maintain what you have gained.

Although exercise alone will not reverse the atherosclerosis in your vessels, it may develop alternate routes of circulation. For additional information, see page 963.

Skin problems

The disorders affecting the skin of the elderly depend, to a great degree, on heredity, complexion, and the amount of exposure to the sun and other damaging conditions. The skin of an elderly person is typically thin, inelastic, wrinkled, and dry. Often it is so thin that it breaks easily, infections heal more slowly, and healing takes longer.

Sun damage causes **actinic keratoses,** a condition in which the skin is dark, rough, scaly, and may bleed. Such lesions often become cancerous (basal cell). Excessive exposure to the sun may also lead to the development of a highly malignant melanoma. Any suspicious lesion should be examined by your physician and should be removed. For a more detailed discussion, see page 996.

There is a decrease in the size and number of sweat glands in elderly people. As a result, the skin is dry, and it itches **(xerotic eczema).** This condition usually affects the legs first, then spreads to the scalp, shoulders, and pelvic area. The itching is more intense at night and is worse in the fall and winter than during the spring and summer. The itching is aggravated by frequent bathing, especially when hot water and detergent soaps are used. Bathing less often and moistening the skin with soothing lotions and bath oils tend to bring relief. Use nondetergent soap only, especially under the arms and in the anal and pubic areas, then rinse all the soap off thoroughly. Humidifying the room air is also helpful (see page 974).

Incontinence

Incontinence is the involuntary loss of urine or bowel contents that develops as a person ages. It is caused by a weakening of the muscles (sphincters) that control the bowel or bladder (see page 1076).

In women, urinary incontinence also results from the weakening of the muscles of the pelvic floor at the time of childbirth. In men, enlargement of the prostate (a gland that surrounds the urethra at the outlet of the bladder) causes difficulty in controlling the flow of urine or even in starting the urinary stream when desired. Three out of every four men who reach the age of eighty have an enlargement of this gland, and in one out of every four, it becomes necessary for the enlarged gland to be treated by surgery.

If you have difficulty emptying your bladder, see your physician. Urine held in the bladder (residual urine) causes irritation of the lining membrane, and not infrequently results in infections. An enlarged prostate should be periodically evaluated by your physician in case the overgrowth becomes malignant.

Declining sexuality

A great deal of speculation and even misinformation prevails regarding the ability of elderly people to engage in sexual intercourse.

The sexual function in both men and women is complicated (see page 1111). Ideal sexual functioning depends on normal, healthy sex organs, which are under the control of the nervous system, and influenced both by conscious thought and the autonomic (automatic) nervous system. Furthermore, the endocrine glands produce hormones that facilitate sexual desire and the capacity to engage in sexual intercourse. Psychological factors such as prejudices, resentments, and taboos may serve as inhibitors.

It is understandable, then, that the sexual experience of one husband and wife may be very different from that of another couple. Thus, in describing, in general, the sexual capacities of elderly people, there will be many individual exceptions, and what is said here will not fit every case.

The desire for sexual intercourse declines slightly but gradually throughout the adult lifetime. The capacity remains, but the nervous energy and vitality needed to perform the sex act gradually diminish. Problems arise when the interest of one partner declines at a faster rate than the interest of the other.

It is a popular belief that a woman's sexual capacity declines rather sharply at the time of her menopause ("change of life" in her late forties or early fifties). While it is true that a woman's ovaries no longer produce sex cells following menopause, thus making it impossible for her to become a mother anymore, the healthy woman of this age does not lose her ability to participate in sexual intercourse. Loss of interest in sex by such a woman usually indicates a

501

psychological rather than a physiological problem, such as the mistaken assumption that she is suddenly old and therefore no longer attractive to her husband.

Barring abnormal attitudes or an exceptional physical problem affecting sexual function, an elderly husband and wife should still be capable of pleasant sexual activity in ways of their own choosing, albeit at a reduced pace. In those problem cases in which a husband and wife do not follow the same pattern of gradual sexual decline, they should seek the advice of a physician or a specialist in gynecology.

Nervous system problems

Certain problems of the nerves and nervous system occur more commonly among old people than in younger people. One of these is **"shingles,"** a painful viral rash. Blisters (which later crust and heal) develop along the course of one or more of the peripheral nerves, causing bouts of intense pain over a period of several months. Approximately 1 percent of older people develop new cases of shingles every year (see page 980).

Stroke is a complication of atherosclerosis that affects the vessels supplying the brain with blood. The tragedy of stroke is that it often leaves the individual handicapped (more so in some cases than in others) because of a loss of control over certain muscles (or arms and legs). For detailed information, see page 1031. Even the elderly person can improve the chances of avoiding stroke by following a fitness program

(see page 1032).

In old age, the supply of blood to the brain gradually diminishes, the availability of oxygen and nutrients to the brain cells is reduced, and the neurons no longer function normally. This problem, which usually begins after the age of sixty-five, is called **senile dementia,** or dementia of the elderly **(senile dementia of the Alzheimer type)**. There is gradually a loss of memory, not of things that happened years ago, but of recent events. Over a period of months or years, the person has an increasing loss of comprehension, is unable to reason, and has mood swings from disinterest in everyday events to overactivity in some particular happening. Attention to personal hygiene disappears, and the personality gradually deteriorates. For a further discussion, see page 1041.

Depression, also common among the elderly, may be a symptom of a more serious problem, such as senile dementia or Alzheimer's disease, or it may be an indication of loneliness—someone who has outlived his relatives and close friends. Looking on the bright side of life; maintaining a fitness program, both physical and mental; developing interests in life, especially in doing something for others; together with faith in God—all of these will go a long way toward helping an older person to avoid melancholy and depression.

Eye and ear problems

Problems related to sight and hearing are much more common as people get older. Fortunately, advances in science and medicine have

502

made these disorders much less serious. Reading glasses are readily available, and **cataracts** rarely pose a problem since new lenses can now be implanted in an outpatient clinic (see page 1136). Hearing aids are available to compensate for **deafness.** See page 1152.

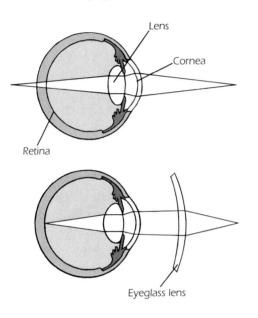

With aging, the lens is unable to focus on near objects.

Cancer

Certain forms of cancer tend to make their appearance as a person gets older. Cancer of the skin (basal cell carcinoma) is common, but it is not dangerous if treated promptly. Lung cancer in both men and women, especially for smokers and heavy past smokers, still remains a major killer. Cancer of the pancreas, colon, rectum, and stomach are also seen more often in older people. For men, cancer of the prostate, and, for women, cancer of the breast and uterus are also common. Because of the advances in medicine and surgery, many of these malignancies can be treated quite successfully. For a more detailed discussion of the different forms of cancer, see page 680.

Diabetes

Type II diabetes—the adult-onset form—occurs frequently among elderly people. Fortunately, it is not as serious as type I diabetes (juvenile-onset form), which begins in childhood. Adult-onset diabetes can be controlled, with or without insulin, by a diet high in fiber and low in sugar. For details, see page 1013.

Outlook for the elderly

The older person who wishes to enjoy health as long as possible will guard against excessive fatigue, irregular hours, an impoverished diet, and indulgence in health-destroying habits. Conversely, intentional efforts should be put forth to maintain a regular exercise program, get plenty of rest and sleep, eat a nutritious diet, keep a positive attitude, and stay involved in church or community programs. These will ensure a longer, healthier, and happier life.

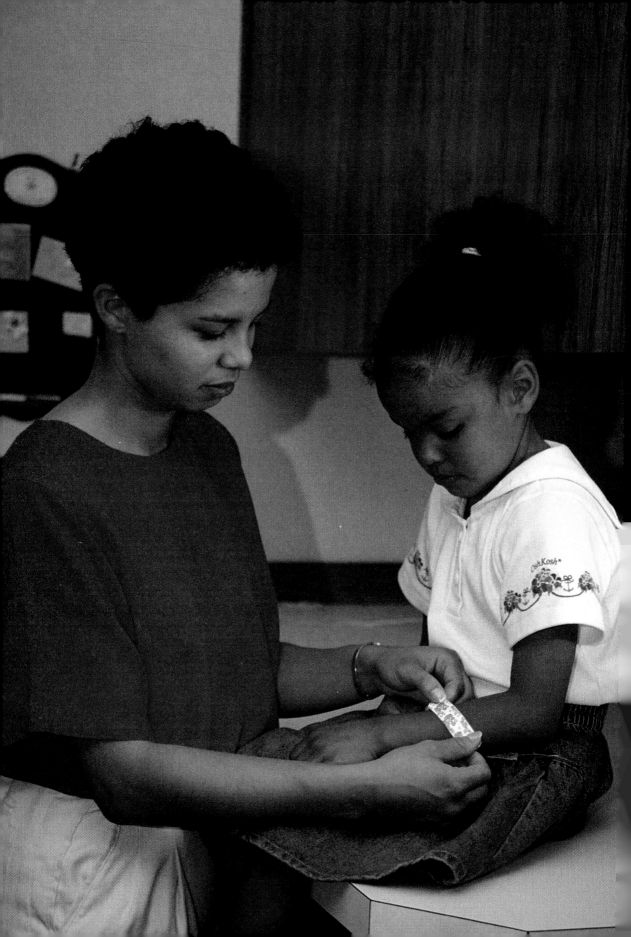

VOL. 2

SECTION 2

MEDICAL CARE AT HOME

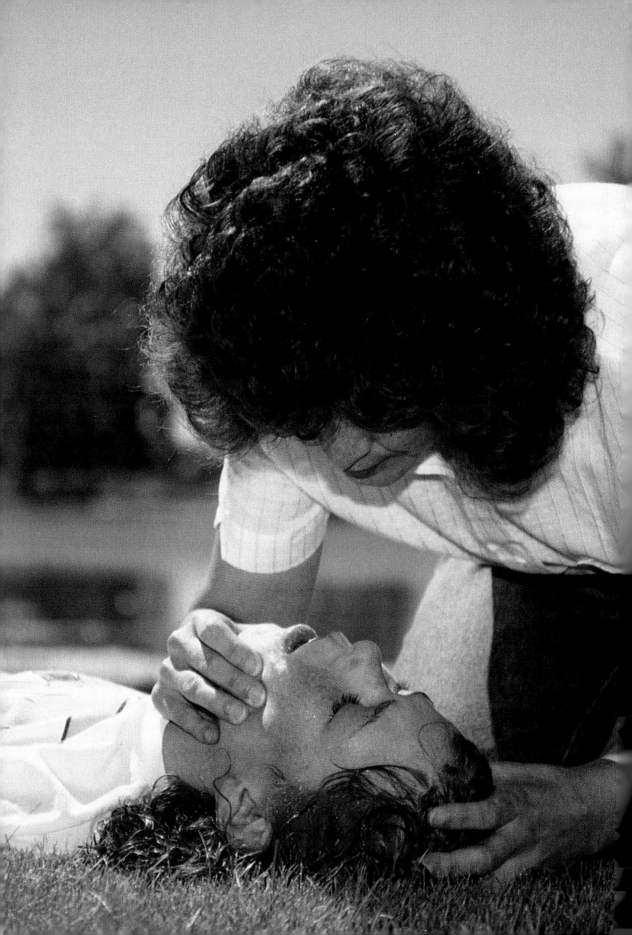

A quick guide to emergency procedures in
LIFE-THREATENING SITUATIONS

Some emergency situations are so critical that, in order to save the victim's life or avoid crippling injury, persons untrained in giving medical treatment must intervene before professional help arrives at the scene. Unfortunately, many people do not know what to do under these circumstances. They need help *fast!* The information for handling these problems is found in the next three chapters, together with a great deal of information about handling emergencies that are not life threatening. The following index of life threatening emergency situations will help you to avoid wasting valuable time searching for the information you need. For information on non-life-threatening emergencies, see the chapter on first aid that begins on page 529, or consult the general index.

POISONING: Where to find help fast

Each state, province, or region of the U.S. and Canada has a poison control center that you can call in an emergency. Usually this number is listed on the inside front cover of your phone book. If poisoning is from a product in a container, have the container available so you can read the brand name and contents to the person you talk to.

CHAPTER 13

Important emergency procedures

Learn them before you need them

The basic support systems of the body are circulation and respiration, for without these functions, life cannot be sustained. To effectively support these systems, **Basic Life Support (BLS)** procedures have been designed to intervene when these systems are assessed to need intervention. Indications for **BLS** are:

- **Primary respiratory arrest.** The heart is able to circulate the blood until all of the oxygen present in the blood and lungs has been depleted, at which time the vital organs, such as the brain and heart, will cease to function, and the heart will stop beating (cardiac arrest). A person will stop breathing (respiratory arrest) from a number of causes. These include drowning, an object in the airway, suffocation, smoke inhalation, stroke, drug overdose, heart attack, injuries, and coma.

- **Primary cardiac arrest.** When the heart stops beating, blood is not circulated, and the oxygen in the blood is used up by the tissues and organs in a matter of seconds. Among the causes for the heart to stop beating are a massive heart attack, fibrillation (twitching) of the ventricles, and beating too fast (tachycardia).

Before instituting any emergency procedure, there must be an **assessment** of the victim. The assessment involves:

1. Response—Is the victim conscious?
2. Breath—Is the victim breathing?
3. Pulse—Is the victim's heart beating?

The major important emergency procedures that are needed from time to time in rendering first aid to someone who is injured or seriously ill are outlined below. They are called the **ABCs** of cardiopulmonary resuscitation (CPR).

1. **A**irway—see that it is open.

2. **B**reathing—give artifical respiration.
3. **C**irculation—provide external chest compression.

Artificial respiration

Artificial respiration can be given, even if breathing has not entirely stopped, but is very slow and weak. Time your breathing **out** with the victim's breathing **in.**

Step 1 **A.** Lay the victim on his back.
B. Establish unresponsiveness. Is the victim unconscious?
C. Look for chest movement, and place your ear to his mouth to check for breathing.
D. Call for help.

Step 2 "Chin lift," *if no neck injury is suspected.*
A. Tilt the victim's head to a "sniffing" position (as when you smell a rose) by lifting up his neck with one hand while pushing back on his forehead with the other.
B. Pinch the victim's tongue and chin between your fingers. Wipe any foreign material from his mouth (using your finger and a handkerchief), and see that his tongue has not fallen backward.

Step 3 Pinch the victim's nose shut, take a deep breath, place your mouth firmly over his mouth, and give two quick breaths in rapid succession. In children cover both nose and mouth with your mouth.

Step 4 Remove your mouth from the victim's face. **Look** toward his chest so you can observe it fall, and **listen** to the sound of escaping air. **Feel** his breath on your face. If you feel none, try exhaling into his mouth again, more vigorously this time. If his chest still does not rise, the windpipe is obstructed. If the victim is a child, slap sharply between the shoulders and clear the mouth of any obstructing material. If the victim is an adult, use the Heimlich maneuver (see page 546).

Step 5 Continue blowing air into the victim's lungs every five seconds (twelve to fourteen times a minute) until he resumes normal breathing or until help arrives.

Caution: When giving mouth-to-mouth respiration to infants or very small children, **remember** that their lung capacity is small. **Do not over-inflate a child's lungs.** Only empty

509

the air you can hold in your cheeks. Give gentle, small exhalations and watch the child's chest rise and fall. If the airway is obstructed, hold the child by the feet and gently thump between the shoulder blades.

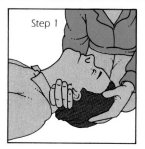
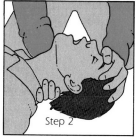
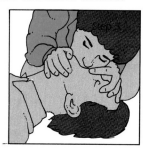

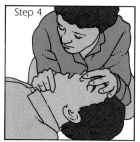
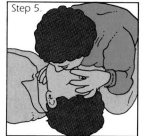

The five main steps in artificial respiration.

Cardiopulmonary resuscitation

When the heart stops beating, the circulation of blood ceases, and soon thereafter breathing terminates. An emergency measure called cardiopulmonary resuscitation (CPR) has saved many lives and is now well established. Everyone should avail himself of the first opportunity to learn from qualified teachers how to conduct this procedure. Many hospitals, fire departments, and the American Red Cross have training programs for the public in CPR. An outline of the procedure is given below, but does not attempt to provide sufficient details to make the reader an efficient CPR operator.

When two rescuers are available, one can administer artificial respiration while the other carries out heart resuscitation. However, there may be only one rescuer who knows the procedure. **Laypersons should do single-rescue technique only.**

Step 1 Establish the victim's unresponsiveness—that he is unconscious: look, listen, feel.

Step 2 Call for help.

Step 3 Lay the victim on his back on a firm surface, such as on the floor. His arms should be parallel to his sides, and his head should be slightly lower than his chest. **Note: If there is a possible neck injury,**

avoid moving the victim's neck as you position him.

Step 4 Tilt the victim's head back, and with one hand behind his neck, raise it upward. This will bring his chin up and open his airway. Clear his mouth of any foreign materials. The ideal head-neck position is "sniffing" (as if smelling a rose).

Step 5 Give two quick breaths.

Step 6 Check the victim's pulse.

Step 7 In adults, place a finger in the notch at the lower end of the victim's breastbone. Place the base of one of your palms 1 inch (2.5 cm) above the finger in the notch. Now remove the finger from the notch and

place that hand on the back of the other hand. Keep your arms straight while kneeling at right angles to the victim.

Step 8 Push straight down, compressing the chest of an **adult** 1-1/2 to 2 inches (4 cm), smoothly and regularly. Between compressions, keep your hands lightly in contact with his chest (so your fingers are raised off the skin). Give eighty compressions per minute. Your timing will be "one-and," "two-and," "three-and"—slightly faster than one per second.

Step 9 **After fifteen compressions, lean forward, tip the victim's head, and give him two full breaths in four seconds.**

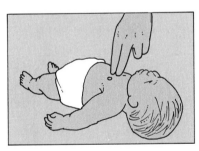
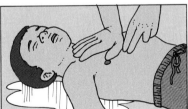

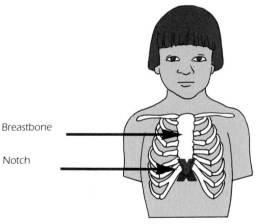

Breastbone

Notch

Cardiopulmonary resuscitation (CPR) in infants and small children. Note the location of the notch just below the breast bone and how the rescuer applies pressure to the chest using only his second and third fingers.

511

Step 10 After every minute or two, check the victim's pulse (preferably in the neck) and breathing for five seconds. Look for the rise of the chest, **listen** to breath sounds, and **feel** his breath on your face. Start each cycle with two breaths.

Evaluation. If on checking you find that the victim is breathing and has a good pulse, keep checking both periodically, and call for help. If you find only a pulse, then give mouth-to-mouth respiration. If you find no pulse, then start CPR. Continue CPR until help arrives or until you are exhausted. If the victim must be moved, do not stop CPR for more than fifteen seconds.

Caution. For infants and small children, the force of compression should not bruise the heart or fracture the ribs. In babies, the pressure should be gentle, exerted through the tips of the operator's index and long fingers. In eight- to ten-year-olds, apply pressure with the heel of one hand.

Initiating vomiting

Vomiting is a way of ridding the stomach of poisonous contents (if induced within thirty minutes).

Caution. Vomiting is not advised if the individual is unconscious or has swallowed a strong acid, a strong alkali, or a petroleum product.

Step 1 If necessary, position the victim so that the vomitus will flow out of his mouth and not be inhaled.

Step 2 Give the victim syrup of ipecac: 1 tablespoonful for children; 2 tablespoonfuls for adults. Follow this with two or more glasses of water or milk. If vomiting does not occur within fifteen minutes, tickle the back of the victim's throat with your finger or with the blunt end of a spoon, fork, or knife.

Combating shock

Shock can result from any number of causes, including a heart attack, severe injuries, acute infections, poisonings, hemorrhage, allergic responses, snakebites, and burns. In shock, there is a sudden collapse of the circulatory system, preventing the body's vital organs (the brain, kidneys, and the heart and blood vessels themselves) from receiving oxygen. If this situation is not corrected immediately, the spiral of failing function continues downward until it becomes irreversible. Following are three major causes of shock and what to do about them:

1. The heart fails to pump sufficient blood, as may occur in an acute coronary attack, heart failure, or cardiac arrest **(cardiogenic shock).**
2. There is insufficient blood in the arteries and veins, making it impossible for the body to maintain blood pressure. This may result from injuries, severe bleeding, burns, and diarrhea **(traumatic or hypovolemic shock).**
3. The blood vessels collapse, which causes them to dilate unduly. The blood pools, and there is insufficient blood to maintain circulation. This is seen in severe infections and in severe allergic reactions **(anaphylactic or distributive shock).**

The common symptoms of shock include generalized weakness; sweating; clammy skin; weak pulse; rapid, shallow breathing; and restlessness. As shock worsens there is mental haziness, lethargy, stupor, and unconsciousness. The victim's body temperature drops, and death ensues. For details, see page 802.

Treating shock

Step 1 Check the victim's circulation and respiration and, if needed, provide life-support procedures. Control any bleeding.

Step 2 Lay the victim down, and if other conditions (injuries) permit, raise his feet and legs about 1 foot (30 cm).

Step 3 Keep the victim warm to prevent loss of body heat.

Step 4 Call for medical help or take the victim to an emergency room.

Step 5 If the victim can cooperate, encourage him to drink water (unless he is vomiting), or, if it is available, a salt-soda solution (salt, 1 teaspoonful [4 gm]; soda, 1/2 teaspoonful [2 gm] to 1 quart [1 liter] of water).

Dressings and bandages

Emergencies frequently involve injuries of the skin and bones. A **dressing** (also called a **compress**), usually composed of a fabric, is applied directly over the wound. While sterile (germ-free) dressings are commercially available, in an emergency, any cloth, or even paper, will do, provided it is relatively clean. Even tissues can be used.

The purpose of a dressing is to control bleeding, prevent further contamination, absorb blood or secretions, and prevent pain.

A **bandage** is a strip of cloth or woven material wrapped around a dressing to hold it in place. Bandages are also used with splints to prevent movement. Adhesive bandages are common examples of a combination dressing and bandage. Sterile gauze bandages of different widths are used to exert firm pressure on underlying tissues, helping to control bleeding.

A bandage should be snug, but not so tight that it will restrict the circulation of blood. After applying a bandage to a limb or finger, check to see that the area beyond the bandage is warm, and, when possible, check the pulse. As an injury swells, a bandage may become too tight and should be loosened.

A bandage must be held in place. A bandage that wraps around a limb or the head can be held in place with safety pins or clips, or, if it is a cloth bandage, it can be split and tied. A bandage can also be affixed directly to the skin with adhesive tape.

Bandages come in a variety of shapes and sizes and must be skillfully applied to conform to the varying contours of different parts of the head, body, and limbs. Common bandages include the sterile gauze roller bandage, the roller elastic bandage, and the triangular bandage (which may be a square folded in half). The stretch in the roller gauze bandage and the elastic bandage allows a snug fit around the varying shapes of the limbs. A triangular bandage can be used as a sling for suspending a limb (see the accompanying illustrations).

Bandaging is a learned skill. The reader is advised to obtain a booklet, the American Red Cross's *Standard First Aid,* and practice bandaging various parts of the body with different bandages. You will then be better prepared to meet an emergency.

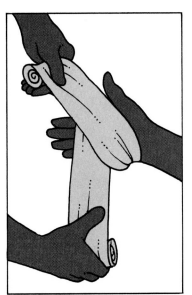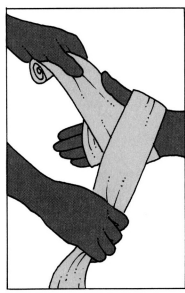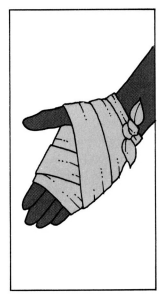

Application of a bandage to the hand.

Scalp/head bandaging

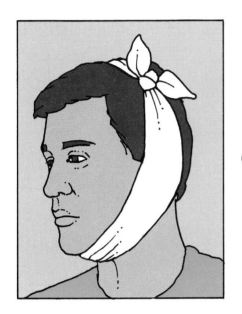

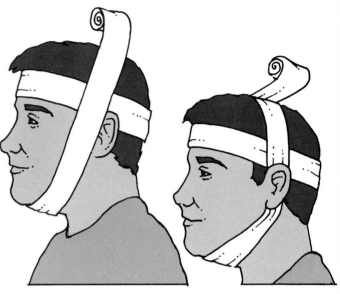

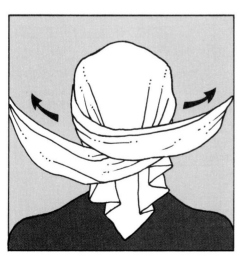

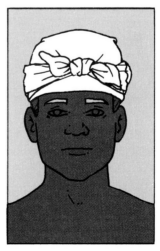

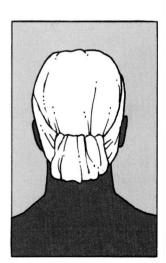

515

Finger and ankle bandages

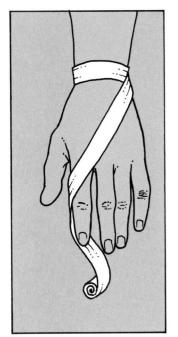
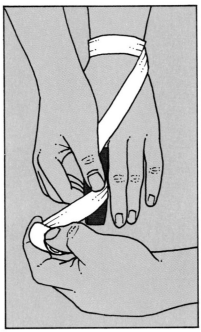
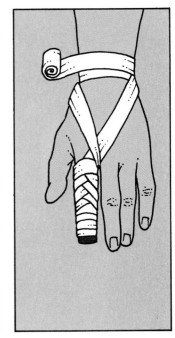

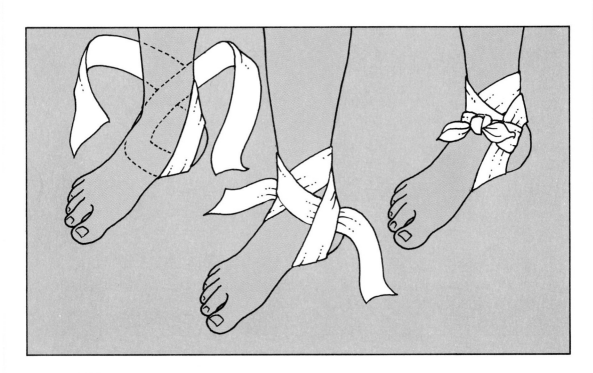

Arm sling

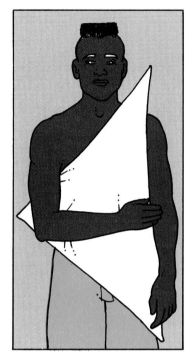

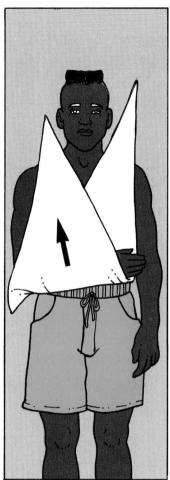

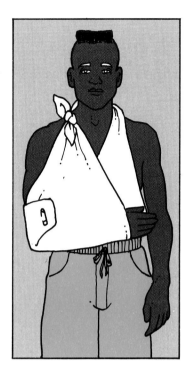

Bleeding

Excessive bleeding (hemorrhaging), both internal and external, are life threatening problems that require immediate attention to prevent death. Internal bleeding requires professional medical attention, and all you will be able to do is watch and give first aid for shock (see page 512). There are several ways to stop the flow of external blood loss, depending on the nature of the injury and where it is located. With the exception of the tourniquet, which is discussed below, the details of how to control bleeding are found on page 541.

A tourniquet is rarely if ever necessary, since direct pressure over the artery proximal to the point of bleeding (nearer the heart) should control the flow of blood. If applied, the condition should be a **life-threatening**

517

hemorrhage, since limbs that are deprived of blood may require amputation. The material required is a wide bandage 2 to 4 inches wide (5 to 10 cm) or cloth torn from a sheet that is folded so it is several layers thick. Wrap the cloth around the bleeding arm or leg twice, just above the bleeding wound, and tie it with an overhand knot. Place a strong, short stick or similar article on the knot, and tie two additional knots on top of the stick. Now twist the stick so that it tightens the tourniquet. It is best to remove a tourniquet only on the advice of a physician.

Write a note indicating the location of the tourniquet and the time it was applied. This note can be written on the victim's forehead or on any writing material that is visible. Use an indelible pen, a pencil, or even lipstick.

Every family should have immediately available a first-aid book published by the American Red Cross. This book describes exactly what should be done under a large variety of emergency situations. It is available at bookstores and at the American Red Cross office nearest your home.

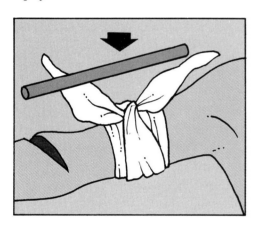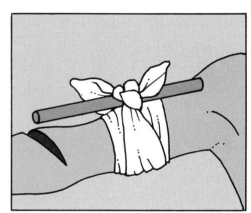

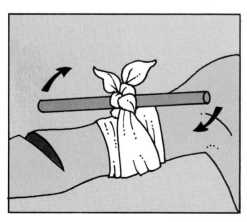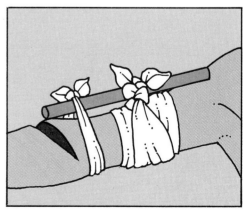

The four steps in applying a tourniquet. A tourniquet should NEVER be used unless the hemorrhage is life threatening.

CHAPTER 14

Poisonings

Millions of poisonings occur each year with over 6,000 deaths, 80 percent of which are children one to four years of age. Medicines lying around the home are common causes, aspirin and iron being among the most common. Pesticides and insecticides also take their toll. The elderly are not immune, since they may forget whether they took their medications and sometimes overdose themselves. With the rampant use of addictive drugs, death from overdosage is all too common.

Fortunately, deaths from accidental poisoning have been greatly reduced in recent years as a result of widespread knowledge about first-aid procedures, prompt and efficient action by physicians in general, and the development in all major cities of poison-control centers. Little children are at high risk, since the medicine cabinets and cupboards in our homes and garages have shelves that are packed with medicines, cosmetics, detergents, bleaches, stain removers, paint thinners, lacquer solvents, insecticides, garden pesticides, and liquid and powder plant foods and fertilizers. Every home should have rules for safeguarding innocent children from needless exposure.

Play it safe—seven important rules

The American Medical Association recommends the following:

1. Keep all drugs, poisonous substances, and household chemicals out of the reach of children. (And remember children can climb.)
2. Do not store nonedible products on shelves that are used for storing food.
3. Keep all poisonous substances and drugs in their original containers; don't transfer them to unlabeled containers.
4. When medicines are discarded, destroy them. Don't throw them where they may be reached by children or pets. Flush them down the toilet, when possible.
5. When giving flavored or brightly colored medicine to children, always refer to it as medicine—never as candy.

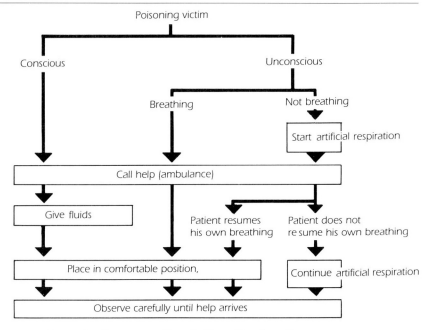

Steps in the care of a victim of poisoning.

6. Do not give or take medicine in the dark.
7. *Read labels* before using chemical products.

First aid for poisoning

The emergency call. Anytime you suspect that you or someone you are with has been poisoned, place an emergency call at once for a physician, the emergency medical squad of the fire department, or the **poison-control center** of the nearest city. In the United States, the number of your local fire department is listed with other emergency numbers on the inside front cover of your telephone directory. **The nationwide telephone number for the U.S. poison-control center is 1-800-632-8000.**

If you are the one who will give immediate first aid till help arrives, try to find someone else to make the call. Give the name, address, telephone number, and the precise location of the victim. Provide as much information as possible as to the nature of the poison, including its name, and if you have the package or bottle, the suggested antidote.

Carefully observe the victim so that you can report all signs and symptoms that might help the first-aid personnel or your physician to advise you. Especially watch for the following: The victim's skin— whether it is dry or moist, cold or clammy, ruddy or blue-colored; the type and rate of his respiration; whether he is vomiting or having diarrhea; whether he is in pain, and if so, where; and his mental state— whether he is confused, conscious or unconscious, or convulsing. Request instructions on caring for the victim until help arrives, or while you are taking him to the emergency room.

Poisons injected through the skin. This includes bites or stings from animals (dogs, cats, squirrels, bats), reptiles (snakes), and insects (spiders, bees, wasps). See pages 530, 535.

Poisoning by skin contact. Many chemicals not only injure the skin but can be absorbed into the bloodstream and affect body organs. See pages 522, 526.

Poisoning by inhalation. Remove a person who has breathed a poisonous gas (such as carbon monoxide) to a place where the air is fresh and administer artificial respiration if necessary. See page 527.

Poisoning by mouth. In ALL cases call for trained help. Gather all the information you possibly can about the identity of the substance, including the container, the label, any remaining poison, and any vomitus.

The two principles underlying any poison treatment are to **decrease further damage** and, when possible, to **remove the poison.** Dilute the poison with water or milk. If the substance is noncorrosive and the victim is conscious, you should induce vomiting (see page 561). However, if the substance that was swallowed burned on the way down, it will also burn on the way up, and you should not induce vomiting.

Five important procedures

Procedure A:

When the victim is unconscious. Administer artificial respiration if needed (see page 509). **Do not give fluids or try to induce vomiting.** If vomiting occurs spontaneously, turn the victim's head so that the vomitus drains freely, and save it for examination.

Procedure B:

When the victim has swallowed a petroleum product. Petroleum products include kerosene, gasoline, benzine, paint thinner, fuel oil, and naphtha. **Do not induce vomiting.** Provide artificial respiration if needed. If the victim is conscious, give him a glass of milk or egg white or crushed banana to soothe the membranes.

Procedure C:

When the victim has swallowed a corrosive poison. These include strong acids or alkalis—battery acid, soldering compound, lye, caustic soda, drain and toilet bowl cleaners, and electric dishwasher detergents. **Do not induce vomiting.** The damage occurs in the mouth and esophagus. Give the victim a glass of milk, or water if no milk is available. Cream, egg white, and cracked ice are also helpful.

Procedure D:

When the poison is causing the victim to convulse. Do not prevent movements, but protect against further injury (see page 558). Loosen the clothing around the victim's neck. Keep your fingers out of victim's mouth to avoid being bitten. **Do not give fluids or try to make the victim vomit.** If vomiting occurs spontaneously, turn the victim's head so the vomitus drains freely, and save it for examination.

521

Procedure E:

When the victim is conscious, is NOT convulsing, and has NOT swallowed a petroleum product or a corrosive poison. Take the following steps: (1) Dilute the poison in the victim's stomach by having him drink milk or water. (2) Induce vomiting to empty the stomach, and collect the vomitus. (3) If it is available, give activated charcoal to absorb any poison that remains.

Specific poisons

Corrosive agents—strong acids and strong alkalis:

Do not induce vomiting. Corrosive agents include strong acids (battery acid, soldering compounds, toilet cleaners), strong alkalis (lye, ammonia, dishwasher detergents, oven cleaners). These cause severe damage to the mouth, esophagus, and stomach, with excruciating pain and rapid onset of shock. Take the victim to a hospital emergency room immediately.

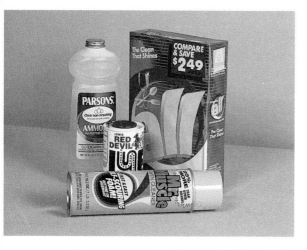

Many common household articles are highly poisonous.

Petroleum products:

Do not induce vomiting. Petroleum products that are frequently found in the home or garage include gasoline, kerosene, benzene, naphtha, turpentine, paint thinners, furniture polishes, lacquer solvent, and carbon tetrachloride. All of these substances should be used in well-ventilated areas. Breathing "dry cleaning solution" or carbon tetrachloride is highly toxic to the liver. Victims who have swallowed any of these chemicals suffer severe pain and distress. If vomited and inhaled, they may cause a serious chemical pneumonia. Take the victim to a hospital emergency room immediately.

Inhaling some of these volatile substances rapidly transfers them to the blood. Young people occasionally "sniff" glue, lacquer thinner, nail polish, and cigarette lighter fluid for a transitory "high." However, these substances irritate the heart, injure the lungs and liver, and if not fatal, may result in permanent damage to these vital organs.

Alcohol (ethyl alcohol; beverage alcohol):

Seek medical help. Symptoms of poisoning from acute overdose or prolonged abuse vary from deep sleep, in which the pulse and respiration are good, to shock and coma. In the latter situation the skin is cold and clammy, the pulse is weak, and respiration is irregular. Death comes from failure to breathe. Keep the victim warm, see that his airway is open, and give mouth-to-mouth resuscitation if needed. If the victim is

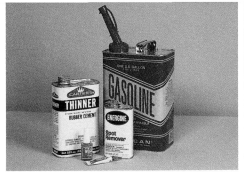
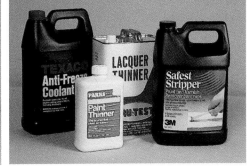
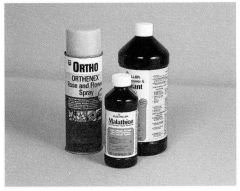
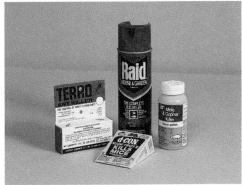

Various poisons commonly used in the home, including gasoline, antifreeze, rubber cement thinner, paint thinners and removers, spot removers, weed killers, insecticides, and rat and mouse poisons.

conscious, induce vomiting (see Procedure E, page 522).

Alcohol (methyl alcohol; wood alcohol):

Seek medical help. Wood alcohol is present in paints, paint thinners, paint removers, and "canned heat." Drinking methyl alcohol causes intoxication, along with headache, pain in the abdomen, nausea, vomiting, and, because of its action on the optic nerve, permanent blindness. If the victim is conscious, institute Procedure E. If he stops breathing, give artificial respiration.

Antifreeze (ethylene glycol):

Seek medical help. Ethylene glycol is used widely in industry as a solvent, and in pure form as a coolant and antifreeze for cars. It is a sweet, colorless, slightly syrupy liquid.

Taken by mouth it produces a form of drunkenness (no odor of liquor on the breath), which may develop into respiratory failure and death. If poisoning is discovered early, **institute vomiting as in Procedure E,** page 522. Since the enzyme that breaks ethylene glycol apart also destroys alcohol, which it prefers, beverage alcohol given in large enough amounts to keep the victim drunk tends to protect the kidney from damage and may be life-saving. Most of the ethylene glycol is not broken down and is excreted, being less toxic than its byproducts.

Medicinal products and drugs of abuse:

Seek medical help. This is a very large class of chemical agents. While each has it own effects in the body, many can be grouped together. Some of the broad classifications, with examples, include: **sedatives** (barbiturates—Seconal, Nembutal, Dolamine, and Halcion); **narcotics** (morphine, codeine, paregoric, heroin, Demerol); **stimulants** (amphetamine, cocaine, "crack," caffeine); **tranquilizers** (Librium, Haldol, Valium); and **antihistamines** (Clor-Trimeton, Benadryl).

The symptoms observed are: with **sedatives, narcotics, tranquilizers, antihistamines**—decreasing alertness, sleep deepening into coma, failure to breathe; with **stimulants**—increased activity, wakefulness, confusion, hallucinations, delusions, antisocial behavior.

Seek medical help first. For those who are depressed, if conscious, institute Procedure E, page 522. If respiration fails—as in cases of severe overdosage—give mouth-to-mouth resuscitation. Keep the victim warm. For those who are excited, prevent injury to themselves and others.

Aspirin and iron are the most common causes of poisoning among children. Symptoms develop slowly for both agents. **Aspirin** may cause vomiting, sweating, fever, mental confusion, unconsciousness, or convulsions. **Iron,** because of its corrosive action on the digestive tract, results in vomiting, diarrhea, abdominal pain, cyanosis (bluing of the skin), and shock. **Seek medical help immediately.** If the intake is discovered early, institute Procedure E, page 522.

Iodine and iodine-containing preparations (Betadine) are commonly used as antiseptics for minor cuts and breaks in the skin. When swallowed, the victim may experience nausea, vomiting, painful urination, blood in the stools, and sometimes convulsions. The mouth is stained brown, and the vomitus is yellow or blue.

Seek medical help. Give plenty of fluid—milk, barley water, a starch solution, or a thin mixture of flour and water. Institute vomiting using Procedure E, page 522.

Hair removers (depilatories):

Preparations for removing superfluous hair commonly contain thallium acetate, which is highly toxic; or barium sulfide and sodium sulfide, which are moderately toxic. Children who drink these products are the usual victims. The symptoms, which appear several hours later, include abdominal pain, vomiting, and diarrhea, which may be bloody. Damage to the nervous system causes unusual symptoms: drooping of the eyelids (one or both), crossing of the eyes, facial paralysis, and possibly delirium and convulsions. The liver and kidneys are injured.

Seek medical help. If the victim has not vomited, give several glasses of milk and induce vomiting as in Procedure E, page 522. Give plenty of water to reduce kidney damage. Keep the victim warm, combat shock, and take him to the hospital.

Pesticides:

Pesticides include a large group of generally highly toxic compounds that are commonly found in the garage, storeroom, or barn. Poisoning by pesticides can occur in one of three ways. Since they are applied as dusts and liquid sprays, they can be inhaled, either in powder or in droplet form. They may come in contact with the skin, from which many can be readily absorbed. They can also be swallowed. They kill pests by deranging certain vital processes (enzymes) within the organisms, and they can derange similar processes in the human body.

Most pesticides used today fall into one of two groups: (1) **chlorinated organic compounds** such as aldrin, benzene hexachloride, chlordane, DDE, DDT, DFDT, dieldrin, heptachlor, lindane, methoxychlor, and toxaphene; and (2) **organic phosphate compounds** such as malathion, parathion, EPN, TEPP, and OMPA.

The symptoms of poisoning from **chlorinated compounds** include aching limbs, nervous irritability, mental confusion, muscle twitching, convulsions, and unconsciousness. Brain and liver damage may occur if treatment is delayed. The symptoms of poisoning from **phosphate compounds** include dizziness, tightness in the chest, and small pupils. About two hours later there develop nausea, vomiting, abdominal cramps, diarrhea, and muscular twitching. This may progress to convulsions, unconsciousness, and death.

Seek medical help. Use rubber gloves while removing contaminated clothes. Wash all skin areas exposed to the pesticide with soap and water. If the victim is conscious, give him several glasses of warm water and induce vomiting as in Procedure E, page 522. If respiration fails, give mouth-to-mouth resuscitation. Certain antidotes are available, but must be given by a physician.

Nicotine, known as "black leaf 40," is a common garden pesticide. Absorption of nicotine is very rapid. It is an extremely poisonous substance, interfering with the transmission of nerve impulses and causing death through stoppage of the heart or respiratory failure. The victim experiences a hot, burning sensation in the upper digestive organs, and convulsions may occur.

Seek medical help. If the victim is conscious, induce vomiting as in Procedure E, page 522 Give activated charcoal, or if that is not available, a strong tea. If breathing stops, start artificial respiration. If the heart stops, begin CPR. Atropine is lifesaving but must be given by a physician.

Insecticides and rodent poisons:

Substances used to kill rodents include phosphorus, arsenic, cyanide, strychnine, and warfarin (Coumadin). Many of the aerosols used to kill flies, wasps, gnats, and ants contain petroleum distillates (see pages 521, 522, 526).

Arsenic is also an active ingredient in insecticides and certain crop sprays. Early symptoms are similar to those of food poisoning, with vomiting, diarrhea, and severe abdominal cramps. Later there are muscle cramps, kidney failure, unconsciousness, convulsions, and collapse.

Seek medical help. If poisoning is detected early, institute vomiting as in Procedure E, page 522. Your physician will administer dimercaprol (BAL), an effective treatment.

Phosphorus, now outlawed in most rodent and roach poisons, is present in many fireworks and causes burning in the mouth, esophagus, and stomach with nausea, vomiting, and diarrhea. The breath has a garlic odor. Damage to the liver and kidneys is extreme. **Seek medical help.** Do not give oily or fatty substances. If there has been skin contact, wash thoroughly. Keep the victim warm, and give artificial respiration if necessary. In the emergency room the stomach may be washed with copper sulfate or potassium permanganate.

Cyanide. Poisoning can result from swallowing, inhaling a vapor, or absorption through the skin of cyanide-containing preparations, including silver polish. Cyanide is extremely rapid in its action, blocking the use of oxygen, and causing respiratory failure and convulsions. Smaller doses cause difficulty in breathing, confusion, vomiting, and diarrhea. **Seek medical help.** Induce vomiting immediately by placing a finger in the victim's throat. If amyl nitrite ampules are available (used to relieve heart cramps), break a vial and have the victim breathe the fumes. Repeat in two minutes. If the victim reaches an emergency room in time, sodium thiosulfate by vein is lifesaving.

Strychnine causes the muscles to contract, resulting in violent convulsions. Death usually is due to inability to breathe because of prolonged muscle spasms. There is no specific antidote. **Seek medical help.** Keep the victim quiet, in a darkened room. An anesthetic or a curarelike compound can be given to prevent convulsions. The stomach may be washed out and activated charcoal administered. Artificial respiration may be needed.

Coumarins (Warfarin) reduce the ability of the blood to clot, and large doses result in internal hemorrhages. Rodents bleed internally and dehydrate (desiccate). **Seek medical help**. If the poisoning is discovered early, institute vomiting as in Procedure E, page 522. In the emergency room a vitamin K product is given orally, and intravenously if needed. In critical situations a fresh whole blood transfusion may be lifesaving.

Food poisoning:

Food poisoning results from eating (1) food which has been contami-

---

Causes of acute food poisoning
(with examples)

Bacteria-contaminated food
Salmonella
Staphylococcus
Shigella

Bacterial toxins in food
Botulin

Foods with natural toxins
certain—
Mushrooms
Fish
Shellfish

---

nated by toxic bacteria, (2) food containing a bacterial toxin, or (3) a food naturally containing a poisonous substance.

Toxic bacteria. The illnesses and treatment of infections of this type are found under s*almonella,* page 713; *shigella,* page 712; and *Giardia,* page 747.

Bacterial toxin. An illness called **botulism** is caused by a toxin produced by a germ that is often present when food is improperly canned, or when it is smoked and preserved without cooking. Examples include canned garden vegetables, turkey loaves, and salted air-dried white fish. The toxin prevents nerve conduction. Symptoms, which occur within eighteen hours after the food is eaten, include visual disturbances and difficulty in talking and swallowing due to muscle weakness. If untreated, paralysis of the breathing muscles will cause death in 70 percent of victims. **Seek medical help.** Artificial respiration may be required. The victim should be hospitalized. An antitoxin is available and can be lifesaving.

Toxic foods. Several varieties of mushrooms contain highly toxic substances. Symptoms, which develop some hours after the mushrooms have been eaten, include vomiting, abdominal pain, diarrhea, prostration progressing to shock, convulsions, unconsciousness, and death in about half the cases. **Seek medical help.** If discovered early and vomiting has not yet occurred, induce vomiting as in Procedure E, page 522. The victim should be hospitalized, where he will be treated

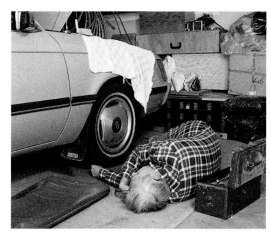

Auto exhaust fumes contain carbon monoxide, which is a deadly poison.

for shock and respiratory failure should these develop.

Carbon monoxide gas:

Some 10,000 cases of carbon monoxide poisoning are reported each year in the United States. Of these, one in seven die accidentally, and one in four are suicide deaths. Carbon monoxide is found in automobile exhaust fumes (reduced appreciably by catalytic converters), inefficiently burning and poorly vented furnaces and stoves (both gas and wood), and in smoke. The gas is colorless and odorless. Hemoglobin's affinity for carbon monoxide is 200 times greater than for oxygen. It not only displaces oxygen from this pigment-carrying protein, but retards the release of oxygen in the tissues. Death is due to oxygen depletion.

Symptoms may come on gradually with headache, faintness, dizziness, weakness, difficulty in breathing, and vomiting, followed by collapse and unconsciousness (coma). Exposure to high concentrations results in unconsciousness, seizures, and

527

death. In a small number of victims the skin has a cherry-red appearance. Prolonged exposure may cause permanent damage to the central nervous system and other organs of the body.

Seek medical help. Call the fire department or police emergency squad. The victim must be removed from the source of poison gas, and if available, given 100 percent oxygen to breathe. Should recovery occur, he should be kept at complete rest for several hours.

CHAPTER 15

First aid

Several basic emergency procedures, needed from time to time in rendering first aid to someone who is badly injured or seriously ill, were presented in an earlier chapter (see page 508). In this chapter a large number of problems that require first aid will be discussed in detail. For convenience they are grouped by categories.

Every family should have at hand a book on emergency procedures and first aid, available in most bookstores. These books concisely present what should be done under a large variety of emergency situations.

It is advised that you be trained in these procedures by taking a course offered by the American Red Cross or a local hospital. The outline below, because of the limitation of space, cannot provide every detail that you might require, but it will help you recall the procedures you have learned.

In this section the various problems you might encounter, which might require first aid, are, for the sake of simplicity, placed in groups.

Allergic reactions

Asthma attack

An asthmatic attack occurs when the air passages in the sufferer's lungs (bronchi) are narrowed as a result of contraction of the bronchial muscles, the swelling of the lining membrane, and the outpouring of mucus. The attack is triggered by sensitivity to some substance, emotional stress, or vigorous exercise. For details, see page 920. The symptoms include difficulty in breathing out (exhaling), tightness in the chest, and wheezing.

First aid
- Remove the asthmatic from any obvious cause of the problem that may be present, such as smoke, pollens, paints, perfumes, dust, animal dander, and molds.
- If the asthmatic has had an attack before, use the medication that was provided. Preparations are

529

available that can be purchased over the counter. These include antihistamines and inhaled bronchodilators.

- If the attack is mild, a warm drink or steam inhalation may bring relief.
- **If the attack is severe, call a physician or go to an emergency room.**
- Usually, the best position for the asthmatic is sitting up and leaning slightly forward. Medications are available (adrenalin, norepinephrine, aminophylline, steroids), and a physician can decide which one is best.

Plant allergies

The three most common plants to which many people are sensitive are poison ivy, poison oak, and poison sumac. The infected area of the skin becomes inflamed, swollen, and covered with blisters, and there is intense itching. A waxy or resinous material causes the irritation. Extracts of these plants have been prepared as vaccines, which for some people are helpful in preventing the problem.

First aid

- The waxy or resinous material that causes the irritation can be removed with soap and water, or it can be destroyed by washing with salt solution or Epsom's salt solution (1 T magnesium sulfate per quart or liter of water).
- Once blistering has occurred, apply dressings wet with saturated solutions of either magnesium sulfate, or baking soda (1 T per quart or liter of water).
- Cover dressings with a piece of plastic to retain moisture. Topical steroid creams will give comfort when blisters begin to dry. Over-the-counter preparations are available at a pharmacy.
- Avoid scratching, as ruptured vesicles spread the rash. Should the lesions become infected, the victim may develop a fever. If the lesions are severe and involve the eyes, mouth, or sex organs, consult a physician immediately.

Bites

Animal bites

Animal bites may result from household pets either at play or when vicious, or from wild animals such as bats, foxes, squirrels, possums, skunks, and others. A bite may be **superficial,** such as a scratch or abrasion from the tooth or claw of a household animal, or it may be **deep**—a puncture wound or large laceration from a domestic or wild animal, possibly transmitting tetanus and rabies.

First aid

- Wash a **superficial bite** with soap and water, and apply an antiseptic (hydrogen peroxide) or antibiotic ointment. Should any lesion show signs of infection, see a physician.

A tetanus shot and an antibiotic may be indicated.

- A **deep bite** should be cleaned with soap and water, and you should go to an emergency room or to a physician. He will give you a tetanus shot, and if the animal inflicting the wound cannot be found, the physician may recommend immunization against rabies. Any bite on the hand should be seen by a physician. See below.

Human bites

All human bites, especially on the hands, whether accidental or intentional, should be taken seriously. Microorganisms in the human mouth can cause very serious infections.

First aid

- Report to a physician immediately. Thorough cleaning and the administration of antibiotics may help prevent grave problems.

Snake bites

Poisonous snakes exist in most major countries of the world, causing many deaths, especially in children. Four kinds of poisonous snakes inhabit the United States: rattlesnakes, water moccasins or cottonmouths, copperheads, and coral snakes. The venom of different snakes varies. Venom not only damages local tissues, but contains toxins that circulate in the blood, injuring the blood cells, the nervous system, the liver, and the kidneys.

Report all snakebites to a physician, whether from a nonpoisonous or poisonous variety. Tetanus shots

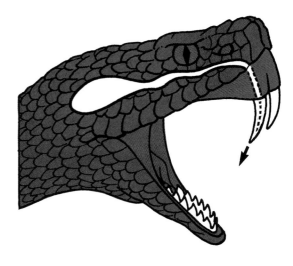

Venom from the poison sac is pumped into the wound via the fangs of a poisonous snake.

and antibiotics may sometimes be given for the bite of a nonpoisonous snake. Prevention is important. Wear high boots and be on the lookout when in snake-infested territory. Do not place your hand in holes or crevices where snakes may be lying.

Antivenoms for a large variety of poisonous snakes are available, but since they are specific for specific snakes, identification of the snake is extremely important.

First aid

- Elevate the part of the body involved, avoid exertion, and see a physician. **Do not cut or suck or use tourniquets.**
- A summary of handling of snake bites has been prepared for your convenience. See next page.

Spider bites

Most spiders are venomous, but lack fangs that can penetrate the

First aid for snakebite

Poisonous or nonpoisonous

All snakebites should be medically treated. Victims should be taken to a hospital, even if the bite is only suspected.

First aid

- Act quickly. Remove the victim from the danger of a second bite.

- Get the victim to a hospital or emergency room as quickly as possible.

- Keep the victim at rest, preferably lying down. Do not allow him to move.

- Splint the limb (arm or leg).

- Keep the bite area below the level of the heart.

- Place a constricting band (*not a tourniquet*) on the heart side of the bite. *Be sure you can feel the pulse below the restricting band.* Loosen the band every fifteen minutes. If swelling occurs at the level of the band, remove and place it a few inches higher. The band should not be placed around a joint, nor around the head, neck, or trunk.

- Reassure the victim.

- If shock develops, keep the victim warm.

- If breathing stops, give artificial respiration. If the heart stops, give cardiopulmonary resuscitation (CPR) if you are trained.

- If there is a snakebite kit available, follow instructions for its proper use. Antivenins are prepared from horse serum. (Hypersensitivity reactions requiring epinephrine [adrenaline] should be anticipated). The epinephrine may have to be given intravenously.

Things to remember

- It is extremely important for you to get the victim to a hospital as soon as possible, even if no symptoms develop.

- Identify the snake if possible. If it can be killed without risk, take it carefully to the hospital for precise identification.

Things not to do

- Do not give the victim food or drink, especially alcohol.

- Do not apply cold to the bitten area, such as cold compresses, ice pack, sprays, etc.

- Do not make incisions or give suction over the wound.

Symptoms

The symptoms will differ, depending on the type of venomous snake. These may include weakness, fainting, sweating, nausea, vomiting, chills, and a drop in blood pressure. There may be swelling of the injured site, drowsiness, difficulty in swallowing, difficulty in breathing, and convulsions.

human skin. The two most common poisonous spiders in the United States are the black widow (widely distributed throughout the Americas) and the brown recluse, found in the southern states. The tarantula, a large, frightening spider, does not inflict a serious bite.

The bite of a **black widow** produces sharp pain locally, followed in about thirty minutes by rigidity of the abdomen and abdominal cramps. Weakness, severe pain in the limbs, and even convulsions (especially in children) may come later.

The bite of the **brown recluse** may not become evident for hours to days. A volcano-shaped ulcer develops at the site of the bite and is accompanied with nausea, vomiting, chills, fever, and a skin rash.

The **tarantula** is not capable of instilling a significant amount of venom. The bite is painful but rarely has any serious aftermath.

First aid
- Take the victim immediately to a physician or to a hospital.
- Do not treat the site of the bite.
- In case of a **black widow** bite, a physician may give calcium gluconate to relax the muscle spasms, and then give the appropriate antivenin. The victim must be observed for a time for developing shock.
- For the bite of a **brown recluse,** some medical authorities advocate surgical removal of the venom-infected site. Others advocate steroids. The attending physician will watch developments closely. Most lesions heal without incident.

- The **tarantula** bites should be observed carefully.

Tick bites
Ticks bury their heads in the skin of warm-blooded animals and drink their blood. Some ticks are harmless, while others carry a variety of diseases, some of which are serious (see pages 720, 734). Do not pull a tick off, because once a tick has become imbedded, it will leave its head in the skin.

First aid
- To remove the tick, place vaseline, oil, or a drop of gasoline, kerosene, or turpentine on the creature. This closes its breathing pores and causes it to dislodge. Or, as a last resort, grasp the tick with tweezers and rotate it counterclockwise.
- Do not touch or crush the tick with your fingers. Following removal, thoroughly cleanse the area with soap and water, then apply alcohol or hydrogen peroxide.
- Report to a physician, especially if you develop a fever within the next few days. Ticks spread rickettsial diseases.

Ant bites
Bites from the many varieties of **common ants** are a frequent experience. The ant injects formic acid into the tissues. For the majority of people, the bite is limited to localized burning, itching, and swelling that spontaneously resolve in a few hours to a day.

The bite of the imported **fire ant**

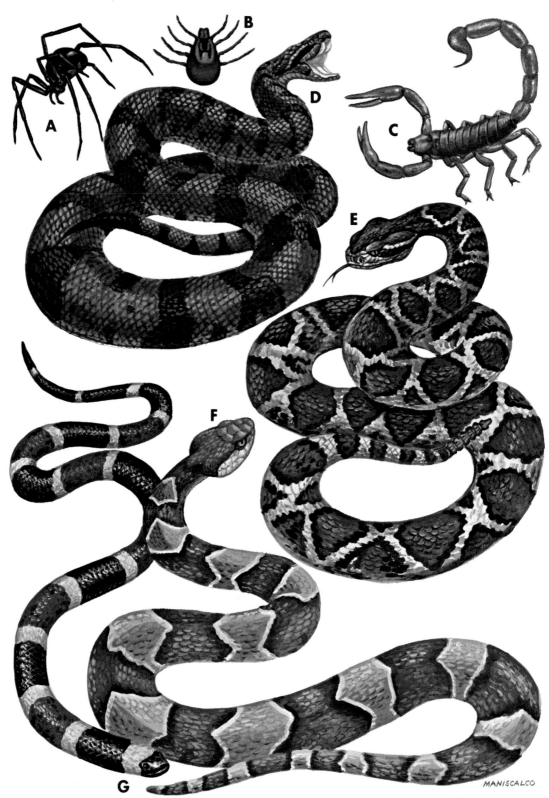

A. Black widow spider (note characteristic red hourglass-shaped mark on underside of the abdomen); B. tick; C. scorpion; D. cottonmouth; E. rattlesnake; F. copperhead; and G. coral snake.

534

(present in the southern United States) evokes a much more serious response. Each bite develops into a painful pustule with localized swelling. The tissues may break down, and scarring occurs on healing.

Some people are hypersensitive to any ant bite, and for them a bite is **a medical emergency.**

First aid
- Clean bites with soap and water. An anesthetic ointment or cala-mine cream will provide some relief.
- Should infection develop (especially after a fire ant bite), see a physician. He may recommend an antibiotic.
- For **anaphylactic reactions** from any ant bite, *rush the victim to the nearest physician's office or hospital emergency room* for an injection of adrenalin (norepinephrine), and antihistamines given orally (see page 679).

Stings

Bee, wasp, hornet, and yellow-jacket stings

The honeybee can sting only once, since it leaves its stinger in the skin. However, other stinging insects are able to sting repeatedly. Usually a single sting, although producing pain, swelling, redness, and itching at the site of the sting, is relatively harmless. On the other hand, several stings at the same time may inject sufficient venom to make the victim quite ill.

A few persons are extremely sensitive to the toxins injected by these insects and develop an **anaphylactic reaction** that may lead to shock and death (see above and page 679).

First aid
- For a **bee sting,** first remove the stinger and venom sac by lifting it off, using a knife blade or long

Note the stinger of a honeybee left in the center of the affected area. The venom produces swelling, redness, and itching.

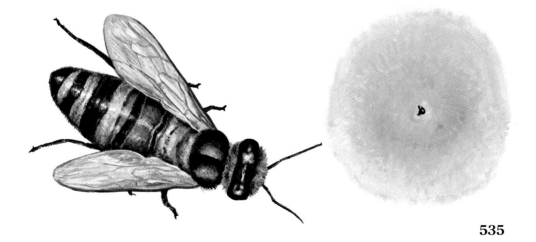

fingernail. Do not grasp the stinger with the finger and thumb as this will inject more venom into the wound.

- For all these stings, apply an ice pack, calamine lotion, or an anesthetic ointment to the sting site to provide relief.
- **For hypersensitive persons: If a bee-sting treatment kit is available,** give an injection of adrenalin (norepinephrine) into a muscle. An antihistamine should then be given by mouth. Watch the victim closely. If reactions develop, give an additional injection of adrenalin and take the victim to an emergency room.
- **If a bee-sting treatment kit is NOT available, rush the victim to the nearest emergency room.**

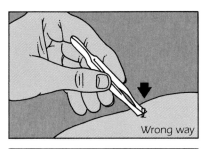

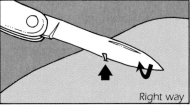

Stinger of a honey bee imbedded in the skin. Removal with a forceps or finger will force the venom into the skin. The stinger should be lifted off with a sharp edge (knife blade or paper edge).

If on the way to the emergency room the victim worsens, place a tourniquet about 3 inches (7.5 cm) above the sting site. Release the tourniquet every ten to fifteen minutes. Be prepared to give artificial respiration or CPR. Treat the victim as for shock, page 512.

Scorpion sting

A scorpion resembles a small lobster and delivers its venom by a stinger at the tip of its tail. Two species of scorpions frequent the southwestern United States, the stings of which are serious but usually not fatal. The stings of scorpions in South America, Africa, and Asia are more serious and often fatal. The most serious situation is for children, and the smaller the child, the greater the danger of death.

First aid
- A physician should be contacted immediately to obtain, if possible, an antivenin, which is the only satisfactory treatment.
- Keep the victim quiet and warm. Some victims experience dizziness, vomiting, salivation, and even shock. The latter should be cared for in a hospital.

Stings by marine animals

A catfish has a barbed stinger on its dorsal fin that is strong enough to penetrate shoe leather. A jellyfish, or Portuguese man-of-war, has long, slender tentacles that stick to the skin. A stingray has a whiplike tail with the stinger located near the base of the tail. A sting from a catfish, jellyfish, or stingray causes severe pain, and may be associated with vomiting, difficulty in breathing, and fainting. The principal danger is an allergic reaction (catfish and jellyfish) or infection (stingray).

First aid

- Because of possible serious responses, it is wise to take the victim of a sting from any of the above creatures to an emergency room.
- Treat the sting of a **catfish** the same as a snakebite (see page 532).
- Remove the tentacles of a **jellyfish** by pulling them off. Some suggest rubbing them off with dry sand. The hand that is used to pull off the tentacles should be protected with a heavy towel or glove. Wash the area and then rub on alcohol. Relief may be obtained by covering the sting with a paste made from baking soda, or soaking an arm or leg in diluted ammonia water, 4 ounces to a gallon (120 ml to 4 liters), or in Epsom salts solution, 6 ounces to a gallon (180 gm to 4 liters). If the glands in the groin or armpit swell, apply an ice bag twenty minutes out of each hour.
- The barbed spine of the **stingray** should be removed by a physician. The venom is quite toxic, so the wound should be irrigated with salt water and then placed in hot water, which destroys the venom. The physician will determine whether an antibiotic is needed to prevent infection.

Burns

A burn is an injury to a tissue, usually skin or mucous membrane, caused by heat, either dry (fire, hot material) or moist (hot liquids, steam), chemicals, electricity, radiation (sun, X-ray, nuclear materials), or friction.

Some two million Americans obtain significant burns each year, of which 75,000 are serious, and of these, 10,000 end fatally. In the United States, burns are the third leading cause of accidental death.

Burns are conveniently classified as to the depth or degree of damage to the skin.

In a **first-degree burn,** only the outer layer of the skin (epidermis) is damaged. The skin is red, tender, and slightly swollen, but there are no blisters. Among the common causes of first-degree burn are mild sunburn and mild exposure to steam, hot water, or direct heat. The skin heals quickly without scarring.

In a **second-degree burn,** both the outer layer and deep layer (dermis) of the skin are injured, causing redness, swelling, blisters, severe pain, and loss of tissue fluid. Causes include severe sunburn, boiling liquids, steam, corrosive chemicals, and electricity. Extensive burns may result in systemic effects, such as shock and infections. The deep layer is not totally destroyed, so the skin will regenerate without extensive scar formation.

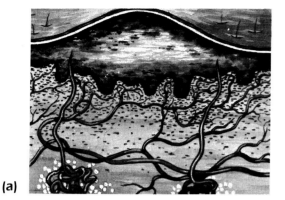

(a)

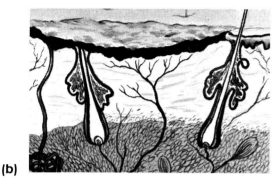

(b)

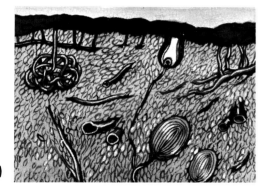

(c)

Diagrammatic views of local burns of the skin: (a) the surface layer of the skin (epidermis) has been separated, and tissue fluid has accumulated to form a blister; (b) a more severe burn has destroyed part of the epidermis; (c) a still more severe burn has destroyed all of the epidermis and some of the dermis; portions of a sweat gland and hair follicle remain.

In a **third-degree burn,** the outer and deep layers of the skin are completely destroyed, and the burned skin is insensitive. In severe cases the underlying tissues, such as muscles, are also damaged. Causes include burning clothes, exposure to flames from fire, ignited gasoline, prolonged contact with hot objects, and electricity. The skin will not regenerate in the center, but only around the edges of the burn. Scarring may be extensive, especially when skin grafting is not successful.

The seriousness of a burn does not depend alone on whether it is a first-, second-, or third-degree burn, but also on the extent of the body's surface that is involved. As a rule, children with burns extending over 10 percent, and adults over 15 percent of their skin surface should be hospitalized. Burns on the face and inhalation burns should receive immediate medical care.

First aid

These suggestions are only for the emergency care of any serious burn. Seriously burned victims should see a physician or be taken to an emergency room.

- For a **first-degree burn,** relief of discomfort is the main goal. Immersing the burned part in cold water gives relief. Applying a nongreasy ointment containing a mild anesthetic will deaden the pain.
- For a **second-degree burn** the object of first aid is to relieve the pain, attempt to control infection, and prevent shock. Pain is most safely relieved by immersing the affected part in cold (not ice)

water for ten to fifteen minutes. If this is not feasible, clean, laundered, and ironed cloths wrung out of ice water may be gently applied over the burn. Blot dry; don't rub. Do not use oil or greasy ointments. A small lesion may be washed with warm, soapy water. Cover the wound with a light cloth to keep it clean.

If the limbs are burned, elevate them slightly. To prevent shock, have the victim recline with his feet elevated. Keep him warm. Remove rings and bracelets that might cause problems should swelling occur. Do not break blisters. Give fluids frequently to replenish fluid lost from the burned area. Salt water, 1 teaspoonful to a quart (4 gm to a liter), can be given by mouth, especially if hospital care is delayed.

- For a **third-degree burn,** the general care is the same as for a second-degree burn, except that shock is much more likely. Do not attempt to clean the wound, and do not expose the burned area to cold water as this may hasten shock. Cover the burn with a sterile cloth. Watch for failure to breathe, and treat shock appropriately (see page 512).

Inhalation burns

Many severe burns resulting from explosions or blasts of hot air, together with smoke inhalation, damage the air passages and lungs, causing persistent coughing, hoarseness, and spitting of blood or particles of carbon. Swelling of the lung tissues may endanger life.

First aid

- Immediately take such victims to a hospital for continued observation, as serious problems may develop days later.

Chemical burns

In the past it was advised to immediately look for an antidote. Do **not** do this, as this takes time.

First aid

- Without any delay, flush the burned area with cool running water for ten to fifteen minutes. If large areas are exposed to the chemical, use a hose or shower.
- Carefully remove all contaminated clothes.
- If one eye is involved, hold the eye open, irrigate continuously with water, being careful to allow the water to run outward, away from the other eye. If both eyes are affected, hold the head forward so as to permit the water to flow off the face.
- For **alkali burns of the eye,** wash as indicated above, cover with a clean, moist cloth, and *go to an emergency room.* A specialist should care for the victim, as serious, long-term damage may occur.
- If the chemical container carries specific first-aid instructions, follow them.
- Cover with a clean, moist cloth and take the victim to an emergency room.
- For acid burns, thoroughly wash the area with water, and, if available, wash with a weak solution of soda (sodium bicarbonate), 1 teaspoonful of soda to a quart of

water (4 gm to a liter).

- For **alkali burns other than in the eye,** wash as above, and take the victim to an emergency room.

Electrical current burns

Serious damage occurs at the point where an electric current enters and leaves the body. The damage is often greater than what appears on the surface and may not become apparent for several days. The most serious problems result from passage of the current through the chest, interfering with the heart action, and through the base of the brain, affecting control of breathing.

First aid

- If the victim is still in contact with the electric current, break the contact, using an insulated tool such as a piece of wood, or some other nonconducting instrument. Take care not to receive the current and become a victim yourself. See page 538 for instructions.
- Give immediate attention to the action of the heart and lungs, and if necessary, institute artificial respiration or CPR (pages 509, 510).
- Call for medical help or take the victim to an emergency room.
- Minor burns can be treated as ordinary burns.

Radiation burns

These occur from overexposure to ultraviolet light (sun, sunlamp, weld-

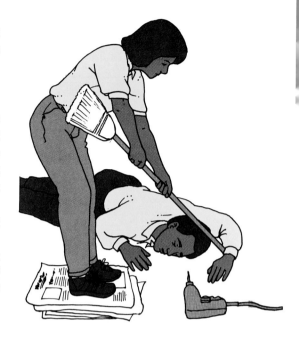

A victim of electrical shock should first be separated from the electric current using some nonconducting instrument (wood, plastic). Otherwise, the rescuer may also become a victim.

ing torch), X-rays, and nuclear materials.

First aid

- For first- and second-degree burns from **ultraviolet light,** treat as for ordinary burns. For the treatment of burns in the eyes from observing arc welding without adequate protection, see page 1129.
- For **X-ray** and nuclear burns, treat superficial skin burns as ordinary burns. Delayed symptoms require expert hospital management.

Acute circulatory problems

Heart attack

A heart attack may come as a surprise, or the person may have been aware of a heart problem. For a complete discussion, see page 783. While occasionally the attack is "silent," the two main symptoms of an acute heart attack are (1) pain in the chest radiating to the neck, one or both shoulders, and the upper abdomen (which is sometimes mistaken for indigestion), and (2) severe shortness of breath. There is pallor, a cold sweat, nausea (sometimes vomiting), extreme apprehension, prostration, and frequently shock.

First aid

- Send someone for emergency help—paramedics or an ambulance—and notify a physician.
- Place the victim in a half-reclining position, and keep him at absolute rest. Loosen clothing around the neck.
- Should respiration stop, start artificial respiration. Should **cardiac arrest** occur (when the heart stops beating), commence CPR.
- If the victim has had previous attacks and has nitroglycerine, place a tablet under his tongue.
- When trained help arrives, follow their instructions. Allow the victim to be taken to a hospital coronary care unit.

Stroke

A stroke results from a hemorrhage into the brain tissues or a clot forming in a brain artery. Strokes may be major, usually causing serious disability, or minor, sometimes called "ministrokes," in which the disability is only slight, and often temporary. The indications of a **ministroke** include headache, confusion, dizziness, speech difficulties, memory loss, and weakness in an arm or leg. If ministrokes occur frequently, personality changes may develop. For details, see page 1033.

The symptoms of a **major stroke** include weakness or paralysis of one side, difficulty in speaking and swallowing, difficulty in breathing, and confusion or unconsciousness. The disability can be serious and is often permanent.

First aid

- For any **stroke,** call a physician or take the victim to a hospital.
- In the meantime, keep the victim warm, quiet, and comfortable, and in a position that will allow saliva or vomitus to flow out of the mouth. If breathing stops, give artificial respiration.
- For a **ministroke,** consult a physician. In the interim, keep the victim quiet, and guard against physical exertion and injuries from falling.

Severe bleeding (hemorrhage)

Rapid loss of blood can lead to death in a short period. Blood lost from the circulation can be external, flowing away from the body, or internal, when blood flows into body cavities.

External bleeding may result from cuts, stab wounds, lacerations, and avulsions (when body parts are torn away). *Blood from an artery* is bright red and may come in spurts (in timing with the heartbeats). *Blood from a vein* is dark red and flows more slowly. *Blood from capillaries* is intermediate in color and oozes out.

First aid

- First, see that the victim is breathing. If necessary, give artificial respiration. If the heart stops, the bleeding will, of course, cease, but attempt CPR (page 510).
- Place a dressing or a thick cloth pad over the wound, hold it firmly in place, and apply sufficient direct pressure with the palm of the hand to control bleeding.
- If this is unsuccessful, try to put pressure on the artery above the site of the hemorrhage. Select the nearest **pressure point,** that is, where the artery can be squeezed against a bone (see diagram). This technique is useful for injuries of the limbs and should not be applied to bleeding in the head or neck.
- A tourniquet should only be used when the victim would die if it were not used (see page 517 for directions). The reason for caution in using a tourniquet is that all tissues below the tourniquet will be deprived of blood, possibly necessitating the amputation of the limb.

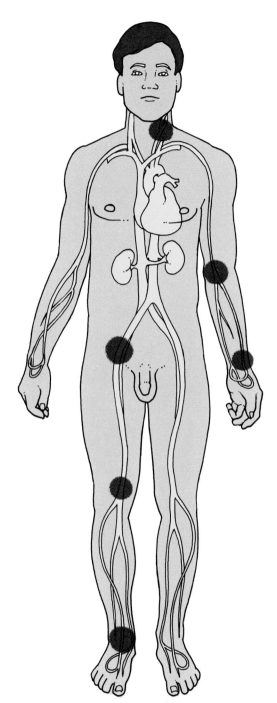

Note the various pressure points—points at which an artery is in close proximity to a bone.

- Treat shock should it develop (see pages 512, 802).
- Where possible, elevate the bleeding area above the level of the heart to make control of bleeding easier.
- If the victim is conscious, encourage him to drink fluids, but do *not* give caffeine-containing drinks, as these will raise his blood pressure, and thus increase the bleeding.
- Take the victim to an emergency room as soon as possible.

Internal bleeding may occur from a torn liver or spleen, ruptured oviduct (tubal pregnancy), stab or gunshot wound, disease within the lung, rupture of varicose veins in the esophagus, or erosion of a peptic ulcer. Bleeding from the lungs may be recognized when bright red, frothy blood is coughed up. Bleeding from sites in the stomach and intestine can be detected when blood is vomited or dark, tarry stools are passed. Signs of shock following a violent injury (such as a car accident or gunshot wound) may also indicate internal hemorrhage.

First aid
- Have the victim lie on his back and keep him warm.
- If breathing stops, give the victim

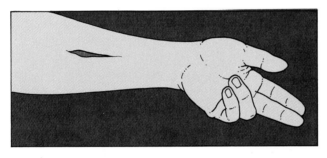
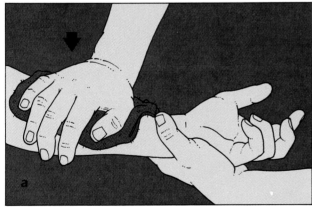
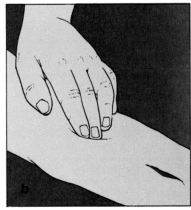

Two methods of controlling bleeding: (a) direct pressure over the bleeding site; (b) indirect pressure applied to the artery above the site of the hemorrhage.

artificial respiration.
- If the victim is conscious, encourage him to drink fluids, but do *not* give him caffeine-containing beverages, as these will raise his blood pressure, and thus in-crease the bleeding.
- Take the victim to an emergency room immediately for surgical intervention.

Nosebleed (see page 907.)

Foreign bodies

Foreign objects may enter the eyes, ears, nose, throat, stomach, and skin. If simple, nonharmful pro-cedures fail to remove the object, immediately see a physician or go to an emergency room.

Ear canal

First aid
- If an **insect** lodges in the ear, take the victim to a dark room and shine a flashlight into the ear canal.
- If this proves to be ineffective, tilt the head so that the affected ear is up, and place a few drops of glycer-ine or oil (cooking or mineral) into the ear canal. This will suffocate the insect. Then, tilt the head the other way and gently irrigate the ear with warm water, using a rub-ber syringe to introduce the water.
- A **hard object** can sometimes be dislodged by tilting the head so the affected ear is directed downward and then pulling the ex-ternal ear in various directions.
- If this fails to dislodge an object that is visible from the outside, place a drop of fast-drying glue on the end of a matchstick. Gently touch the object with the glued end of the match and wait till the glue dries, then withdraw the match. The object should come with it. This should **not** be at-tempted if the object cannot be easily seen.
- If you are unsuccessful in remov-ing the insect or object, see a phys-ician.

The eye

Consult a physician immediately if a splinter of steel or any other foreign material has penetrated the eyeball. Dust particles, sawdust, and similar objects may be removed from the surface of the eye as follows.

First aid
- Do not rub. Close the affected eye for a few minutes. The extra flow of tears may wash out the particle.
- If this is unsuccessful, pull the lower lid down so its lining is vis-ible. Have the person roll the eye up. Remove the object with the tip of a clean handkerchief or a moistened cotton swab.
- If the object is not found, grasp the lashes of the upper eyelid and draw the lid out and down over the lashes of the lower lid. Release the upper lid so that the lower lashes can brush out the foreign particles.
- If this procedure is ineffective, fill a

544

medicine dropper with plain water or commercial eyewash solution, and, by grasping the eyelashes, draw the lids outward. Gently flush the undersurface of the lids.

- If the object still remains, invert the upper eyelid. This is accomplished by taking a wooden matchstick and pressing backward and downward on the upper eyelid while pulling the eyelid (by means of the lashes) outward and upward. Use the tip of a handkerchief to wipe the object off.
- If this is unsuccessful, or vision is blurred, or pain persists, apply an interim pressure patch to the eye and immediately take the victim to an emergency room.

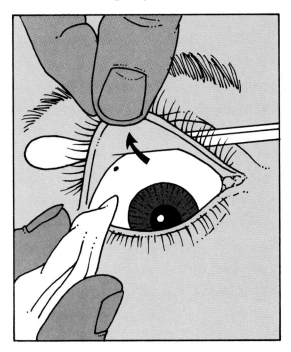

Eversion of the upper eyelid. A match or applicator stick is placed over the fold of the eyelid. By grasping the eyelashes the lid can be pulled outward and then upward.

The nose

Children will sometimes force beans, kernels of corn, or objects of similar size into their nostrils.

First aid

- Often, simply blowing the nose, one nostril at a time, will dislodge the object.
- The nasal cavity is narrow from side to side but tall in the vertical direction. If the object can be seen by having the child tip the head backward, slip a curved loop of thin wire (a loop, **not** a bent wire with a sharp end), either over or under the object, and draw it out.
- If this is unsuccessful, see a physician.

The throat

Choking or strangling is the sixth most common cause of accidental death in the United States, causing more deaths than firearms or airplane accidents. Children often inhale an object while at play, or a bite of food too large to swallow lodges in the throat (pharynx) and completely blocks the air passageway.

First aid

- If the person has inhaled an object but can breathe, take him to an emergency room immediately. Do not attempt to dislodge the object.
- If the obstruction has completely blocked breathing and the victim is **choking** or **strangling,** attempt one or all of the following three approved procedures.

Back blows. The victim can be standing, sitting, or lying on his side.

545

Place yourself in position to deliver a series of four quickly repeated, sharp blows between the shoulder blades with the heel of your hand. The blows should be forceful enough to jar the victim's body. For an infant, support the child, face down, on your forearm or knee and deliver appropriate blows (but not as strong as with an older child or adult).

Epigastric thrust (Heimlich maneuver). If the victim is conscious, have him stand or sit. Position yourself behind him and place the thumb side of your fist against his abdomen, just above the umbilicus but below the lower end of the breastbone. Grasp your fist with your other hand, and, pulling inward, give four quick, upward thrusts. If the victim is lying on his back, straddle the hips or a thigh. With one hand on top of the other, place the heel of the lower hand just above the navel and below the breastbone. Using the weight of your shoulders, give four quick, upward thrusts toward the diaphragm.

Finger sweep. Raise the chin upwards, grasp the tongue with a handkerchief, and pull it forward. Pass the forefinger of the other hand over the tongue and along the side of the throat (not the middle, as this may push the object further in) to reach the edge of the object. With a sweeping movement, bring the object forward into the mouth.

Even after breathing has been re-established, the victim should be seen by a physician to determine whether any tissue damage has occurred.

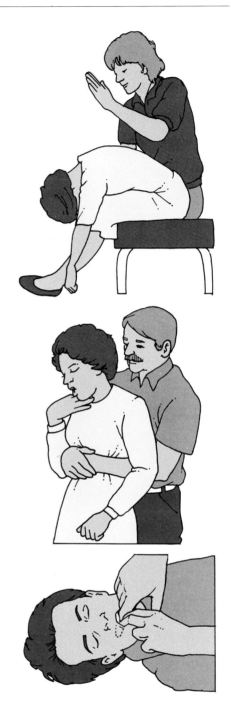

Three ways of removing an object from a blocked airway: back blows; epigastric thrust (Heimlich maneuver); and finger sweep.

The stomach

It is common for small children to swallow coins, marbles, keys, seeds, bobby pins, and even safety pins. An object without sharp points will usually pass out in the stool within a day or two. The danger is that open safety pins and bobby pins may become lodged in the intestine and perforate its wall.

First aid

● See a physician immediately if an open safety pin or other sharp-pointed object has been swallowed. X-rays will reveal the object and its location. It can then be determined whether it should be removed surgically or by means of an instrument.

The skin

Usually the foreign object is a thorn, a splinter of wood, glass, or metal, or a fishhook. If the object goes underneath the fingernail or toenail or is deep in the tissues, see a physician. A booster shot for tetanus may be wise.

First aid for a splinter

● Clean the skin area with soap and water, sterilize the ends of a sharp-pointed pair of tweezers and a needle, passing them rapidly through a flame, and enlarge the opening in the skin with the needle until enough of the splinter is exposed that you can grasp it with the tweezers. Withdraw it and cover the wound with an adhesive bandage.

First aid for a fishhook

● If the barb has not penetrated the skin, simply withdraw the hook.
● If the barb has penetrated the tissues, see a physician.
● If a physician is not readily available, thoroughly cleanse the site. Push the hook on through the tissue until the point of the barb appears, then cut off either end of the hook with a wire cutter and withdraw the remainder of the hook. Cleanse the wound thoroughly, apply an adhesive bandage, and see a physician for a tetanus shot. Watch for possible infection.

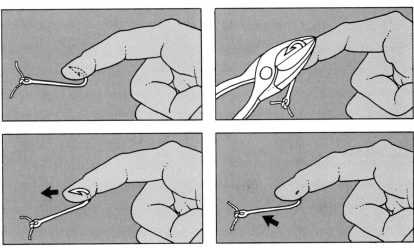

The four steps for removing an embedded fishhook.

Fractures

A fracture is a break in a bone. In a **simple** or **closed** fracture, the broken bone does not protrude through the skin, as it does in an **open** or **compound** fracture. A **dislocation** occurs when joint structures (joint and socket) are torn apart, displacing at least one of the bones of the joint. For details, see page 941. Broken bones and dislocated joints are painful, often misshapen, and cannot be used. A broken bone may injure adjacent structures and cause bleeding, as may happen with rib fractures.

The purpose of first aid is to protect the fracture and body structures from further injury, and, when necessary, to prepare the victim for transport and to provide whatever support care is needed.

General principles of first-aid care

- See that the victim is breathing, and give artificial respiration if needed. Check the pulse, and, should the heart stop, start CPR (see page 510).
- Keep the victim warm and watch for signs of shock.
- If there is severe bleeding, place a gauze or cloth pad over the wound and apply necessary pressure.
- If the conditions warrant it, call for medical assistance or an ambulance.
- Do not let the victim use or move a possible fracture, as this may make the condition worse.

- Do not try to set or reduce a fracture or dislocation.
- Do not attempt to move a victim or splint a fracture if trained medical help is on the way, unless the circumstances demand that this be done.

Simple fractures

First aid

- If medical help is on the way, make the victim as comfortable as possible.
- If medical help is not immediately available or if the patient has to be moved, immobilize the fracture. Depending on the fracture site, this may be done with a sling but is usually done with a splint. **Splints** can be made from whatever material is available, including boards, sticks, magazines, or cardboard. The splint should reach beyond the joints above and below the injury to prevent movement of the fractured bones. An arm may be splinted to the body or a leg to the other leg (if only one is broken). Strips of cloth, neckties, leather belts, or bandages may be used to fasten the splint in place.
- It is sometimes necessary to straighten an arm or leg in order to apply a splint. Support the fracture, holding the bone above and below the break. For fractures of the lower limb, pull steadily and gently until the splint is in place.

Open (compound) fractures
First aid
- The clothing at the fracture site should be cut away and removed.
- Staunch any bleeding with a sterile (clean) pad and appropriate pressure.
- Cover the area with a clean bandage or cloth.
- If the victim must be moved, splint the fracture as necessary (see below).

Dislocations
These are handled as are simple fractures.

Special situations
Fractures of the neck, spine, head, ribs, and pelvis may require additional precautions. Fractures in these sites should be suspected after observing bumps and abrasions, abnormal positions of body parts, the type of accident, and the victim's complaints of pain, numbness, or paralysis.

Neck or spine fracture
These usually result from automobile accidents, whiplashes, falling from a ladder, jumping from too high a height, and diving incorrectly into a shallow pool.

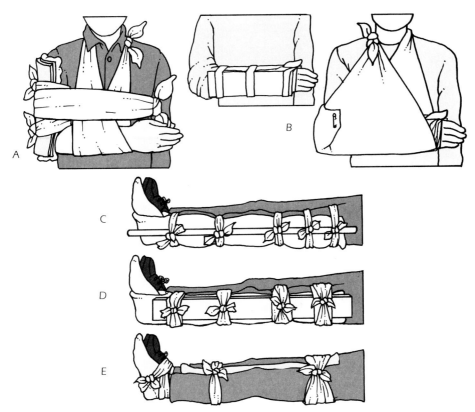

Methods of splinting: (a) arm in a sling, both strapped to the body; (b) splinted arm held in a sling; (c) leg in a padded splint, made rigid with a stick; (d) leg splinted between two padded boards; and (e) injured leg is "splinted" to the good leg.

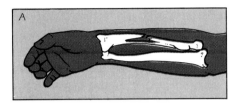

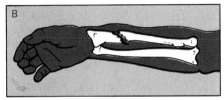

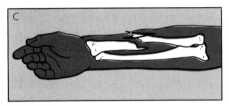

Types of fractures: (a) incomplete or "greenstick"; (b) closed; and (c) open.

First aid
- Keep the victim absolutely motionless. Place clothes, blankets, or any suitable materials on either side of the head or back to prevent movement.
- Move the victim only if necessary, when there is danger of fire or explosion. Obtain the help of several people to lift the victim (or to turn him when this is necessary for breathing), so that many hands, working together, prevent the back, neck, or head from bending or moving in any direction. Lift the victim onto a stretcher, board, door, or any available rigid material. If the victim sustains injuries in a swimming pool, float him to the side and get adequate help before lifting him out of the water.

- While waiting for emergency help to arrive, check the pulse and respiration periodically, watch for shock, and keep the victim warm. Elevate his legs if signs of shock develop.

Skull fractures
A skull fracture, which could include brain injury, should be suspected if the victim has lacerations on the face or head, if he received a blow on the head, lost consciousness, is mentally confused or lethargic, has memory loss or speech disturbances, is paralyzed or convulses, or if the pupils are of unequal size. Another sign of skull fracture is blood or clear fluid trickling from the nose or ears.

First aid
- Treat the injury as though a neck fracture existed, since head and neck fractures may occur simultaneously.
- Check the pulse and respiration, and administer artificial respiration or CPR as needed.
- Control bleeding by placing a sterile gauze (or clean cloth pad) over the injury and applying appropriate pressure.
- Check for signs of shock. Do not give fluids.
- Do not move the victim. Seek professional help immediately.

Pelvic or hip fractures
These fractures occur from falls, especially in the elderly, and not infrequently happen spontaneously because of weakened bones (osteoporosis). Symptoms include pain in

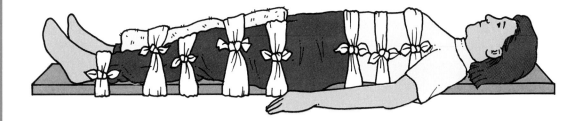

Fractures of the neck and spine require splinting to prevent any movement. A full-length board is

the low back, accentuated by movement of the leg, and pain in the hip, groin, and pubic area.

First aid
- Do not move the victim. Movement may cause injury to the pelvic organs.
- If it becomes necessary to move the victim, use the same method as for fractures of the back.
- While waiting for medical help to arrive, keep the victim as comfortable as possible, and watch for signs of shock.

Rib fractures

Rib fractures result from falls, car accidents, or banging into a sharp object. Should the broken end of a rib pierce the lung or heart, or the blood vessels within the chest be ruptured, the victim's life is threatened. When a rib pierces a lung, the lung may collapse, and red, frothy blood may be coughed up.

When many ribs on one side are fractured, that part of the chest wall loses its rigidity **(flail chest).** When

appropriate for these and certain fractures of the lower limb.

the victim inhales, the injured area sinks in, inhibiting his ability to fill his lungs with air. When he exhales, the area bulges out. The victim also avoids breathing, and especially coughing, because of the severe pain these cause.

First aid
- Check the victim's pulse and respiration, and watch for signs of shock. Take any appropriate steps.
- Evaluate the victim's problems. If pain is the principal symptom, or if the victim has a flail chest (see above), the chest should be stabilized with a firm-fitting binder (a broad bandage or a series of bandages) placed snugly around the chest (beginning below the armpits) so he can breathe more freely and the weakened area of the chest wall does not bulge with each exhalation.
- Place the victim in a slightly reclining position to make breathing easier.
- See your physician or go to a hospital emergency room.

551

Wounds and injuries

A wound is an injury to the body in which the normal relationship of tissues is broken. If the break is in the covering tissues, such as the skin and mucous membranes, it is called an **open wound.** If it occurs in underlying tissues, it is spoken of as a **closed wound.**

There are a number of types of wounds: **abrasions,** in which the skin or membranes have been rubbed or scraped; **incisions,** in which the tissues have been cut with a knife or other sharp material such as glass or plastic; **lacerations,** in which the tissues have been torn apart by a blunt object, the edges being irregular; **punctures,** in which a hard object (a knife, bullet, nail, or thorn) makes a hole as it penetrates the skin or membrane and the underlying tissues; and **avulsions,** in which the tissues have been torn away from their supporting structures, such as loss of the scalp from hair being caught in a drill, or a leg lost in an explosion.

Any part or organ of the body can sustain one or more of these wounds. Many of the specific injuries that the body experiences have already been described, and their care has been outlined.

Space does not permit a description of every type of injury to every organ and body structure. Here we will discuss the general principles of first-aid care for wounds and injuries that have not yet been described.

The first-aid care of wounds and injuries

- Do only that which preserves life, prevents further injury, and promotes healing.
- For any serious injury, call for trained medical help immediately, and when necessary, transport the victim to a physician, an emergency room, or a hospital.
- Keep the airway open, check for breathing and pulse, and when needed, administer artificial respiration or CPR (pages 509, 510).
- Watch for shock, and give shock care if needed (page 512).
- Stop bleeding immediately. Place a sterile gauze or clean cloth pad over the lesion, and apply pressure. If this fails, apply pressure to the blood vessels supplying the area at suitable pressure points. If this is unsuccessful and the wound is on one of the limbs, apply a tourniquet as a last resort.
- If the wound is on a limb and there is no fracture, elevate the limb to reduce bleeding.
- Do not try to clean the wound, except for irrigation with cool water to remove foreign bodies and to relieve pain. Cover the area with sterile gauze, a clean cloth, a piece of plastic, or even tinfoil.
- Immobilize the injured area.
- If the victim has sustained a back, neck, or head injury, do not move him except to save his life from a fire, explosion, drowning, etc., and then follow specific procedures.

552

Abdominal injuries

Injuries in which the abdomen has been torn open or received a stab or gunshot wound are gravely serious, as hemorrhage and infection may both occur.

First aid
- Keep the victim lying on his back. Place a pad under the knees to keep them bent and to relax the abdominal muscles.
- If the intestines protrude, do not try to replace them. Cover them with a clean cloth or a piece of plastic or tinfoil.
- Control bleeding with a pressure pad.

Abrasions

Here the skin has been forcefully scuffed or scraped off. Frequently, small particles of dirt, sand, and other foreign material have been ground in.

First aid
- Remove the clothing covering the injured area, and gently clean the wound with soap and water, removing as much of the dirt that has been ground in as possible. Cover the wound with a sterile gauze or clean cloth.
- Check with a physician about the advisability of a tetanus toxoid booster.

Bruises (contusions)

A bruise is an injury to tissues deep to (underneath) the skin in which the skin itself is usually not broken. Bruises are caused by a blow, falling against a hard object, or being struck by a solid object. The small blood vessels rupture and bleed into the tissues. Disintegrating blood causes the familiar "black and blue" discoloration that is evident as the lesion heals.

First aid
- Cold compresses during the first twenty-four hours tend to reduce swelling.
- Contrasting hot-and-cold applications thereafter increase circulation and promote healing.

Black eye

Treat as a bruise (contusion). If the victim has double vision, consult a physician.

Bruised fingertip (fingernail)

Fingertips are often caught in a door or smashed with a hammer. Blood often accumulates under the nail, and because of intense pressure from within, the pain is excruciating.

First aid
- Treat as a bruise (contusion).
- To relieve the intense pain from blood accumulating beneath the nail, heat a paper clip or wire (the thickness of a pencil lead) in a flame till it is red hot, then gently press the red-hot end on the nail above the accumulated blood. A hole will be formed and the blood released.

Penetrating chest wound

These are made by a knife, bullet, or any object that passes through the chest wall. Air can be sucked into the space around the lung, and the lung may collapse.

First aid

- Ask the victim to forcefully breathe out, and immediately apply a pressure dressing (gauze or pad of clean cloth) over the wound. Hold the dressing in place till professional help arrives, or, if such help is not immediately available, secure it with a snug bandage. Go to an emergency room.

Cuts and lacerations

Cuts are openings made in the skin or mucous membrane by a sharp instrument (knife, glass, metal, wood). Cuts open and bleed easily. Lacerations are tears caused by blunt objects that leave jagged edges.

First aid

- The edges of a superficial cut can be drawn together with adhesive tape or band-aids, and pressure applied till bleeding stops.
- For a cut that has passed through the deep layer of the skin and entered underlying tissues, suturing may be necessary. This is especially true of lacerations in which the edges may have to be trimmed. See a physician or go to an emergency room.

Sprains

Sprains are caused by a sudden and forceful twisting and wrenching of a joint, accompanied by stretching or tearing of the surrounding ligaments, tendons, muscles, and blood vessels. The ankles, fingers, wrists, and knees are most frequently involved. The usual symptoms are immediate pain, especially when moving the affected part, with swelling and tenderness.

First aid

- For a **mild sprain,** keep the injured part raised and apply cold or ice packs for the first day to reduce swelling.
- For a **severe sprain,** provide similar first aid as for a fracture, as one cannot be distinguished from the other. See a physician or go to an emergency room. An X-ray will determine the type of injury and the appropriate treatment. Severe sprains often require immobilization similar to fractures.
- Medication may be given for severe pain.

Strains

Strains result from overuse or overexertion of a muscle, which causes its fibers to excessively stretch and sometimes rupture. A strain may occur from improperly lifting a heavy weight, from athletic activities, from carrying a heavy suitcase without sufficient rest periods, or even from missing a step while descending a stairway.

First aid

- Treat **back strains** with bed rest on a very firm mattress and the application of heat. Should pain persist or the back strain be severe, consult a physician, as the problem may be a herniated disc (see page 951).

- For strains of the arm or leg muscles, rest, together with warm, wet applications, should bring significant relief.
- Medication may be given for severe pain.

Environmental overexposure

Excessive exposure to cold, heat, or sun can cause serious damage to tissues of the body and may have life-threatening consequences if the whole body is involved. Body heat generated from intense exercise may have similar effects.

Frostbite (cold injury)

Frostbite is the actual freezing of the tissues of some part of the body, most often of the toes, fingers, ears, nose, and cheeks. Just before freezing, the skin appears violet-red, but changes to gray-yellow once it has frozen. A common sign of frostbite is gradual loss of pain, feeling, and function. **Do not rub or massage the frozen parts with snow. This results in greater tissue loss.**

First aid
- If the first aid is given out-of-doors, wrap the frozen part with a dry coat, blanket, or even several layers of newspaper.
- If help is rendered outside a hospital, in a house, warm the frozen area immediately by soaking it in **warm** water (101° to 105°F or 38° to 40°C). Do **not** use a heat lamp, hot water bottle, or heat from a stove. Warming may take up to an hour. The victim will experience pain, possibly severe, as the frozen tissue warms and as feeling and function return. Blisters may form, but should not be broken, and the area will swell severely.
- Elevate the affected part. Do not put pressure on it, but gently exercise it.
- Cover with a sterile bandage or clean cloth.
- Go immediately to an emergency room. Be careful not to allow refreezing, as this seriously damages the tissues. It is better to delay thawing if refreezing is possible.

Hypothermia

Hypothermia refers to a condition in which the body temperature drops below normal (98.6°F or 37°C). When more body heat is lost than is replaced (as during prolonged exposure to very cold, windy conditions), body temperature gradually falls, and physical and mental functions slow down. The elderly, the very young, alcoholics, and persons taking psychotropic medications are most susceptible. The victim progressively exhibits shivering, numbness, stumbling, slurred speech, mental confusion, drowsiness, and coma, terminating in cardiac arrest and death.

First aid
- Check the victim's vital signs and give artificial respiration if needed.

- Wrap the victim in blankets or warm clothes, and promptly take him to a shelter or emergency room. Hot-water bottles will provide additional heat, but do **not** use them in areas that may be frostbitten.
- Remove wet or damp clothes, and if the hypothermia is mild (the person is mentally alert but extremely cold), give a hot drink, **but NO alcohol.**
- If the hypothermia is severe, wrap the victim in warm blankets, or immerse him in a tub of water that is warm to the skin of the elbow. The water must **not** be hot. Rewarming may take several hours.
- Some victims go into shock during rewarming, and for that reason it is best if the rewarming can be done in a hospital or emergency room. If this is impossible (as on a camping trip), put the victim in a sleeping bag with a normally warm (euthermic) second person.

Heat cramps

Heat cramps, seen during intense exercise, are painful contractions of the muscles. It has long been held that the primary cause was salt depletion. Evidence now suggests that dehydration is the real cause and that salt depletion rarely occurs.

First aid
- Massage and gently stretch the cramped muscles. Contracting the opposing group of muscles appears to be quite effective.
- Have the victim drink lots of water. Salt should not be required unless the victim drinks more

than 10 quarts (9 liters). Drinking generously before, during, and after strenuous exercise will generally prevent these painful cramps.

Heat exhaustion (heat prostration)

Heat exhaustion may develop from prolonged exposure to excessive heat and high humidity or from intense exercise (more commonly in a hot, humid environment), because the body's heat-dissipating mechanisms are inadequate to remove the heat being produced. The symptoms include a moderate rise in body temperature (102°F or 39°C), profuse sweating, clammy skin, fatigue, rapid breathing, headache, heat cramps, and the tendency to faint. Dehydration is common.

First aid
- Give plenty of water, and if the victim feels nauseated, have him sip the water.
- Take the victim to a cool environment. Place moist cloths on his forehead and wrists, and turn a fan on him if one is available.
- Have the victim lie down and raise his feet a foot (30 cm) above the level of his head.
- If the victim is unconscious, take him to a hospital immediately. If the hospital is some distance away, give a retention enema of plain water, which will be absorbed.

Heatstroke (sunstroke)

Heatstroke is the most serious form of heat injury. Young people are most likely to experience heatstroke when undergoing strenuous exercise. However, elderly persons and those who are ill may develop heatstroke without active exercise. The precipitating cause is high environmental temperature and humidity. The symptoms, which come on abruptly, include flushed, hot, dry skin; no sweating; mental confusion; lethargy; and rapid onset of coma. Body temperature may rise to 106°F (41°C) or higher. If treatment is not instituted immediately, the victim will go into shock. The higher the body temperature, the worse the prognosis.

First aid

- Heatstroke is a medical emergency. Take the victim to the nearest hospital or emergency room. When this is not possible, the following will be helpful.
- Cool the victim to lower his body temperature. Placing the victim in a tub of ice-cold water has long been recommended. This, however, tends to induce shivering, which, in turn, raises the body's core temperature. Better results have been obtained by continuously sponging the face, body, and limbs with cool water. A fan blowing on the victim will aid cooling. Reduce the cooling measures when the body temperature has fallen to 102°F (39°C) to keep the victim's temperature from dropping too low.
- If the victim is in a hospital, fluids can be given intravenously. When this is not possible and the victim is conscious, have him drink a glass of water (8 oz or 250 ml) every twenty minutes.
- When the body temperature has reached normal, dry the victim off. However, check his body temperature for a while, and if it starts to rise again, resume cooling measures.
- **Do NOT give alcoholic beverages.**

Unconsciousness (coma)

A number of conditions may cause unconsciousness. A few of the more common ones include heart attack, stroke, diabetic coma (too little insulin and too much blood sugar), hypoglycemia (too much insulin and too little blood sugar), a head injury, uremia, poisoning, or a drug overdose, and cardiac arrest.

First aid

- In all cases, summon medical help or take the victim to an emergency room.
- In the meantime, keep him warm, keep his airway open, and, should breathing cease, give artificial respiration. If the heart stops, start CPR.

Fainting

Fainting is a temporary loss of consciousness due to a reduction of blood flowing to the brain. A common cause is emotional concern. For a detailed discussion, see page 803.

First aid

- Have the victim lie on the floor and elevate his feet. Consciousness will usually be regained quickly. If it does not return within one or two minutes, call a physician.

- If a person is about to faint, have him sit down and lean forward, putting his head between his knees. Then have him try to raise his head while someone else is pushing his head downward. This will force blood to the brain, which should prevent fainting.

Convulsions

A convulsion is a sudden onset of unconsciousness accompanied by rigidity, followed by jerky contractions of the body muscles **(seizure).** While the muscles are rigid, the victim stops breathing, loses control of his bladder and bowel, and may bite his tongue. The many causes of convulsions include **epilepsy,** head injury, stroke, meningitis, withdrawal from alcohol or drugs, drug overdose, poisonings, and, in children, high fever.

First aid

- Protect the victim against injury. Lay him down on a soft surface if one is available. Place a rolled-up handkerchief between his upper and lower jaws (teeth), **not** a hard, blunt object.
- Allow the victim to convulse. Do **not** restrain his movements.
- Do **not** put a child with a high fever in a tub of water, but sponge him down with lukewarm water.
- Do not try to give fluids, but provide artificial respiration or CPR if needed (pages 509, 510).
- Following the seizure, allow the victim to sleep and rest.
- Seek medical help.

Delirium

Delirium is a state of mental haziness ("out of his head") in which the victim is confused, restless, anxious, and unable to cooperate, and his imagination is out of control. Causes include high fever, acute intoxication with alcohol or other drugs, poisonings, and many serious illnesses.

First aid

- Protect the victim from injury and keep him in a quiet environment.
- Seek medical help. If this is delayed and the victim can cooperate, encourage him to drink water.

Drowning and near-drowning

Drowning occurs when water enters the voice box (larynx), which then goes into spasm, or when water floods the lungs (air passageways). If he is not rescued within minutes, the victim will sustain permanent damage to his brain and other organs from a lack of oxygen. If he is deprived of oxygen too long, he will die.

Drownings are America's fourth leading cause of accidental deaths, the highest drowning rate being among infants less than one year of age. Of these, some 70 percent drown in the bathtub. A growing number of children die in outdoor hot tubs. Fifty percent of drownings among youth and adults are related to the use of alcohol. Drowning is a serious concern of water-related recreational sports.

The steps in drowning may vary, but they commonly follow this sequence: the victim panics, and while struggling to stay above water, breathes rapidly and deeply. He then becomes exhausted and holds his breath as his head goes down. He swallows water, vomits, and then coughs violently. Eventually he gasps, and his lungs fill with water. This is followed by unconsciousnes, convulsions, and death.

Cautions

- Unless he is trained and capable of assisting a drowning person, an inexperienced observer should not jump into the water to save the victim, but should **summon help.** Far too many would-be rescuers have drowned with their drowning victims.
- Throw the victim a life jacket, a plastic bottle, a rope—anything that will float or that he can grasp onto while being pulled to shore.
- If a boat is available, row out to the victim and tow him to shore. Do not try to pull the victim aboard, as the boat may capsize.
- If the incident resulted from a water accident that may have caused neck or back injuries, do not lift the victim directly out of the water. Float him to shore, or place a board or stretcher underneath him and then lift him out of the water.
- If the victim has fallen through thin ice, have him place his arms and chest on the edge of the ice, then throw him a rope or extend a long board to him and pull him onto the ice. If enough rescuers are available, have them lie face down on the ice and form a human chain out to the victim.

First aid

- If the victim's breathing has stopped, give mouth-to-mouth respiration, if possible while he is still in the water. If his chest does not inflate, do not drain water from his lungs, but blow more forcibly into his lungs. Take special precaution not to overinflate the lungs of an infant or small child.
- Once the victim is on shore, if he has no pulse, start CPR (page 510). Continue for one hour unless he revives sooner. Take him to a hospital immediately, as serious complications may develop following a near-drowning.

Diving emergencies

Diving. Serious injuries to the head and neck may result from diving and striking one's head against a rock or the floor of a swimming pool.

Deep diving. With scuba-diving equipment, swimmers can dive to depths of more than 100 feet (30 m). Drowning can result from failure of equipment to provide air or oxygen and from the lines becoming entangled in weeds or rocks.

Decompression sickness, "the bends." Divers who remain too long at depths greater than 30 feet (10 m) and then ascend to the surface without allowing enough time for the gases dissolved in the blood and body fluids to reach a new equilibrium (decompression) develop gas bubbles in their tissues, with serious aftereffects.

Symptoms occurring soon after emerging from the water include pain in the joints, pain in the chest with cough and difficult breathing, paralysis of certain muscles, disturbances of vision, and dizziness.

First aid
- For striking one's head when **diving,** see "neck fracture," page 549.
- For **drowning** or **near-drowning** when deep diving, see "drowning," page 558.
- For **decompression sickness,** special pressure equipment is required. Ask official lifeguards where such equipment is available and call for professional help. If the help is delayed very long, the victim, if physically able, may dive to depths that will redissolve the gas bubbles and then ascend more deliberately.

Hernia
A hernia is a protrusion of the bowel through a weakness in the abdominal wall. (For details, see page 862.)

First aid
- It is usually simple, especially to begin with, to push a hernia back into the abdomen (reduce) by applying pressure on the protrusion with the fingers. Having the victim lie on his back, with his hips slightly elevated and his knees drawn up to his shoulders, will aid in the procedure. If this is unsuccessful, have the victim consult a physician immediately.

Hiccup
A hiccup is a sudden, uncontrolled, fitful contraction of the diaphragm, during which inhalation is abruptly stopped by closure of the larynx. Hiccups usually occur at intervals of a few seconds, and most attacks end in a few minutes. Sometimes, however, especially following abdominal surgery or in connection with serious illnesses, an attack may last hours or even days, and become life threatening.

First aid
- A number of simple, harmless procedures are advocated to end a hiccup: drinking water; while stooping forward, drinking water from the side of the glass away from you; holding your breath; sucking ice; and breathing into a paper sack held over your nose and mouth.
- If these simple measures are ineffective, see a physician.

Alcoholic intoxication
An individual's capacity to function physically and mentally is impaired when he is intoxicated with alcohol. He is sluggish, uncoordinated, and clumsy. He is mentally dull, his judgment is faulty, and his understanding is distorted. At times he may be violent, and he can be dangerous. Or he may go into a stupor and lapse into a coma.

First aid
- Should the intoxicated person show signs of shock (cold, clammy skin; rapid, weak pulse; and irregular breathing), seek professional medical help.
- If the victim's breathing becomes inhibited, give him artificial res-

piration (page 509). Keep his airway open, turning his head to one side so that vomitus will flow out of his mouth.

- Keep the victim warm. Intoxicated persons lose heat more rapidly than normal individuals.

Vomiting

Vomiting may be due to dietary indiscretion or a temporary gastrointestinal infection, or it may indicate a serious illness. If simple measures do not relieve the problem within a day, see a physician.

First aid

- Put the victim to bed and keep him warm.
- Encourage him to drink plenty of fluids. Give him sips of ice-cold water or have him suck ice or give him hot, clear broth to drink, again in sips.
- If vomiting continues, call a physician, who will determine the underlying cause and may prescribe an antivomiting medication.
- If the victim is unconscious, keep his airway clear of the vomitus and get medical help.

561

CHAPTER 16

The home medicine chest and first-aid kits

Surveys have shown that nine out of ten aches and pains, together with minor injuries, are brushed off or treated by the sufferer with some readily available medication or simple procedure. Of the remaining problems, less than half are cared for by trained health professionals. The home medicine chest is usually a ready source of band-aids and bandages, ointments, disinfectants, and remedies for headaches, upset stomachs, colds, coughs, diarrhea, and constipation.

Precautions

The most important rule for your medicine cabinet is "Be Careful!" Parents and guardians of small children should be aware that aspirin and iron are among the most common forms of poisoning among children. Children like to play doctor and nurse, and when parents are not watching, they sometimes frequent the medicine cabinet. The result is often tragic. Medicines should be kept away from little hands, even when secured in child-resistant bottles. Children should be taught from babyhood never to take medicine unless it is given to them by a parent, nurse, or teacher. Do not encourage a child to take a medicine by telling him that it's "candy." It may taste sweet, but it is *not* candy.

Note the expiration date of all medications that you purchase, whether with a prescription or over-the-counter. If you are in doubt about a medicine that has been around for a while, check with your pharmacist before using it. Your pharmacist can advise you as to which medicines should be stored in the refrigerator and which will keep well in a drawer or cupboard. All medicines should be labeled. *Never use medicine from a container that has no label.* Medicines should be kept out of reach of children or in a locked container or cupboard.

It is unwise to prescribe leftover medicines for another member of the family, or for a neighbor who appears to have the same problem you or someone in your family had. Before retaking a medication, check with your physician.

Do not discard tablets, capsules, injectables, or ointments in places where children may find them. Wherever possible, flush old medicines down the toilet. Otherwise, seal them in a childproof container and place them in the garbage. Always break off the needles on disposable syringes before throwing them away.

Contents of a medicine chest

It is important to stock your medicine cabinet ahead of time with certain basic items so that in a time of emergency you won't have to waste precious time going to the store to purchase what you need. The following list should be adequate as a start. You will, of course, add to it as time goes on. But always be sure you have an adequate supply of these items on hand:

Equipment

Scissors—medium size.
Medicine droppers—two.
Tweezers—sharp pointed.
Rubber syringe—soft, small.
Disposable syringes with needles (1 ml)—five.
Sewing needle—medium size.
Teaspoon or measuring cup—small.
Hot-water bottle.
Safety pins—six medium, six large.
Ice bag.
Razor blades—stiff-backed.
Clinical thermometers—

- oral—one.
- rectal—one.

Flashlight.
Safety matches.
Bedpan (optional).

Supplies

Absorbent cotton—sterile, small roll.
Cotton balls—sterile, small bag.
Sterile gauze pads—prepackaged.

- four 2 inches (5 cm) square.
- four 4 inches (20 cm) square.

Cotton tip applicators—small package.
Adhesive tape—one roll, 1-inch (2.5 cm) wide.
Band-aids—one box, assorted sizes.
Roller bandages, gauze—

- one roll, 1 inch (2.5 cm) wide.
- one roll, 2 inch (5 cm) wide.

Ace bandage—one 3 inch (7.5 cm) wide.
Enema kit (chemical)—one.
Rubbing alcohol—
16 ounce (500 ml), one bottle,

563

baby oil, small bottle.

Petrolatum (Vaseline)—4 oz (100 gm).

Glycerin—8 oz (200 ml).

Activated charcoal—
- powder, 4 oz (100 gm)
- tablets, bottle of fifty.

Antiseptic soap—bar or liquid.

Antiseptic—small bottle (for skin).

Milk of magnesia—medium bottle.

Medications

Boric acid ointment—5 percent.

Zinc oxide ointment—small tube.

Eyewash—small bottle with eye-cup.

Eucalyptus oil—small bottle.

Antihistamine—Chlor-Trimeton, twenty-five tablets.

Nitroglycerin—sublingual 0.3 mg, ten tablets.

Adrenalin (norepinephrine)—injection five 1-ml vials with five 1-ml disposable syringes.

Milk of magnesia, medium bottle.

Epsom salts—1 lb (500 gm).

Syrup of ipecac—2 oz (50 ml).

Earache drops—small bottle.

Calamine lotion—4 oz (100 ml).

Antacids—aluminum or magnesium hydroxide, twenty-five tablets.

Cough syrup—small bottle.

Tylenol—120 mg, ten tablets.

Common uses of medications

Glycerin: moisten lips or around mouth.

Charcoal: powder for poisonings; tablets for indigestion.

Boric acid ointment: prevent infection.

Zinc ointment: skin-drying effect, prevents infection.

Eucalyptus oil: for vaporizer.

Antihistamines: hay fever, sensitivity reaction.

Nitroglycerin: angina chest pain.

Adrenalin: for sensitivity to insect bite or sting.

Milk of magnesia: milk laxative.

Epsom salts: for catharsis, or arm or leg bath.

Syrup of ipecac: for controlled vomiting.

Ear drops: mild outer-ear infection.

Calamine lotion: for itching skin rash (see page 973).

Antacids: occasional indigestion.

Cough syrup: for nonproductive cough.

Tylenol: mild muscle pains or transient headache.

Medicines for emergency use

Antiseptics: For any superficial wound that may become infected. It is perhaps more important to thoroughly cleanse the lesion with mild soap and water.

Emetics: These agents produce vomiting. Syrup of ipecac, when used, produces prompt vomiting. To induce vomiting, use Procedure E, pages 512, 522 .

Nitroglycerin: For relief of an anginal attack. See page 782.

Adrenalin: To be injected only in

the event of a severe allergic reaction or anaphylactic shock. See page 535.

Antihistamine: Given in conjunction with adrenalin for a severe allergic reaction, or in case of stings of certain insects. See page 677.

First-aid kits

Various manufacturers put together special first-aid packages or kits, often of sizes and shapes that are convenient for packing into a case. These kits are also packaged to prevent contamination or spoilage, and generally have printed directions for use on the outside. The extra cost of obtaining your first-aid kit in such form will probably repay you in the long run. Your pharmacist will doubtless be able to show you samples.

It would obviously be impossible to take along your entire medicine cabinet on a trip away from home. However, it is wise to take along those first-aid articles that you feel might be needed. If you are going into a country where poisonous snakes abound, be sure to add to your arsenal a snakebite kit (available commercially). If you have in your party someone who might suffer an angina attack, nitroglycerin tablets would be a wise choice. You might wish to prepare your own first-aid supplies and carry them in a small toolbox or a fisherman's tackle box.

Every family should have available for immediate use a book put out by the American Red Cross on first aid. This book presents very concisely what should be done under a large variety of emergency situations. The book is available at many bookstores and at the American Red Cross office nearest you.

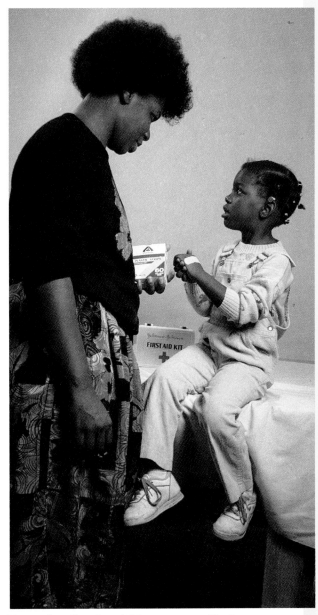

Every family should have a medical kit and a first-aid manual.

CHAPTER 17

Home care of the sick

While for certain illnesses it is best that sick people be cared for in a hospital or a nursing home, sometimes they can receive better care at home, where they can feel the assurance of a warm, loving atmosphere. Home care allows the sick person to maintain his place in the family. Also, the cost of his health care is kept to a minimum, and hospital beds are left free for those who are more critically ill. Recovery is often hastened by home care, because the support network is better in the informal setting.

Home care varies from situation to situation. Some illnesses are short, others of long duration. Some patients are largely able to care for their own needs, such as eating and drinking and using the commode, while others require that someone else take care of most or all of their needs. There are also the elderly, taken into the home for a prolonged period to be cared for by their adult children.

As hospital costs rise, difficult procedures and highly technical equipment are increasingly being used in the home under the supervision of professional home-care teams. The family members are taught the care of the machines as well as the treatment. Your physician will advise you about the appropriateness and availability of such assistance in your situation.

However, the essence of home care for a sick person is to provide an environment that speeds recovery or rehabilitation, or that provides continuing comfort and support for a patient who is chronically and perhaps terminally ill. For those who have had no specific training in either medicine or nursing, the most important skills for giving adequate home care are common sense and a desire to meet the patient's needs.

This chapter outlines the basic principles of home care for those who are ill. It is assumed that in most instances the person reading this chapter will be the care giver, and for that reason the chapter has been written in the second person, addressing the care giver as "you." Even though you probably are not a doctor and may not be a nurse, the sick person will be referred to as "your patient."

The health team

Most communities have a number of organizations whose purpose is to help those needing specialty health care. The visiting nurse association, together with the city or county health department, will either provide, or at least assist you in receiving, the services recommended by your physician. The visiting nurse, the physical therapist, the occupational therapist, the speech therapist, the psychologist, the social service worker, the vocational counselor, and others will, as needed, become involved in assisting you in meeting the needs of your ill family member.

The social worker will help you determine such needs as financial requirements, special equipment, special foods and dressings, and he or she will aid you in obtaining any assistance you lack.

The visiting dietitian will suggest ways to provide the special diet your patient needs. The visiting nurse may dress wounds and give injections, and, if needed, show you how to do these things. An occupational therapist will set up activities that can hasten rehabilitation for a stroke victim or for someone whose recovery requires special movements.

Should your patient be terminally ill, an organization called a **hospice** can help you and the ill family member better understand and plan for death. This helps to bring sympathy and comfort into the home.

Numerous **professional and voluntary organizations** are prepared to help sick people with specific problems. Among these are the American Red Cross, the American Heart Association, the American Cancer Society, and the American Lung Association. Others relate to specific diseases, such as diabetes, blindness, arthritis, kidney diseases, muscular dystrophy, epilepsy, mental retardation, multiple sclerosis, alcoholism, and Parkinson's disease. They provide information and help that otherwise might not be available.

Many **services** exist that can be of great assistance, including door-to-door transportation, adult day-care programs, hospital day-care programs, home-health aides, and homemakers. Churches and other agencies may provide such things as "meals-on-wheels."

The sick room

Choosing the room

While the exact arrangement must be adapted to the circumstances in each home, you should keep certain principles in mind as you make the choice. The room should make it as easy as possible for you to care for your patient and provide him with comfort and encouragement. Ideally,

567

the room will be pleasantly decorated and admit sunlight when it is desired. In any case, it must provide for heating and cooling, and it should be near a bathroom.

Home activities provide interest to sick people and distract them from their own concerns. For that reason, in most cases, a downstairs room is preferable to one on the second floor, since it will bring the sick person closer to the activities of the home. Also, a downstairs room will save you as the care giver much time and effort.

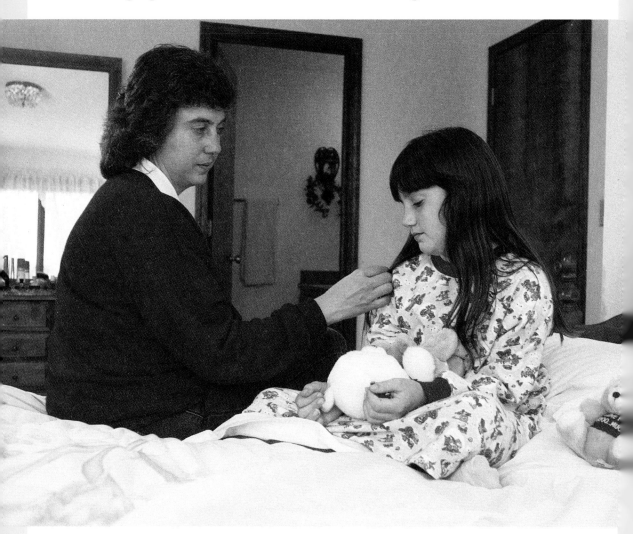

The patient's room should be bright and comfortable.

Maintaining the room

The room should be clean and in order, with each needed article in its designated place so that its access is comfortable for the patient and convenient for you. You should air the room once or twice a day, even in cold weather, by opening the doors or windows. At such times the sick person, if he is bedfast, should be well covered and, if he is sitting up or able to walk about the room, should wear adequate clothing. It is better not to keep food in the room. A potted plant or a few flowers, together with a pleasing view out of a window, will bring a great deal of cheer and can help to speed recovery.

The kind of bed to use

A comfortable bed is extremely important. If the care will be prolonged, it may be advisable to rent or purchase a hospital bed that can be raised and lowered. You can handle the needs of a bedfast person much more easily if his bed is higher than the conventional bed. You can raise a regular bed by placing the legs on sturdy blocks. For children and helpless older people, you may need to attach side rails to the bed, or by some other means prevent the patient from falling out of bed.

You can make a bed firm by placing a sheet of plywood under the mattress. The mattress should be firm but comfortable, with no lumps or hollows. Turning the mattress periodically keeps it from becoming misshapen. The mattress should be protected by a full-size pad or blanket that can be easily washed.

Bed making

The sheets should be made out of an absorbent material, preferably cotton. They should be enough wider and longer than the mattress that they can be tucked in securely. Place the lower sheet over the mattress pad and snugly tuck it in at the top, bottom, and sides with smooth, square corners. Be sure to make this sheet tight, or it will tend to wrinkle and feel very uncomfortable.

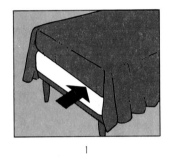
1

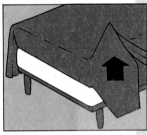
2

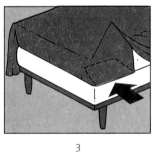
3

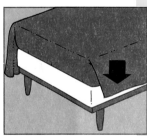
4

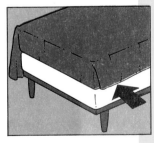
5

Five steps in mitering the sheet at the corner of a mattress.

Should the mattress need to be protected from discharges, place a smaller plastic sheet over the bottom sheet and cover it with a narrow **drawsheet** that is slightly wider than the plastic. These need cover only the midportion of the bed (see illustration below). Be sure that the plastic sheet and the drawsheet are kept free of wrinkles.

The drawsheet can be an ordinary sheet that has been folded once lengthwise. Place the folded edge toward the head, crosswise of the

inconvenience to your patient and without remaking the entire bed.

Fit the top sheet to the bed with the upper end 6 to 8 inches above the head of the mattress. Smooth it carefully and tuck it in at the bottom with smooth, square corners. Fit the blankets with the upper ends a few inches below the top of the mattress, depending on the patient's height. You can then arrange the bedspread with its upper end about 3 inches above the upper end of the blankets and the lower end tucked under the

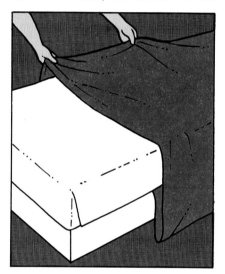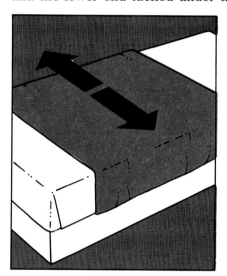

A drawsheet is placed crosswise on a bed.

bed, and over the plastic sheet, overlapping the plastic a few inches above and below. Leave the end on one side of the bed longer than the other.

Even when no plastic sheet is needed, a drawsheet is still a great convenience. You can draw it to one side or the other, giving the patient a cool, smooth spot on which to lie, or, in case of accidental soiling of the bed, you can change it with little

mattress, with square corners, and the sides left hanging. Finally, turn the upper sheet back over the bedspread and blankets about 1 foot. With well-shaken pillows in place, the bed is ready for use. You may need to loosen the covers at the foot of the bed to give room for the patient's feet when he lies face up and when he turns. A device called a cradle will help to keep the bedding off his feet.

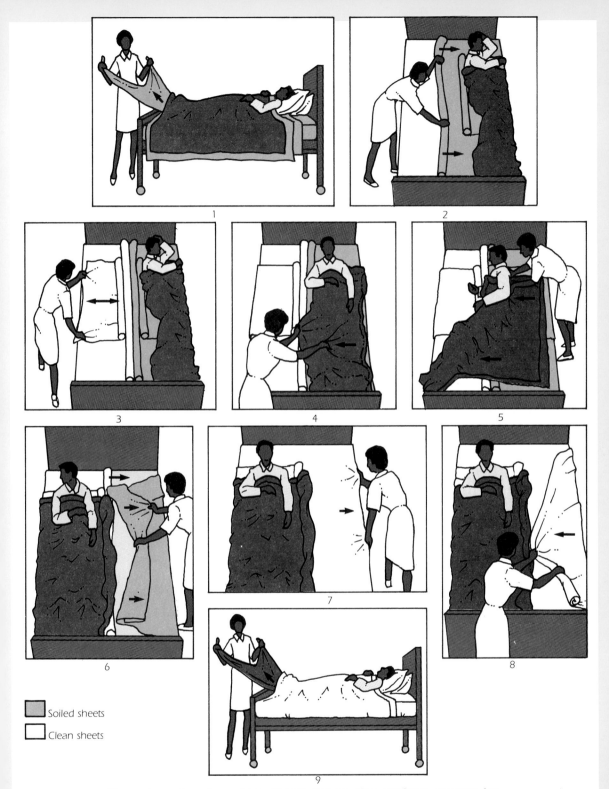

Soiled sheets

Clean sheets

Procedure for changing sheets when the patient cannot be moved from the bed. Note the progressive steps.

Changing bed linen for bedfast patients

The secret to changing the linens when the patient cannot get out of bed is to make half of the bed at a time. Loosen the drawsheet on the long side, then go to the opposite side and, reaching over the patient, grasp the drawsheet on the other side (which was longer) and pull it toward you. The patient will roll on his side to your half of the bed. Now go to the opposite side, loosen the bottom sheet, and roll it lengthwise toward the middle of the bed (toward the patient's back).

Place a clean sheet lengthwise along the bed and make that half of the bed, rolling the unused half of the clean sheet toward the middle of the bed. If you wish to use a drawsheet, place it above the clean sheet and roll them together toward the center. Now roll the patient onto the clean half of the bed. Remove the soiled linen, unroll the clean sheets, and draw them tightly across the rest of the bed, tucking them in snugly along both sides and the top and bottom.

Pillows of various sizes make comfortable positions possible by reducing muscular tension. When the patient is lying on his back with his knees bent, a pillow under the knees and another to rest his feet against are helpful. A weak or helpless patient turned on one side appreciates a pillow tucked against his back for support, and a small pillow slipped under the abdomen also helps. When the patient is lying on his side, flexing the upper knee a little more than the lower one and placing a pillow between them helps him to feel rested and relaxed.

When a patient is able to sit up in bed, a kitchen chair serves nicely as a back support. Turn it upside down with the legs against the head of the bed so that the back forms an inclining plane (see illustration on page 578). Pad it with pillows. If the patient is weak, a pillow under each arm will make sitting more comfortable. However, while pillows as knee supports and footrests are very comfortable, patients must be forced, if necessary, to change positions. Habitually held positions contribute to the shortening of muscles and tendons, which, in turn, lead to deformities. Also, constant pressure of the bed on one area of skin is the main cause of bedsores.

Caring for the patient

Patient care begins in the morning when you wash his face and hands, help him clean his teeth, and brush his hair. The patient may also use the toilet. You should smooth his bed and shake his pillows, and he will be ready for breakfast.

It is a good idea to keep a record of your patient's temperature, pulse rate, and bowel movements. The temperature and pulse of a seriously ill person should be taken and recorded before breakfast, midmorning, midafternoon, and in the evening. These procedures are quite simple. One of the most convenient ways to keep these records is with a sheet of paper on a clipboard that you hang at the foot of the patient's bed.

The temperature

The temperature is taken with a thermometer. Those most commonly used in a sick room are a calibrated glass tube with a mercury bulb at one end. As the bulb warms, the mercury expands and rises in the tube to indicate the patient's "heat" or temperature. A person with a temperature reading above normal during illness is said to have a "fever." To determine a person's temperature, place the bulb of the thermometer in the patient's mouth, in the armpit (axilla), or in the rectum (through the anal opening).

Thermometers for rectal use have a rounded bulb, while those for taking readings in the mouth or armpit have a long, slender bulb. The oral method of determining temperature is the most common. The average normal oral temperature is 98.6° Fahrenheit (37° Celsius), plus or minus a degree or two, depending on the individual and the time of day. Most thermometers indicate the normal body temperature with an arrow. Temperatures generally tend to be a little lower in the early morning and may be a little higher in the afternoon. The temperature of the same person taken under the arm is usually 1°F (0.5°C) lower than the oral temperature, while the rectal reading is one degree higher.

Electronic and temperature strip thermometers are usually used in institutions but are, of course, more expensive.

Do not take a temperature reading until at least fifteen minutes after the patient has had a drink, eaten a meal, had a bath, or smoked a cigarette. Breathing through the mouth or breathing cold air will also affect the temperature reading. Before using a mercury thermometer, be sure that it has been shaken down at least two degrees below normal (below the arrow). Place the bulb under the patient's tongue and have him hold it in place with his lips firmly closed. Take a reading after two minutes, then shake down the column, rinse the thermometer in cool water, disinfect it in alcohol, and put it away.

If your patient is unconscious, it is easier to take his temperature under the arm or in the rectum. The latter is the preferred method for infants and little children. Do not place a mercury bulb in a child's mouth. If he should crush it, he could be injured by the glass, either in his mouth or in the intestinal tract if he should swallow the glass, and the mercury is poisonous.

The pulse

You can determine a patient's heart rate by "taking his pulse." The most convenient place to do that is on the thumb side of one of his arms, just above the wrist. Place two of your fingers over this area so that you can easily feel his heartbeat. Another method is to place the palm of your hand behind the patient's wrist (on the back side), then curve your fingers around his wrist to the point just above the thumb side where you can feel his pulse. Watch the second hand of your watch and count his heartbeats for thirty seconds. Double your count, and you will have the number of beats per minute. Record this on the chart, noting any irregularities, which should be reported to the patient's physician. While the pulse rate varies with different individuals, the usual is sixty-six to eighty beats each minute. The pulse rate tends to go up about ten beats per minute each time the temperature goes up one degree.

Respiration

Sometimes it is important to know the rate of a patient's respiration. Normally an adult breathes between twelve and twenty times a minute, though with pneumonia the rate may go as high as forty or fifty breaths per minute. Respirations are best counted for a full minute.

The bowel movement

Bowel movements are important both for the patient's comfort and for his health. Because partially or completely bedridden patients get little or no exercise and because they tend to drink less water and to eat foods that are low in fiber, they tend to have constipation or little to no bowel movement.

Encourage regular bowel movements. If possible, have your patient go to the bathroom or use a commode. Encourage him to drink plenty of water. A good drinking schedule is a glass on awakening, one between breakfast and lunch, one between lunch and the evening meal, and one before bedtime unless bed-wetting is a problem.

If at all possible, your patient's diet should be high in unrefined foods: whole grain cereals, fruits (rather than fruit purees and juices), and vegetables. If this is not possible, give him a commercial fiber preparation (Metamucil) and a medication to soften his stool.

The bedpan

Today, portable toilets are available for campers and trailers, and these make excellent substitutes for a commode. When the patient is unable to get out of bed, a bedpan and, for a man, a **urinal** are necessary equipment for evacuating the bowels and bladder. A metal bedpan should be warmed before it is used. Sprinkling talcum powder on the rim will make sliding the pan under the patient's buttocks easier. If the patient is unable to lift his own hips, roll him on his side, push the bedpan against his lower hip with the open end directed toward his feet, and roll him back onto the pan. Following the bowel movement, hold the bedpan in place and roll the patient onto his side. Be sure to have toilet paper available to clean the patient.

Use the bedpan for ordinary bowel movements and also for emptying the bladder of women patients. Keep in mind, though, that lying on a bedpan is an abnormal position for emptying the bowels or the bladder, and often more straining and effort are required than in the normal sitting position. So, do not rush your patient, but give him time to relax.

Enemas

Occasionally it may be necessary to give an enema to avoid (or treat) severe constipation. Prepared chemical enemas are available at any drugstore. They are compact, convenient, and require a minimum of time and effort to use. The enema fluid is contained in a plastic bottle that has a tube on one end to insert into the patient's rectum. The contents of the bottle are emptied into the patient's lower colon by squeezing on the bottle. This stimulates the bowel to action.

If at all possible, the patient should use the bathroom or a commode as the enema is given. If this cannot be done, protect the bed with a plastic sheet beneath and above the patient—anywhere discharge is likely to spill. It is most convenient if the patient can lie on one side, with his upper leg drawn toward his abdomen. Immediately after the water has entered the patient's rectum, turn him on a bedpan and place a pillow under his back for support. If the patient cannot be turned on his side but must remain on his back, place him on the bedpan first, with his knees flexed.

A water enema requires an enema kit—a rubber or soft plastic water bag with a hose running out the bottom end and a tube at the other end of the hose for inserting into the patient's rectum. These are available at any drugstore. These bags generally hold a quart of water. The water in the bag (or commercial enema) should be about 100°F (38°C). If a saline enema is recommended, use about 2 teaspoons of salt per quart of water.

To administer a water enema, lubricate the end that will be inserted into the patient's rectum with vaseline (commercial enemas come with a prelubricated end). Hold the enema bag no more than 2 or 3 feet above the patient's hips, insert the tube into the patient's rectum, and allow the solution to flow into the patient's colon at a moderate rate. Do not rush the procedure. Because a patient's skin tends to adhere to a bedpan, you should always lift his hips with one hand before removing the bedpan. Cover the bedpan and empty it immediately.

People tolerate varying amounts of fluid. The average adult can take up to 2 quarts of water. Better results are obtained if the patient can hold the enema solution for a few minutes and expel it gradually. Give another enema if the results of the first one are not satisfactory.

Baths

The best time to give a bath is in the morning, about an hour after breakfast, just before remaking your patient's bed. Be sure the room is warm. Unless a patient is unable to leave his bed, he should be encouraged to shower or bathe every day. This gets him out of bed, gives him exercise and relief from lying, and is simple and easy. Removable tub attachments are available that make it easier for a patient to get in and out without danger of slipping or falling. If the patient needs to sit while taking a shower, place a stool in the tub. If the patient can take his bath alone, this is a good time for you to make his bed.

Your patient will feel clean after his shower. This helps to raise his spirit,

575

gives him a feeling of well-being, and speeds his recovery. Be sure to wash the face, hands, and teeth of a bed patient twice a day. Give him a plain bath of warm or cool water every other day, and a soap bath on alternate days. Giving a patient a bath in bed is not difficult if you follow these simple steps.

- You will need two large towels or light blankets. Place one towel or blanket over the upper sheet, and, holding it at the top with one hand, draw the sheet out from below with the other hand. Arrange the other blanket or towel under the patient the same way you would when changing a lower sheet. The patient is now between the two blankets or towels.

- Bring two basins of warm-to-hot water to the bedside, along with two washcloths, a face towel, one or two bath towels, soap, a nail file, scissors, rubbing alcohol, talcum powder, and the patient's clean gown and bed linen. Remove the patient's gown or sleeping attire, but keep him covered with the top blanket. Wash and dry a small area of his body at a time—his face and neck, one arm and then another, and so on. Use a face cloth with soap first, and then rinse with the other cloth. Gently but thoroughly dry the patient's skin.

- Areas that need special attention are the underarms, the navel, between the toes, between the thighs, the rectal area, and the external genital organs. Have the patient roll on his side (or use the drawsheet technique) to wash his back and rectal area. Most patients can clean their own genitals if given the washcloths. The hands and feet may be placed in a

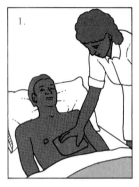
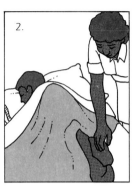
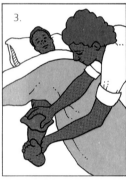
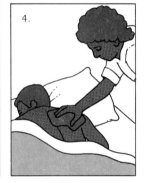
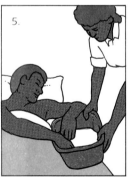
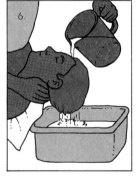

The major steps in giving a bed bath, and in washing the hair of a bedfast patient.

basin for washing, if this is desired.

- While the patient is on his back, give him an alcohol rub over the pressure points of the back (see below) and follow with a general rub with talcum powder. Inspect other pressure points and rub with alcohol, followed by talcum powder. This adds greatly to the patient's comfort. Then put on his clean gown or pajamas. Make his bed, and he will be ready for the day.

- You should wash the patient's hair from time to time. Begin by moving him down in the bed and raising his shoulders with pillows so that his head is tilted backward. Protect the pillows and bedsheet with a sheet of plastic. Place a large pan beneath the patient's head, pour water on his hair, shampoo it, and then rinse it thoroughly. Dry the hair with a towel first, and then with a blow-dryer.

Food and drink

The monotony of a patient's day can be broken by appetizing meals. Unless his physician has indicated a special diet, small servings of simple, nutritious food, arranged attractively and served at regular mealtimes, is best. Remember that sick people tend to lose their appetites, so do not overload the tray. If your patient can talk, ask him what his favorite foods are. This is especially important for children.

Before bringing your patient his tray, place him in a comfortable position so he won't get tired before the end of the meal. Cups and dishes should not be so full that the contents are likely to spill. Serve hot foods hot and cold foods cold, always checking to see that the temperature of the food will not burn a very sick patient. Liquid foods may be served through a drinking tube. Straws are available that can be bent to make it easier for the patient to drink while he is reclining. Patients with fevers especially enjoy fruit juices, broths, and soups.

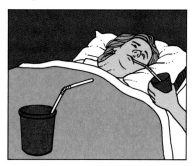

A bent straw is a good way to give a drink to a patient.

You may have to spoon-feed a very sick patient or an elderly person, and this, of course, takes time. You can keep food hot with a child's dish that has a hollow bottom, filling the bottom with hot water. Allow plenty of time between mouthfuls. Give the patient liquids through a bent straw. If he is suffering from a prolonged illness, ask his physician for advice about the best diet.

Preventing bedsores

Patients who seldom or never change position in bed because of weakness or a lack of feeling in the skin tend to develop bedsores at the points where the body exerts the greatest pressure against the bed:

577

the back, hips, buttocks, shoulder blades, elbows, and heels. Fortunately, these sores are easily preventable by moving the patient frequently. Do not allow the patient to remain in any one position longer than two hours. Alternate positions to which you can turn the patient include lying on the back, face down, on either side, and a variety of positions in between. Because friction can damage the skin, you should avoid dragging your patient over the sheet.

Be sure that the patient's sheets are always clean, dry, crumb free, and pulled tight to prevent wrinkling. Air pillows and sheepskin pads help to prevent bedsores in patients who require prolonged bed rest. Because a nutritious diet promotes general resistance, it also aids in preventing bedsores.

Preventing stiff joints

Unless a long-term bed patient is paralyzed, you should encourage him to exercise every hour to prevent his joints from getting stiff, especially the limbs. Have the patient wiggle his toes, extend his feet and rotate his ankles, and bend and extend his legs at the knee and his thighs at the hip. He should also open and close each hand, bend his elbows, and rotate his arms and forearms. Even if a particular part of the body cannot be moved (such as the part of the body that is in a cast), contracting and relaxing the muscles will strengthen the muscles and the bones to which they attach. Wherever possible, every joint of the body should be moved through its range of motion each day. If the patient is unable to do this for himself, you should do it for him.

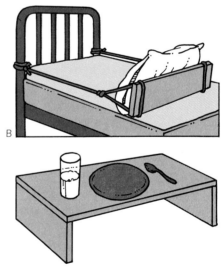

Provide the following comforts for a bedfast patient: (a) an inverted chair for a backrest; (b) a simple home-made footrest; (c) a device to remove pressure from the feet; and (d) a removable table.

This will prevent stiffening or contracture.

Medications

All medicines must be given on the order of the patient's physician and according to the directions on the labels of the containers. Follow all directions carefully, such as, "Do not take on an empty stomach." Liquid medicines must be accurately measured. Use a medicine glass with a graduated scale or a specially designed measuring spoon. Check and recheck the amount of medicine to be given or the number of tablets or capsules to be taken.

When pouring medicine from a bottle, hold the bottle with the label side up. This will protect the label from being soiled and possibly obliterated. After counting tablets or capsules, give them to the patient in a spoon or small dish, along with water to help him swallow them. An unconscious patient should not be given tablets or capsules, as they may cause choking or suffocation. Liquid medications should be dropped far back on the tongue of an unconscious patient to compel swallowing.

Acid medicines and those containing iron should be given through a drinking tube to prevent injury to the teeth. In giving oils, such as castor oil, first rinse the glass in very cold water, leaving a little water in the bottom. Then add the dose of oil and a little more water. The cold water prevents the oil from sticking to the teeth and tongue and enables the patient to take it in one swallow. Sucking a lemon or an orange im-mediately afterward takes away the taste of oil. Glasses, spoons, and tubes should always be thoroughly cleaned after use.

Medications can have undesirable side effects. Ask your patient's physician what toxic responses you might expect. If the patient develops symptoms unrelated to his illness or to those the drug may produce, report it to the physician immediately. Some patients are allergic to certain medications (such as penicillin), responding with itching, hives, rash, difficulty in breathing, and wheezing. If any of these develop, call the physician immediately. See under "allergic reactions," pages 676, 677.

You must be very careful any time you give medicines, because a mistake can have serious results. Nurses who work with patients in hospitals always check what they call the "five rights" before giving any patient a medication. You can check yourself on these five points and avoid medication errors. The "five rights" are:

1. Be sure you are giving the *right* medication.
2. Be sure you are giving the medication to the *right* patient. (Most people have only one patient to care for at home, but if you have more than one, then you need to be sure you give the right medication to the right patient.)
3. Be sure you are giving the medication at the *right* time.
4. Be sure you are giving the *right* dose (amount).
5. Be sure you are giving the

medication by the *right* method—oral, injection, rectal, etc.

Several additional precautions will protect the patient and others from the harm that medicines can do if they are not administered properly:

- Never give medicine from an unlabeled box or bottle.
- Never give medicine selected in poor light or in the dark.
- Never leave medicine within the reach of children, uncooperative patients, or the elderly.
- Never leave disinfectants standing in drinking glasses or near medicines.
- If for any reason a dose of medicine has been omitted, do not increase the next dose. Inform the patient's doctor and ask him what to do.

Home care for contagious diseases

Infectious diseases that can be transmitted from person to person are called **contagious** or **communicable** diseases. Some contagious diseases are often spoken of as "childhood diseases" because children are affected more frequently than adults. Among these are mumps, measles, chickenpox, and whooping cough.

Contagious diseases are caused by the entry of germs and viruses into the body. These microorganisms can be transmitted from person to person in a variety of ways: on tiny droplets of moisture expelled from the nose or mouth during a sneeze or cough, in contaminated food, by body discharges (sputum, urine, feces) and wound discharges, and by insect carriers (such as contaminated flies that land on food). Everyone should cover his nose and mouth with a handkerchief or paper tissue any time he sneezes or coughs. In most Western countries, paper tissues are so easy to obtain that boxes of them should be kept readily available in the home and office. This is doubly important for the one who is sick with a contagious disease, and the patient should be so instructed. You should try to remain out of the path of the current of air coming from your patient's nose and mouth. If the patient does not or cannot cooperate by covering his nose and mouth when sneezing and coughing (and this is especially difficult for little children), you should wear a surgical mask while caring for him.

Because infectious agents may be carried in the patient's sputum, in discharges from his nose and open wounds, and in his urine and feces, these body discharges must be discarded appropriately and the hands washed thoroughly to prevent contamination of objects and persons in the home.

Hand washing

As the patient's care giver, your hands are the first to become contaminated. Your hands will then carry the infectious agents (germs or viruses) to objects about the room, to other parts of the house, and to other people in the home. Anyone caring for a sick person should develop the habit of never touching his own mouth, face, and hair.

After each contact with a person who has an infectious disease, you should wash your hands carefully under warm running water, using plenty of soap. Take time to work the suds in between your fingers and high onto your wrists. Clean your fingernails with a nail brush or with a blunt instrument. Paper towels are preferable for drying because they are disposable. If frequent washing tends to irritate the skin of your hands, apply a mild hand lotion after each washing.

Wearing a gown

By wearing a gown when you care for a person with a contagious disease, you will not only keep your clothes clean, but you will also prevent infection from being carried to other parts of the house and to other people. It is not necessary, of course, to put on a gown simply to hand the patient a book or a drink of water, but it is advisable to do so when caring for your patient in ways that require you to come in physical contact with him or his bedclothing.

Many styles of gowns are available. You should choose one that has long sleeves and fully covers your body. Leave it hanging near the door to the patient's room as you leave, and it will be readily available when you return. Wash your hands each time you remove the gown. If you wear a short-sleeved gown, you should wash your forearms up to your elbows.

The patient's dishes

You should discard all food that remains on the dishes of a patient with a contagious disease. If your kitchen sink is equipped with a disposer, rinse the food down the drain and wash the sink with soap and a little liquid bleach. You can also flush the leftover food down the toilet. If you must place the discarded food in a garbage can, put it in a plastic sack first and close the sack tightly. This will keep flies and other insects from becoming carriers of the infection.

Disposable plastic or paper dishes and plastic spoons, forks, and knives will save you time. These also should be disposed of in a plastic sack. If you feed your patient with regular dishes, you must wash all his dishes separately from the dishes used by the rest of the family. Be sure to use lots of hot water and detergent when you wash the patient's dishes. A little bleach in the water will help to kill the patient's germs.

Waste disposal

The safest way to dispose of discharges from the patient's nose, mouth, or infected wounds is to collect them with paper tissue over your hands so you don't come in contact with them, and place them in a tightly closed plastic sack that you burn, either in a stove or outside. If local laws prohibit outdoor burning, call your fire department and ask how to dispose of the soiled materials of a contagious person.

581

You should never dispose of a contagious person's urine and feces in a stream or lake. However, you can safely flush them down the toilet, provided your home has a properly functioning septic tank or is connected to a city sewer system in which the sewage is scientifically treated. If your circumstances do not permit these safe disposal methods, you must treat the patient's urine and feces with a disinfectant before emptying them. Disinfectants such as phenol or cresol, which are used in portable toilets, are available at drugstores and many supermarkets. Be sure you use these preparations according to the instructions.

The patient's laundry

You should wash your patient's clothing, bed linen, and towels as soon as possible after removing them from the sickroom. You can wash them in your home washing machine, but separately from other laundry. Use hot water and lots of soap or detergent. Any laundry that has been heavily contaminated by the patient's discharges should be boiled for five minutes before laundering. If you are accustomed to sending the wash from your home to a commercial laundry, items from the patient's room should be packaged separately with an affixed label informing the laundry that it contains contaminated articles.

Cleaning the sickroom

Depending on the illness, germs may still linger in the sickroom after the patient has recovered. Clothing and linens should be laundered, and other washable items should be thoroughly cleansed with water and detergent. Rent a carpet cleaner to clean the carpets and larger rugs. Nonwashable bedspreads, drapes, and similar articles may be dry-cleaned or aired in the sunlight for six or more hours. The household thermometer should be washed in soap and cold water, soaked in alcohol (70 percent), and then stored for future use.

Importance of good nursing

The healing processes of a body that has been afflicted by disease or injury are greatly influenced by the patient's mental attitude. His comfort and optimistic attitude depend on your patient, loving care. Often such care is even more effective in promoting his recovery than the treatment prescribed by the physician. Good nursing care should also be provided to the patient with a terminal illness.

All of us will die sooner or later. The only difference is when. Think of the Golden Rule: How would I want to be treated in the same situation?

Learn to anticipate your patient's needs. Look for little things you can do without being asked that will help him feel comfortable, and protect him from being wearied by visitors or annoyed by gossip. Try to remember simple things like rubbing your patient's back, hips, and heels with alcohol and dusting them with talcum powder to prevent bedsores.

Keep the home free of excitement in the evening, and make early preparations for the night's rest. Wash your patient's face and hands, clean his mouth, and change his gown if that is needed. A hot footbath may quiet your patient. Help him to use the toilet or bedpan before going to bed. Turn him on his side, and brush crumbs and any other irritating material from his bed. Loosen his lower sheet one side at a time and pull it tight to remove all wrinkles, and retuck it under the mattress.

Rub the patient's back and hips, using firm, circular strokes to the general area and finishing with long, soothing strokes down the spine. Shake his pillows and readjust them. Loosen the covers at the foot of his bed. Straighten the upper sheet and the blankets. Adjust his pajamas. End by asking if there is anything more he wants. Then, turning out or adjusting the light, say "good night," and leave the room so your patient can go to sleep. This will keep him from lying awake, expecting you to return, or thinking that something more is to be done.

The following advice on the care of patients in the home, published years ago, has an up-to-date ring and provides an excellent summary:

"Those who minister to the sick should understand the importance of careful attention to the laws of health. Nowhere is obedience to these laws more important than in the sickroom. Nowhere does so much depend upon faithfulness in little things on the part of the attendants. In cases of serious illness, a little neglect, a slight inattention to a patient's special needs or dangers, the manifestation of fear, excitement, or petulance, even a lack of sympathy, may turn the scale that is balancing life and death, and cause to go down to the grave a patient who otherwise might have recovered.

"The efficiency of the nurse depends, to a great degree, upon physical vigor. The better the health, the better will she be able to endure the strain of attendance upon the sick, and the more successfully can she

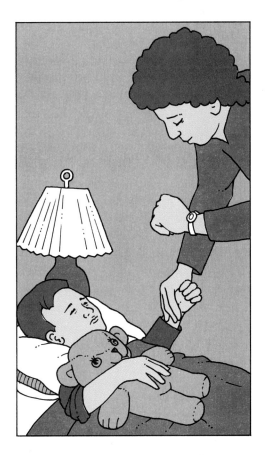

Little things that provide comfort encourage recovery.

583

perform her duties. Those who care for the sick should give special attention to diet, cleanliness, fresh air, and exercise. . . .

"Where the illness is serious, requiring the attendance of a nurse night and day, the work should be shared by at least two efficient nurses, so that each may have opportunity for rest and for exercise in the open air. . . .

"Nurses, and all who have to do with the sickroom, should be cheerful, calm, and self-possessed. All hurry, excitement, or confusion, should be avoided. Doors should be opened and shut with care, and the whole household be kept quiet. In cases of fever, special care is needed when the crisis comes and the fever is passing away. Then constant watching is often necessary. Ignorance, forgetfulness, and recklessness have caused the death of many who might have lived had they re-ceived proper care from judicious, thoughtful nurses."[1]

Anticipating the possibility that you might need to care for a sick person in your home someday, and especially in preparing for a specific situation, it would be a good idea to take advantage of the courses in home nursing that are offered by the American Red Cross and other community or church agencies. Every homemaker is likely to become a home nurse sometime during his or her life.

Help with specific problems and situations is available from community agencies such as public health departments, visiting nurses' associations, and the home-care services offered by many medical centers today.

---

1. Ellen G. White, *The Ministry of Healing* (Boise, Idaho: Pacific Press) pp. 219-222.

CHAPTER 18

Simple home treatments

The human body—your body—is undoubtedly the most remarkable and intricate living "machine" in this world. If you have not already read the descriptions of the many systems that make up your body, it would be time well spent for you to do so (see vol. 3). It will also be profitable for you to read those parts of these medical books that outline the simple measures you must take to preserve the efficient functioning of your body's systems. Living healthfully will enable you to keep your performance at top level for the longest period, and at the same time postpone the onset of disease and the frailties of old age.

But each person has a different background and has inherited a different constitution. We have also lived different lifestyles—either a lifestyle that has minimized the wear and tear of everyday living, or one that has neglected the principles of good maintenance. We have each been given a body that must last us a lifetime, and, sad to say, there are no trade-ins. There is just one per customer.

But the time comes, sooner or later, and sometimes sooner than later, when things go wrong. Structures wear out, inherited defects make their appearance, faulty health habits take their toll, our resistance drops, and we become sick. What should we do then? Call a physician? Rush to a hospital? The answer is Yes and No.

It would be ridiculous, if not impossible, for you to call a physician about every slight ache or pain. Reasonable people use simple remedies for the relief and cure of minor injuries and illnesses. Actually, such a practice is encouraged by the medical profession. The average person is no more skilled in determining what is wrong with himself than he is in knowing what is wrong with his computer. However, just as there are a number of simple things you can do to solve computer problems, so there are several simple things you might do to solve illness problems.

The difficult decision is in knowing when to treat yourself and when to call a skilled professional. Here are a few suggestions that may prove helpful.

When to get medical help

You should always seek medical help, and not just use home treatments, under any of the following conditions:

- When a symptom is severe.
- When it persists.
- When it returns frequently.
- When you have any question as to its significance.
- When you are doubtful about what you are doing.

Unfortunately, the bathroom cabinets in many homes are stocked with medicines for headache, acid stomach, sleeplessness, and on and on, which family members use rather indiscriminately. Self-medication is encouraged by advertisements on television and radio, in the press, and in the drugstore. People are all too ready to take chemicals that provide temporary relief of the uncomfortable symptoms, while doing permanent damage to their bodies.

On the other hand, simple procedures and remedies that leave no harmful residual effects are available to everyone. These remedies make use of simple agencies such as water, light, controlled exercise, and rest. Their results depend on the body's natural response to its surroundings and to its own activity. While it is true that the use of these procedures should be restricted to minor ills, they often bring benefit with a relatively small expenditure of time and money, and without the harmful side effects of drugs and medications. Keep in mind that **any major treatment suggested in this book should be carried out with the approval of your physician.**

Readers who wish to become skilled in the use of the simple home procedures outlined in this chapter should take a course in these methods, or at least purchase a book about them. We especially recommend *Simple Remedies for the Home* by Clarence Dail and Charles Thomas, Preventive Health Care and Education Center, 4027 W. George Street, Banning, California 92220. The authors of this medical set drew heavily on the work of these men in writing this chapter.

Applying heat and cold (thermotherapy)

Skin and mucous membranes cover the structures (tissues and organs) that make up our bodies. However, these are much more than mere coverings. The skin and mucous membranes are equipped with detectors for heat, cold, touch, pressure, and pain. The skin also plays a major role in regulating the temperature of the body.

With few exceptions, the application of heat and cold as a medical treatment is made on the skin. As heat and cold pass through the skin (or mucous membrane), the temperatures of the underlying structures are altered, and ultimately the temperature of the body as a whole is affected.

The body is designed to maintain the equilibrium of its various systems. That is, it resists changes in temperature or any of its other myriad functions. This resistance to change is called *homeostasis*. However, you can stimulate chemical and physiological changes by applying heat and cold, and often as heat and cold penetrate the tissues, they have a healing effect. In addition, through nerve connections, reactions to heat and cold in the skin may reflexively affect organs deep within the body, initiating responses that are favorable to recovery.

Sources of heat and cold

Heat and cold can be applied to the body in a number of ways. The most common sources are water (hot or cold), infrared lamp or heater, sunshine, and things as simple as a heating pad or hot-water bottle. Heat and cold enter or leave the body by radiation, conduction, convection, evaporation, and friction. The application of heat and cold can be wet, such as a hot foot bath, hot shower, steam inhalation, alcohol rub, or cold shower; or the application may be dry, as with a heat lamp, electric-light cabinet, sunshine, or an ice pack.

Effects of heat and cold

The application of heat and cold affects the circulation of the blood. It also causes certain chemical responses to occur within the blood and produces a number of chemical responses within the affected tissues.

Heat dilates blood vessels and increases the circulation of blood, both in the local area where the heat is applied and, in general, throughout the body. It also increases the congestion (accumulation) of blood near the skin and decreases its congestion deeper within the body. It accelerates the clotting of blood and increases white blood cell activity (phagocytosis). Heat warms local tissues and the whole body and increases swelling in the area where it is applied by drawing blood and tissue fluids into the area. Finally, heat increases glandular activity and muscular relaxation, and stimulates the body's chemical and physiological activity.

For the most part, the effects of **cold** are the opposite of those caused by heat. The blood vessels constrict, local and general circulation slows down, and congestion (accumulation) of blood deeper within the body is increased. Blood clotting is prolonged, and white cell activity decreases. The body as a whole is cooled, swelling in local tissues is diminished, muscles contract, and chemical and physiological activities are slowed down.

Alternating heat and cold generally increases local circulation, increases white blood cell activity, probably accelerates the clotting of blood, constricts blood vessels, and increases muscular activity.

With this understanding of the effects of heat and cold, we can make

587

applications in specific ways to help the body's recovery processes. For example, immediately after a person has sprained his ankle, the application of cold will cause the flow of blood and other tissue fluids through the area to diminish, thus helping to keep the swelling down.

Breathing warm, moist air from a steam inhalator helps to relieve throat irritation and loosens secretions in the trachea and bronchi. It soothes the inflamed membranes, and, interestingly, at first facilitates coughing, but later relieves it.

Most of these effects are due to the direct action of either heating or cooling the tissues. However, as already mentioned, the body resists changes that tend to upset its normal equilibrium (homeostasis). It tries to prevent change by doing things that react against it. For example, sweating is one of the body's common reactions to heat, which is the body's effort to stay cool. On the other hand, shivering is a typical reaction to cold—the body's effort to stay warm. The body's reaction to heat may produce a sedative effect in the patient, as with a warm bath; its reaction to cold may be tonic, as with a short, cold shower. The desired effect is obtained by applying heat and cold in the right way. It is therefore important that hot and cold treatments be given properly and with skill.

Important considerations

Heat and *cold* are comparative terms and must be defined. This, unfortunately, cannot be done with accuracy, since people differ in their tolerance to heat and cold. The temperature sensation produced by water varies according to the condition of the skin, its previous temperature, the vigor of blood circulation, and even the season of the year. Testing the temperature of water to be used in treatment, therefore, should be done *with a thermometer* as well as with the hand.

When applying heat and cold, great care must be exercised to avoid damage to the skin and underlying tissues. Patients must not be chilled or overheated, nor, of course, should they be burned.

Careful, thoughtful consideration must be given as to what the particular procedure will do to the patient. Take, for example, the case of a diabetic with atherosclerosis to whom you are considering giving a hot foot bath. Locally applied heat increases the tissue's need for oxygen, and therefore for more blood. The fact that he has atherosclerosis may mean that the circulation in his feet is impaired, limiting the amount of blood that can be drawn to his feet should heat be applied. Giving a hot foot bath to such an individual would increase the demand for oxygen and for increased blood flow. Since it may not be possible to provide sufficient blood, tissue damage is likely to occur, and even gangrene may be precipitated.

The treatments described on the following pages use water and other simple means. Note the different uses and precautions (contraindications—when not to use a procedure), and follow the directions carefully.

Hydrotherapy procedures

Hot foot bath

The hot foot bath is one of the most useful of all water treatments. It is simple to do and produces several beneficial effects. The blood flow is increased locally, and if the foot bath is prolonged, there is general warming and increased blood flow in distant parts of the body. Congestion in the pelvic organs, chest, and head is decreased.

Uses. A number of conditions are benefited. These include a head cold, sore throat, cough, and bronchitis. Cramps in the pelvic organs may be relieved, as well as headache. There is generalized muscular relaxation. It is quite effective for nosebleed.

Contraindications. Do not apply heat to the feet or legs in any condition in which the circulation is poor, such as diabetes, atherosclerosis of the lower limbs, and diseases of the peripheral blood vessels. Nor should heat be applied to the feet or legs when there is acute swelling from a sprain or arthritis, loss of feeling in the legs and feet, or when the patient is unconscious.

Procedure. Use a container (plastic or metal) sufficiently large to accommodate the feet, that will allow water to cover the ankles. The water temperature should range between 104 and 112°F (40 to 44°C). Begin the treatment at a lower temperature, and periodically add hot water, thus gradually increasing the bath temperature according to the tolerance of the patient. The treatment should last ten to fifteen minutes. Encourage the drinking of cool or warm water. Be sure to place your hand between the hot water and the patient's feet any time you pour more hot water into the container.

The treatment can be given while the patient is lying in bed (bedclothes should be protected with a plastic) or while he is sitting in a chair. Small children can place their feet in a kitchen sink. Keep the upper body warm with a light blanket or large bath towel. Apply a cold compress to the patient's head, and replace it every two or three minutes. When the treatment is over, lift the feet out of the water, pour cold water over them, and dry them thoroughly. Should the patient be sweating generally, dry him with a towel, followed by an alcohol rub. Let the patient rest, lightly covered, for about twenty minutes before getting up.

Hot-and-cold immersion baths (for arm/hand and leg/foot)

In this treatment, a part of the patient's body is alternately immersed in hot and then cold water. This increases the circulation in the area, first causing dilation of the blood vessels, then contraction. Swelling is reduced, and phagocytic activity (destruction of foreign microorganisms by white blood cells) is increased.

Uses. Similar to those of a hot foot

589

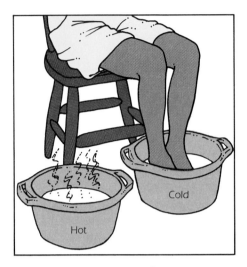

Hot and cold leg and foot bath.

bath, but also very effective in reducing the swelling from a sprained ankle or wrist, twenty-four hours after the accident occurred. (Initially a cold compress or cold foot bath is indicated.) It is also useful for an infection in the extremities.

Contraindications. Similar contraindications as for a hot foot bath, but not as stringent.

Procedure. Obtain plastic or metal containers sufficiently large and deep to immerse a foot and leg or a hand and arm. Fill one with hot water (see hot foot bath), and the other with cold or ice water. Place the patient's foot and leg into the hot water (as hot as can be tolerated without burning) for three minutes, then plunge it into the cold water for thirty seconds.

While the limb is in the cold water, pour additional hot water into the hot tub to maintain or raise the temperature, taking care not to make it so hot that it will burn the patient. This should be done four or five times for a complete treatment. A towel should be handy to dry the extremity, which should not be allowed to chill. Often the heat causes the entire body to be warmed, making the patient perspire. If this begins to happen, apply a cold compress to the forehead during the treatment. When the procedure is complete, the patient may take a warm shower and dry off, or, if he is in bed, he can be dried off and have a brisk alcohol rub.

Fomentations

A fomentation is the application of moist heat to some area of the skin by means of a heated, moistened cloth pad. This localized, sudden application of heat increases surface blood flow, relieves internal congestion, increases the circulation of white blood cells, relieves muscle spasm and certain types of pain, promotes sweating, and causes generalized relaxation.

Uses. Fomentations are often helpful for the common cold, coughs, bronchitis, and influenza. They also provide relief from the pain of neuralgia and certain forms of arthritis. Applied to the spine (warm, not hot), fomentations produce sedation and help to combat insomnia.

Contraindications. Do not apply fomentations to the limbs of those with peripheral vascular disorders or to diabetics. Neither should fomentations be used on an unconscious or paralyzed person. If given to a patient who has recently had a heart attack, check with his physician first, and if administered, place an ice bag over the heart.

Procedure. The fomentation pad

is best made of blanket material that consists of 50 percent wool to retain heat and 50 percent cotton to hold water. A thick Turkish towel or thick terry cloth may also be used. Six pads are made from cut material, 30 x 36 inches (75 x 90 cm), folded in thirds, and then sewn so that the finished pad is 12 x 30 inches (30 x 75 cm). Have available some eight to ten light, medium-sized towels, two large bath towels, four washcloths,

ened pads in a microwave oven until they are heated. This is the most convenient method.

When the heated pad is wrung dry or removed from the steamer or microwave oven, wrap it in a light towel, fold it double, and roll it up to retain the heat. You may make three of these heated rolled-up pads in quick succession.

Before beginning the treatment, see that the room is comfortably

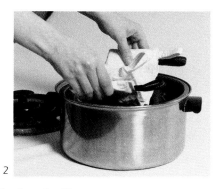

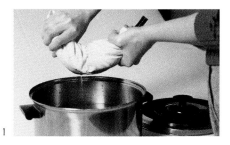

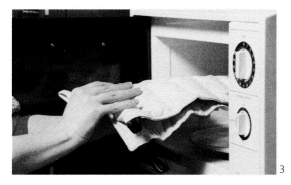

Three ways of preparing fomentation cloths: (1) wringing cloths out of hot water; (2) steaming moistened cloths in a kettle; and (3) heating damp cloths in a microwave oven.

and a bowl of ice water.

The pads may be heated in one of three ways: (1) Fold a pad in thirds and twist it into a loose roll. Holding the two ends, immerse the middle portion in a large kettle of boiling water. Then pull the ends, twisting at the same time to wring the pad as dry as possible. (2) Moisten the pads and place them in a steam boiler (not in water) until they are thoroughly heated. (3) Place moist-

warm. It is extremely important that the patient not be chilled at any time. Have the patient disrobe and lie down. Place a large bath towel underneath and another over the patient, then cover him with a blanket. Place a light towel over the area to which the hot fomentation pad is to be applied—the chest, for example. Place a heated fomentation cloth on the towel covering the chest. A few moments later lift one side of the pad and then the other, and wipe the chest with a dry face cloth to prevent burning. If the pad is too hot, place an additional light towel between the pad and the patient. Place extra coverings (face cloths), if needed, over bony prominences or the nipples, lest they burn.

As soon as the patient is reasonably comfortable, place the second fomentation underneath him, lengthwise along the spine. Then wrap one around the feet, unless contraindicated, and wrap it in a towel. This may be done in place of a hot foot bath.

Prepare additional hot fomentations to replace the one on the chest every three to five minutes—three in all. Fomentations should be tolerable but not necessarily comfortable. Before replacing a fomentation pad, dry the heated skin quickly. (Removing the moisture remaining on the skin makes it easier to endure the heat of the newly prepared fomentation.) A fresh, dry, light towel should replace the one on the skin each time a fomentation pad is changed. Fomentations on the spine and feet are not changed.

Keep a cold, folded, wet face cloth on the forehead during the procedure, recooling it frequently. Allow the patient to drink as much cool water as he desires through a bent straw. After the fomentation is removed the last time, wipe the skin briskly with a cold, wet face cloth. Dry the patient immediately, and cover him with a blanket to prevent chilling. Following the complete treatment, allow the patient to lie quietly for at least thirty minutes.

Hot and cold to the chest

This application is similar to the fomentation, with one important modification.

Uses. Aids in the treatment of chest colds, coughs, and bronchitis. Stimulates deep breathing.

Contraindications. These include: recent surgery, malignancy, pleurisy, impaired sensation, and impaired circulation. Also excluded are children under twelve, and patients who are paralyzed or unconscious.

Procedure. Start a fomentation to the chest as described above. When the fomentation is removed, dry the chest immediately. Have the patient take a deep breath, and rub his chest briskly with ice, covering the area twice. This should be done at the end of each chest fomentation. Otherwise follow the routine for fomentations.

Cold mitten friction

With this procedure, cold is rapidly applied section by section to the skin, using cold wet face cloths or cold wet mitts.

Uses. Cold mitten friction builds resistance to cold as well as general body resistance. Phagocytic action is increased, as is antibody production. This treatment stimulates the circulation and is useful in terminating a fomentation. It can also be used to end the morning shower.

Contraindications. Do not use this procedure when the patient is chilled, nor should friction be applied to skin lesions or eruptions.

Procedure. A face cloth that has been folded in half and sewed on two sides makes an excellent bag or mitt into which the hand can be placed.

The patient should be warm, undressed, and lying between two light blankets or large bath towels. Dip the mitt in cold water, wring out any excess water, and put it on your hands. Start with the extremities, then the chest, and finally the back. Vigorously rub the skin of one arm for five to eight seconds. Dry the arm immediately, and cover it to keep it warm. Follow with the other arm, then the lower extremities, and finally the chest and back. Apply a cold compress to the forehead during the procedure.

Hot mitten friction

The method of application is similar to that of cold mitten friction, except that hot water is used instead of cold. This procedure is excellent for warming a chilled patient and for producing relaxation and inducing sleep. Do not apply this treatment on skin lesions or to an overheated patient.

Cold compress

A cold compress is a cold or ice cold wet cloth applied to some part of the body. It deceases the local flow of blood, prevents congestion in a limited area, and relieves pain due to swelling or injury. When applied over the heart, it slows the rate of the heartbeat.

Uses. A cold compress lessens the pain and swelling of a sprain of the wrist or ankle when applied immediately after the injury has occurred. It relieves sinus congestion and headaches, slows the heart rate in tachycardia, and provides relief when applied to the forehead during fever, or when general body warming pro-

cedures are being employed.

Contraindications. Cold compresses should not be used on patients with diabetes, skin diseases, or those who have an intolerance to cold or who are chilled.

Procedure. Use an ordinary small hand towel or face cloth, fold it to the desired size, and wet it in cold or ice water. Wring out the water just enough so that it does not drip. Renew every two to five minutes. Apply the compress firmly to the patient's forehead, ankle, heart, or wherever desired. Be sure the patient is warm before starting the treatment.

Heating compress

A **wet heating compress** is a cold, wet, lightweight cloth or several layers of wet gauze applied to a localized area of the body, covered with a wool (or similar material) bandage, and held in place for several hours, allowing the body to first warm and later dry the compress. It initially produces constriction of the blood vessels, followed by dilation. Depending on the location and size of the compress, it may produce general warming and sweating.

Uses. The wet heating compress helps to relieve the pain of acute sore throat (pharyngitis, laryngitis, tonsillitis), joint pain from arthritis and rheumatic fever, chest cold, cough, chronic bronchitis, and asthma. For pleurisy, use a "dry" heating compress.

Contraindications. Do not use this procedure if the patient is unable to warm up the compress (may use a heat lamp or hot-water bottle to facil-

593

itate warming). Do not allow chilling. If chilling seems likely, discontinue the procedure and use a "dry" heating compress instead.

Procedure. Heating compresses can be applied to the neck, ankle, wrists, and other desired parts. Dip a piece of cotton cloth in cold water and wring it dry. Quickly place the cloth around the desired area, wrap it with a wool (or similar) bandage, fastening it with safety pins. Allow it to remain in place for several hours or overnight. On removal, wipe the area with a cool, damp cloth, then dry thoroughly.

The strip of wool cloth should be 3 to 4 inches wide (7.5 to 12 cm) and about 6 inches (15 cm) longer than the cotton cloth strip. The width and length of the bandages are determined by their use. For a neck compress, the cloth strip should be about 3 x 30 inches (7.5 x 75 cm), while the wool strip should be about 4 x 36 inches (12 x 90 cm). For the chest, the strips should be proportionately wider and longer. Always see that the cold wet strip is well covered by the dry wool cloth.

The method for using a **dry heating compress** is identical to that of the wet heating compress, except that the thin cotton cloth is **not wet,** but is applied **dry.** For example, if a dry heating compress is to be applied to the chest, a thin cotton undershirt can be worn and covered with a long-sleeved wool sweater.

Steam inhalation

This application provides warm, moist air to the respiratory passageways that relieves inflammation and congestion, loosens secretions, prompts discharge from the throat and lungs, and prevents drying of the respiratory membranes.

Uses. Steam inhalation relieves coughing and congestion of the nose, throat, and bronchi. It loosens dry and thick secretions in the airways, and soothes a dry, irritated throat.

Contraindications. Infants, very young children, and the very aged may not be able to handle the heat.

Procedure. There are a number of ways in which moist, warm air can be provided to a patient. Commercial steam inhalators are available at moderate expense and are very convenient. Directions require filling a small container with water and plugging in the device. In a few minutes steam is projected through a small aperture. Most brands will function continuously for eight or more hours. The inhalator can be placed on the floor or on a stool near the head of the bed. Children should not be able to reach the inhalator, as steam may burn their hands. The patient does not need to be placed in a tent.

If you do not have access to a commercial inhalator, you can boil water on the kitchen stove and inhale the steam (beware of burns from getting too close to the boiling water), or boil water in a tea kettle on an electric portable burner in the bedroom. If concentrated steam is desired, the steam from the inhalator or kettle can be directed toward the patient with a newspaper that has been rolled into a cone shape. Another way to concentrate the warm vapor is to erect a "tent" over the bed with a

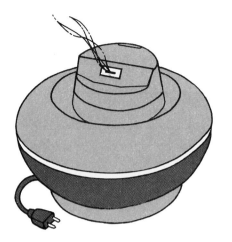

Warm, moist air from a commercial vaporizer soothes the respiratory passageways.

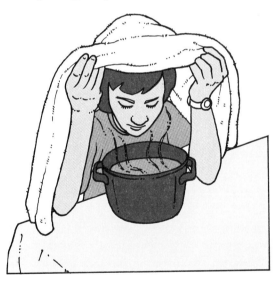

Warm, moist air rising from a pan of hot water may be inhaled, reducing congestion.

sheet and allow the steam to flow into the tent.

You can medicate the water with a few drops of pine oil or eucalyptus oil. However, remember that some people are allergic to these oils, especially to pine oil.

Showers

A shower is a device by which multiple small streams of water are directed under pressure onto some surface of the body. It is one of the cheapest and best forms of home therapy. Depending on the temperature of the water, a shower can be relaxing or stimulating, warming or cooling. It can improve the general circulation. It can be used for ambulatory patients, and even for those who can sit while the shower is running.

Uses. A shower will relieve the pain from bruises and muscle spasms. It can warm a chilled person or preheat for a cold application, such as a cold shower. It is refreshing and cleansing. The common cold and bronchitis are helped.

Contraindications. Persons with heart disease, advanced atherosclerosis, certain kidney diseases, high blood pressure, and hyperthyroidism should avoid showers. A cold shower is especially not suitable for a rheumatic patient.

Procedure. A shower can be taken in a number of ways. If a person is chilled, a warm to hot shower will produce general warming. Hot and cold showers are stimulating. Bring the water to body temperature for a minute or so before ending the shower. Gradually increase the temperature to tolerance, and then abruptly turn the hot water off, allowing the cold water to strike the skin for about ten seconds. Over time, healthy people can learn to tolerate cold for longer and longer periods. Some like to take a hot shower and

595

end by giving a cold mitten friction. Plain cold showers can be used for their stimulating action.

Precautions. Have a stool available in case the patient should feel faint. Care should be taken that the patient does not slip or fall. Do not allow the patient to become chilled after a shower.

Tub bath

Immersing the entire body in water is a simple but effective means of altering the function of major body systems. A **hot tub bath** increases the general circulation, raises body temperature, and is relaxing. A **graduated tub bath** is effective in lowering body temperature. A **neutral bath** is calming.

Uses. A hot bath improves the general circulation, relieving the congestion of the internal organs. Also, it alleviates stiffness and pain in the muscles and lessens fatigue. A graduated bath is effective in lowering elevated body temperature, as in a fever. A neutral bath aids in calming an agitated patient and relieves nervous tension.

Contraindications. People with heart and valvular diseases, vascular disorders, high blood pressure, diabetes, and cancers should avoid hot tub baths. Also, elderly and frail persons do not tolerate a hot bath.

Procedure. For a **hot tub bath,** obtain the consent of the patient's physician. The tub should be two-thirds full of water at about 101 to 103°F (38 to 39.5°C). Assist the patient into the tub. Have him lie down so that water covers his chest. Place a cold compress on his fore-head and cover his knees (if they are exposed above the water) with a towel. Encourage him to drink a glass of water. The initial bath should be no longer than ten minutes, with a rise in body temperature of no more than one degree. If well tolerated, subsequent baths can be longer (not to exceed twenty minutes), with water temperature somewhat higher (not to exceed 106°F. [41°C]). Patients should be watched closely, as they sometimes feel faint. Following the bath, dry the skin thoroughly, and finish with an alcohol rub or a cool sponge. During the treatment take the patient's pulse and temperature at five-minute intervals.

For a **graduated bath,** commence with a water temperature of approximately 100°F (38°C). Maintain this temperature for three minutes, then gradually lower the temperature with cold water to about 94°F (34°C) over a period of five minutes. If the patient tolerates the cooler water, gradually lower the temperature to 90°F (32°C). If the patient feels chilly or develops goose pimples, rub his skin constantly with a face cloth. Do not allow him to become chilled. At the end of the bath, dry the patient promptly and thoroughly, and wrap him in a warm blanket.

For a **neutral bath,** maintain the water temperature at slightly below normal body temperature—approximately 97°F (36°C)—for at least twenty to thirty minutes, longer if well tolerated. Do not allow the patient to chill. Keep the room warm. Following the bath, dry the patient thoroughly but avoid unnecessary rubbing. Do not excite the patient as this destroys the sedative effect. Have the patient rest in bed following the bath for at least thirty minutes.

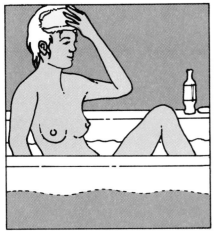

A hot half-bath may be taken in a bathtub. Note the cold compress to the forehead.

Hot half-bath

The person sits in the tub with water covering the legs, hips, and lower trunk. Blood is drawn from the upper to the lower body, and from the internal organs to the skin.

Uses. This procedure relieves congestion in the bronchi and sinuses, and pain in the low back and pelvic area. It may be used to raise the body temperature (artificial fever). Higher water temperatures can be tolerated than in a full tub bath since only part of the body is submerged.

Contraindications. Avoid this procedure on patients who have heart disease, diabetes, and atherosclerosis, especially of the legs and feet.

Procedure. The person sits in a tub of water that has been heated initially to 101°F (38°C). Cover his legs, hips, and lower trunk. Gradu-

ally raise the temperature of the water by adding hot water and removing tub water. The water temperature should be raised to tolerance, not to exceed 112°F (44° C). The bath should last from five to twenty minutes. Apply a cold compress to the forehead and drape a towel over the exposed shoulders. The bath may be ended by dashing a pail of cold water over the lower body and limbs, or by using a cold sponge. Dry the patient promptly. When the patient first stands up, watch closely for possible fainting. Take his pulse and mouth temperature at five-minute intervals.

The **sitz bath** is a version of the hot half-bath in which the patient sits in a tub of hot water with his feet outside, placed in a hot foot bath. The water in the tub should cover the patient's hips. Higher water temperatures can be maintained in the pelvic area without causing as much general heating of the body. The other procedures are similar to those described under the hot half-bath. It has been used effectively in relieving menstrual cramps and in treating (or as an adjunct treatment) for inflammatory conditions of the pelvis.

Ice water or ice pack

The application of ice water or an ice pack to a local area or to parts of a limb causes the contraction of blood vessels, slows down the oozing of blood, and prevents edema.

Uses. This procedure diminishes the swelling from bruises and sprains and also gives relief in conditions such as rheumatic fever, rheumatoid arthritis, and acute infectious arthritis. Ice water or an ice pack will also lessen the pain of acute bursitis and the pain from an inflamed joint. The pain and swelling of a small burn are reduced when cold water is applied immediately after the burn has occurred.

Procedure. Commercially-made ice bags are available from a pharmacy, and are both convenient and effective. However, the following method can be successfully used. Spread crushed ice over a towel or piece of flannel so that it makes a 1-foot square (30 x 30 cm) of ice 1 inch deep (2.5 cm). The towel or cloth should be folded and safety pinned to hold the ice in place. Place the ice bag (or the towel or flannel containing the ice) on the part to be treated. Cover the area with plastic, then a towel. *Check periodically to avoid tissue injury. Do not let melted ice water soak onto the skin.* If well tolerated, the pack may be held in place with a bandage. The application may be continued up to thirty minutes. Remove the pack, dry the patient thoroughly, and cover him to keep warm.

Immediately following the spraining of an ankle or wrist, the foot or ankle may be gradually submerged in a bucket of cold or ice cold water. If the patient complains of the water being too cold, remove the limb momentarily and resubmerge it. The application may be continued for up to thirty minutes, depending on the patient's tolerance. These applications can be made for thirty minutes out of every two hours for up to six treatments.

For a small burn (finger, hand, etc.) place the affected area under cold running tap water or submerge it in a pan of ice cold water. Allow it to remain in the cold water until the pain is relieved, or for thirty minutes.

Sponge or rub

Sponging consists of applying water with a sponge, washcloth, or the bare hand, with little if any friction. A treatment in which water or some other liquid (lotion or cream) is applied with the bare hand is called a "rub," although little actual rubbing is done.

Uses. This treatment moistens the skin, soothes the patient, lowers body temperature, and reduces fever.

Procedure. Generally a washcloth is used, dipped in cool, tepid, or warm water, and squeezed out enough to prevent dripping. Each part of the body is gone over lightly, back and forth, until it is perceptibly cooler. Each part is then dried lightly, not rubbed. Hot sponging is used in fevers where there is chilliness, the same methods being followed as with cool or tepid sponging, except that less water is applied. Keep the patient covered except for the part being sponged.

Alcohol rub

Rubbing alcohol is applied to the skin with the hand. Alcohol has a drying action on the skin, precipitating the protein in the superficial cells. It evaporates rapidly, thus lowering body temperature.

Uses. This application cools the body, lowers the temperature, and refreshes the patient. It also toughens the skin, and is especially useful when applied to pressure points to prevent bedsores. It is very effective in terminating warming procedures such as hot showers, fomentations, hot tub baths, etc.

Contraindications. Do not use this treatment on infants and small children because of absorption through the skin and lungs (vapors inhaled).

Procedure. Rubbing alcohol (isopropyl alcohol) can be purchased from a drugstore for this purpose. **Wood alcohol (methyl alcohol) should never be used.** Regular alcohol (ethyl alcohol) can be used but should be diluted to 70 percent. A small amount of rubbing alcohol is poured into the palm of the hand and quickly rubbed over a portion of the patient's skin. Use both hands, spreading the alcohol over the arms, legs, chest, abdomen, and back. Keep the patient covered except where the alcohol is being applied.

Applications of dry heat

Hot-water bottle

A hot-water bottle is a most useful article in the sick room. Its warmth can be applied to many parts of the body.

Uses. A hot water bottle relaxes, warms, and relieves congestion and pains. It will produce relaxation and induce sleep. It can augment the heating action of a hot compress or fomentation.

Contraindications. Never use a hot water bottle with patients who have impaired sensation, who are paralyzed or unconscious, or who have poor circulation.

Procedure. Fill the bottle to two-thirds full with hot but not boiling water. Screw the top on lightly and expel the air by squeezing the bottle until the water reaches the neck. The stopper should then be screwed tight and the bottle held upside down to check for leaks. Place the bottle in a bag made from flannel or Turkish toweling and position it on the desired area of the patient. **Never use an unprotected hot-water bottle.**

Electric heating pad

The uses and contraindications of a heating pad are similar to those of a hot-water bottle. Pads come with a temperature range—mild, moderate, or high heat.

Radiant heat

Radiant heat is long infrared waves emanating from a heat source such as an electric heater, wood stove, or heat lamp. The waves strike the skin, warming it, and the heat gradually penetrates to the deeper tissues.

Uses. Heating pad treatments are similar to those of a hot-water bottle. In many cases, radiant heat benefits sufferers with neuralgia, neuritis, arthritis, and sinusitis.

Contraindications. Same as those for a hot-water bottle.

Procedure. Radiant heaters can be purchased from a medical supply store. However, an electric bathroom heater without a fan is an excellent source, as is an infrared bulb (appropriately mounted), available in most department stores. Heat can be applied for thirty minutes or longer, taking care to place the device at an appropriate distance from the part of the patient being treated. Do not overheat, as this may cause burns.

Sun bath

In a sun bath, areas of the skin are exposed to the direct rays of the sun (solar radiation) for varying lengths of time. The three types of light waves—ultraviolet, visible, and infrared—all have different effects on the skin and body as a whole. The skin may be both benefited or harmed, depending on the length of exposure.

Uses. Solar radiation toughens and thickens the skin, initiates the production of vitamin D, kills bacteria, modifies the activity of certain endocrine glands, and warms and relaxes the muscles. It also aids in the treatment of many nonpulmonary forms of tuberculosis.

Contraindications. Avoid sunbaths in cases of pulmonary tuberculosis and certain drugs that photosensitize the skin. If you are taking medications, check with your physician before taking a sun bath.

Procedure. In general, the sun bath is best taken before nine o'clock in the morning and after three o'clock in the afternoon. First expose a limited part of your skin for five minutes to direct sunlight and observe the next day if any burning has occurred. If you were sunburned, decrease the time of exposure; if not,

increase the area exposed and the duration of exposure by one minute each day, exposing first the front of the body and then the back for the same length of time. It is unnecessary to expose the head, and the eyes should be shielded from direct exposure. Patients should be guarded from chilling, overheating, and overexposure.

It has been shown that fifteen minutes of daily exposure to the sun three times a week will provide all the vitamin D required by the body. Unfortunately, the same wavelengths that activate the production of vitamin D also cause aging of the skin and skin cancer. For this reason, a sunscreen (suntan lotion—available in drugstores) should be applied if longer and more frequent exposure is desired. However, it should be noted that sunscreens may effectively block the ultraviolet rays from penetrating the skin.

Dark-skinned persons require, on the average, six times the exposure to obtain the same physiological benefit as do light-skinned people. Blond, blue-eyed, and very fair-skinned people are the most susceptible to the sun's effects.

Sunlamps (ultraviolet lamps)

If it is not feasible to give a patient sun baths, but the effects of sun baths are desired, sunlamps, which provide the light spectrum desired, are available from *reliable* medical supply companies. The directions for their use should be followed carefully. Beware of the pseudoscientific claims made for various lamps on the market. Check with a physical therapist before making your purchase.

The uses, contraindications, and procedure for use are otherwise similar to those described under "sun baths." For a detailed discussion of the effects and general benefits of sunlight, see page 68.

Massage

Massage is a system of remedial or hygienic manipulations of the body tissues with the hand or some instrument. It consists of rubbing, stroking, kneading, vibrating, or tapping. Although it is natural for a person to rub a part that may feel uncomfortable, the procedures of massage for the treatment of disease or injury are too complicated for a person to administer unless he has had proper training in an accredited institution. Massage by a well-trained therapist should be given only with the consent of a physician, and limited to the patient's specific needs.

Progressive relaxation

Here is a simple way you can learn to relax overly tense muscles. Each learning session should last about twenty minutes. One or two sessions a day is sufficient.

Step 1. Lie on your back on a firm mattress or carpeted floor with your arms resting along your sides. Try to be as comfortable as possible.

Step 2. Relax your right hand at the wrist if you are right-handed, or your left hand if you are left-handed. This may take some time to learn. Some find that clenching the fist allows them to "feel" the muscles relax. When you think you have

mastered this procedure, have a friend pick up your relaxed hand by a finger and let it go. If it fails to flop down, you are not ready to go on to the next step.

Step 3. Now relax your hand at the wrist and your forearm at the elbow. At each step, check to be sure you are really relaxed. Don't rush. It may take you several days to achieve the first step or two. Once you have mastered these, the others will come more rapidly.

Step 4. Now relax your hand at the wrist, your forearm at the elbow, and your arm at the shoulder. This will relax an entire upper limb.

Step 5. When you have accomplished the above, start on the opposite limb—hand at the wrist, forearm at the elbow, and arm at the shoulder. At the end of each session, relax both limbs together.

Step 6. Start on one of your lower limbs—the foot at the ankle, the leg at the knee, and the thigh at the hip, then the full lower limb. Now relax both upper limbs and the lower limb.

Step 7. Now do the other lower limb in the same step-by-step manner, relaxing all four limbs.

Step 8. Next concentrate on relaxing the muscles of your back. Follow this by relaxing the muscles of your abdomen and chest.

Step 9. Then relax the muscles of your neck so that your head is completely relaxed at the neck and shoulders.

Step 10. The final groups of muscles to relax are those of the face, scalp, and lower jaw (mandible). You should now be able to relax your entire body.

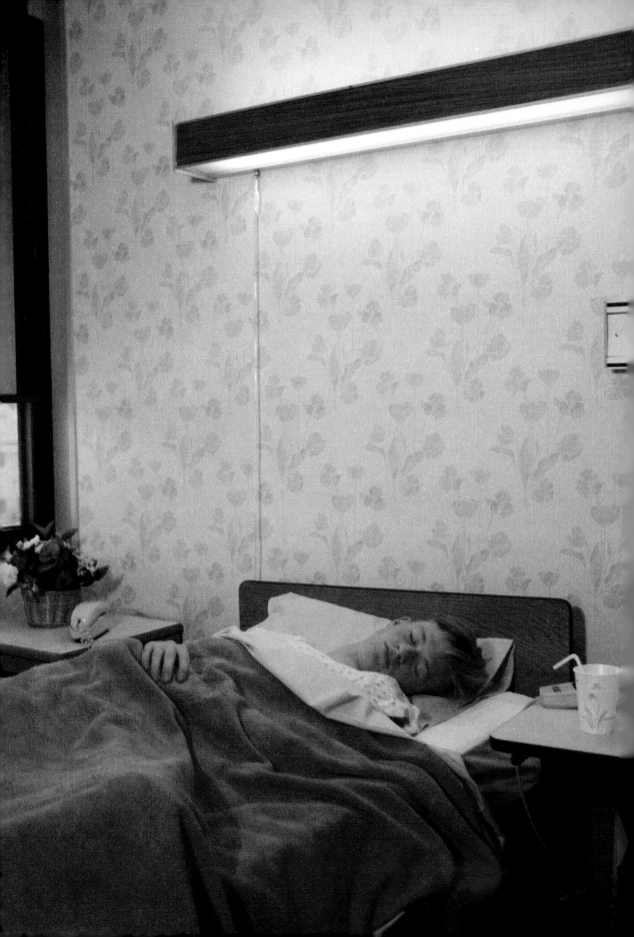

VOL. 2

SECTION 3

GENERAL DISEASES

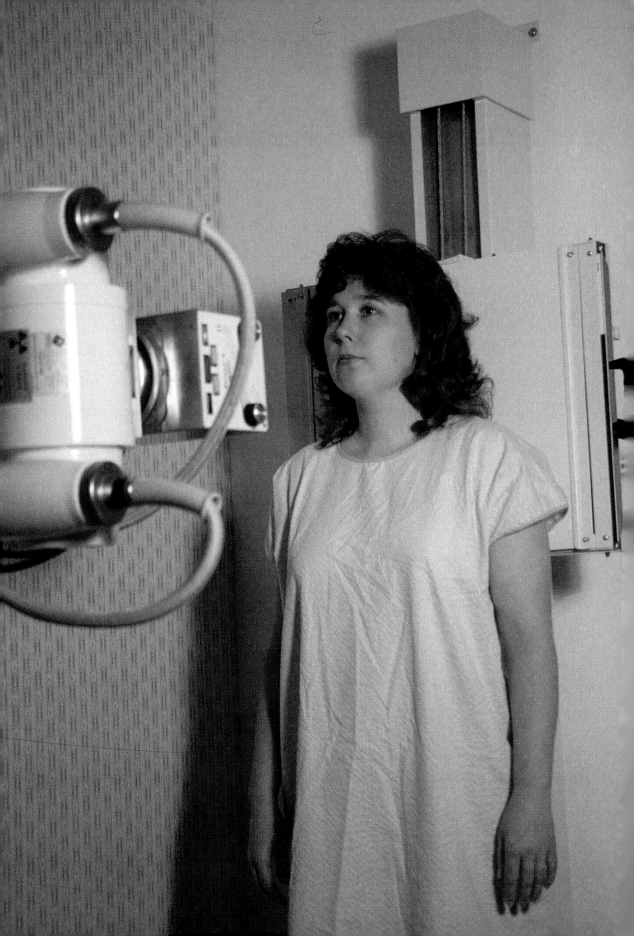

CHAPTER 19

Why disease?

Disease is the loss of health. Health, as already pointed out, is (1) the efficient functioning of every system of the body, (2) adequate support from all that is required for its smooth operation, and (3) every process appropriately directed to carry out its designed activity. Problems arise when something interferes with any of these three aspects of functioning.

Your body puts forth every effort to keep each of its systems performing at its best. When something gets in the way, for whatever reason, the initial effect is a **functional change**—first a loss in the *quantity* of output, followed by a loss in *quality* of the product if the interference continues. If the interference is not removed, a **structural change** will occur in the system, and the malfunction will have become an illness or disease.

Perhaps an example will help to make the point more clear. Take the case of a person with iron-deficient anemia. Because his iron intake was inadequate, his body's iron reserves were used up, and the *quantity* of red blood cells manufactured by his bone marrow decreased. This is a **functional change.** As the shortage of iron got worse, his bone marrow released cells with an inadequate amount of iron (reduced *quality*), which caused the anemia.

As the deficiency continues, the body releases immature, defective red blood cells in an effort to meet the need. Thus a problem of *structural change* has developed.

Every disease has its cause. As the Scripture says: "The curse causeless shall not come" (Proverbs 26:2). As medical science advances and the functioning of the human body is better understood, the causes of disease, which are multiple, are becoming more clear. For a disease process to become established in your body, its defenses must be overwhelmed, and this is no easy matter. It is a formidable undertaking.

Your body's defenses

Your body is like a citadel under attack—a citadel with walls, moats, and guards within. Hostile microbes—bacteria, viruses, fungi, and parasites—surround you on every side. They are on everything you touch and wear and eat. They are in the very air you breathe. But in order to gain even a toehold, these organisms must first breach "the walls": your skin and mucous membranes. And this is no easy task.

Even if they break through the "walls," these invaders must still cross the moat. Deep under the skin, the enemy faces huge "tanks," or phagocytes—cells that will swallow up any invader. Also, your body manufactures antibodies—custom-made chemicals that are specifically designed to neutralize and destroy each enemy soldier. (For a full discussion, see "infections," page 700.) Your body's immune system is a highly sophisticated "chemical warfare" unit, employing every possible strategy to thwart the enemy forces (see page 828).

The enemies without

The air carries disease-producing germs. Some ride in the tiny droplets that are discharged each time you cough or sneeze. Others are carried on the dust particles that originate in your house, on the street, and many other places in the environment where you live.

Flies may transport these germs to your food from the excreta in a barnyard. Insects, such as mosquitoes, may inject them directly into your blood, causing you to come down with malaria or yellow fever.

Microbes that produce disease in humans thrive best at about the same temperature as that of the human body (98°F or 37°C). Very few grow at temperatures below 50°F (10°C). That's why refrigeration of food is such an effective way to prevent disease. On the other end of the scale,

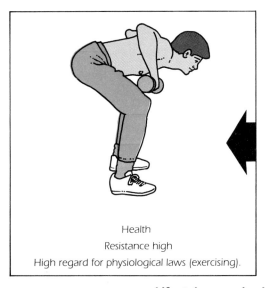

Health
Resistance high
High regard for physiological laws (exercising).

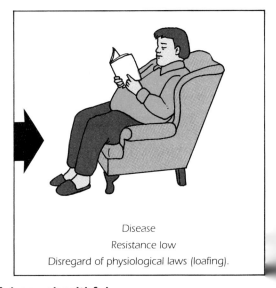

Disease
Resistance low
Disregard of physiological laws (loafing).

Lifestyles can be healthful or unhealthful.

germs do not grow well in temperatures above 115°F (46°C), and most are killed above 170°F (77°C). That is why sterile medications, dressings, and instruments make possible the countless lifesaving procedures that are performed every day in hospitals, clinics, and doctors' offices.

A variety of chemicals are also available that effectively control many infectious organisms that otherwise might do us harm: antiseptics and disinfectants, and even home detergents.

The enemies within

Sometimes, as history has repeatedly recorded, the worst enemies of a nation are those who reside within its borders. This analogy holds true for the human body. Hereditary and cultivated weaknesses will make your body citadel more vulnerable to the disease organisms from without.

Hereditary weaknesses

Your genes carry the chemical information that you inherited from your parents, and they not only determine the design of every structure in your body, but also whether you will be susceptible to certain diseases and resistant to others. Scientists have identified thousands of genetic disorders, from which millions of people suffer. Among the many hereditary disorders, we will mention the following here:

Physical defects. Cleft palate, open spine (spina bifida), hydrocephalus, extra fingers and toes (polydactylism), and defects of the heart.

Functional disorders. These include insulin-dependent diabetes (in children and youth); chronic glaucoma (a common cause of childhood blindness); cystic fibrosis (atrophy of the sweat glands in the skin and of the mucus-secreting glands in the respiratory and digestive systems); sickle cell anemia (abnormal hemoglobin molecules); hemophilia (a defect in the blood's clotting mechanism); lactose intolerance (the inability to digest milk sugar); and color blindness (the inability to distinguish between certain colors).

Cultivated weaknesses

Beginning about fifty years ago, it became evident that many of the diseases from which people suffered and died were due neither to infectious organisms nor to inherited defects, but were the result of the way they lived. In time these became known as lifestyle diseases. It is now recognized that the majority of illnesses are largely due to the way people eat, work, and interact with one another. This is true in both the developed and the less developed countries (for a more complete discussion, see page 124). The following habits that make people either resistant or susceptible to disease are only a few of the many that might be mentioned:

Diet. Food provides the raw material from which the body's tissues are made, repaired, and maintained. Food also contains certain elements essential for the efficient functioning of its organ systems and the energy with which to drive these systems. Deficiencies in one or more of these nutrients will bring on malfunction, disease, and even death. However, a nutritious diet will prevent these disorders and provide all that the body needs.

But both the quality and quantity of the food consumed is important. Excessive intake of even the best food can bring on obesity, a condition that lowers resistance and paves the way for high blood pressure, heart disease, cancer, diabetes, arthritis—and a shortened life span. On the other hand, persons of ideal weight live longer and have fewer of the many diseases from which overweight people suffer.

A diet high in fat, mainly animal fat (saturated fat), especially in the presence of high intakes of cholesterol, lays the foundation for atherosclerosis, which, in turn, contributes to coronary heart disease, stroke, and certain forms of cancer. The generous use of refined sugar contributes to the development of dental caries (tooth decay), hypoglycemia, and diabetes. Excessive consumption of salt (salty foods) is the basis for hypertension in a large share of the population. Diets low in fiber are now known to increase the possibility of developing cancers of the colon and rectum. Such diets also tend to raise blood cholesterol levels.

It has been clearly shown that a low-fat diet (especially when the fat used comes from plant sources) that is also low in refined sugar and high in fiber reduces the risk of all the diseases listed in the previous paragraph.

Unhealthful habits. Physical inactivity, or the lack of muscular exercise, is a major contributing factor to many of the so-called "wear-out diseases." The world today is increasingly mechanized, with machines

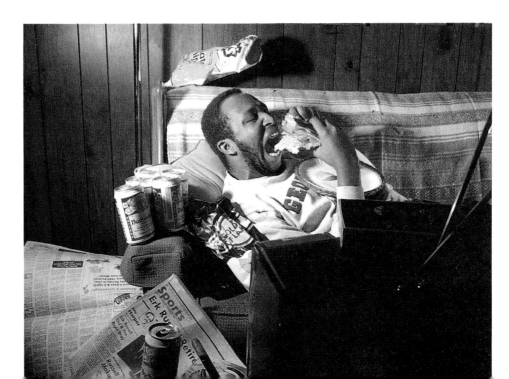

doing what muscles were designed to do. A physical fitness program will significantly reduce the risk of atherosclerosis, coronary heart disease, stroke, and noninsulin dependent diabetes. Exercise is also, without a doubt, the most important single factor in preventing or improving osteoporosis (demineralization of the bones). Exercise eases muscular and emotional tensions and sharpens the mind for mental activity. It has a powerful healing effect on anxiety and depression.

The pressures of a technologically advanced society tend to rob people of adequate relaxation, rest, and sleep. Fatigue lowers a person's resistance to disease, impairs his capacity to perform, and reduces his ability to control his emotions.

Injurious habits. Every society today is plagued with problems caused by the use of drugs, both legal and illegal. The accepted use of **beverage alcohol** contributes to thousands of deaths each year on the highways. More than 50 percent of all automobile accidents in which there is a fatality involve the use of alcohol. The chronic use of alcohol injures the heart, destroys the liver, and accelerates the natural degeneration of the brain cells (neurons).

Tobacco, when smoked, injures both the smoker and the innocent nonsmoker who is exposed to the smoker's smoke. Cancer of the lung is one of the primary causes of death in both men and women in the United States. More than three-fourths of all deaths from coronary heart diseases occur among those who smoke. Chewing or smoking tobacco affects those areas exposed to either the juices of tobacco or its smoke. Cancer of the mouth, tongue, larynx, and esophagus are significantly increased among those who chew or smoke. Chronic lung diseases, like chronic bronchitis and emphysema, are greatly increased in smokers. Children born to smoking mothers weigh less at birth than the babies of nonsmoking mothers, and infants and children grow more slowly in homes where one or both parents smoke.

Caffeine, obtained in the drinks of millions around the world, contributes its share of illness (see page 261). And, of course, little need be said of the ravaging effects of **drugs of abuse** in all societies where they are used. In addition to their destructive effects on body and mind, illegal drugs tend to spread such diseases as hepatitis and AIDS and the sexually transmitted diseases.

Mental attitudes

A person's thoughts and emotions, when conflicting or out of perspective, interfere with his state of health. The close relationship between the mind and the body is well understood today. Emotional stress and tension trigger the body's "alarm reaction" at varying levels of intensity. Sometimes called the "fight or flight mechanism," the alarm reaction is an emergency response that helps people to put forth extraordinary efforts in order to save their lives. It is intended to be used only in short bursts. However, anxiety, frustration, and anger can keep this mechanism active at a low level for hours or

609

days, and perhaps even for months. The result is a wide spectrum of physical and mental illnesses.

Worry, emotional conflict, and a sense of guilt predispose to many of the diseases affecting the heart, blood vessels, digestive organs, and the endocrine glands. At least half of the common illnesses from which people suffer are caused, or at least aggravated, by unhappy thoughts and uncontrolled emotions. Emotional stress will increase the flow of gastric acid in the stomach (contributing to peptic ulcer), raise blood pressure, and heighten the risk of angina and coronary heart disease.

Why disease?

No two people are alike. Each one of us has a different inherited and environmental background. It has been well said that health is like a chain, which, when exposed to wear and tear, will always break at its weakest link. Or to put it a slightly different way, a chain is no stronger than its weakest link. And, like a chain, every human being will eventually "break" at his or her weakest "link."

As we have seen, disease can result from many factors. But in most cases, sickness does not arbitrarily overtake a person, descending "out of a clear sky" to bring illness here and sudden death there. Unhealthful habits of eating, thinking, and living lower our immune mechanisms and weaken our defenses. While some are afflicted by diseases they have inherited, the vast majority suffer because of their own way of life.

Fortunately, many of the most prevalent diseases can be prevented. Then why should not each of us adopt habits and patterns of life that will prevent illness and postpone aging? This is the best guarantee of a long, healthy, and happy life.

Yet each person has that weak link, and despite the most healthful way of life, the time comes when functions begin to fail and disease reveals its ugly face. That is why periodic checkups by a physician are a wise precaution. Many problems that will cause irreparable damage if they are allowed to progress can be easily remedied if they are detected early.

CHAPTER 20

Common problems and symptoms

When your car makes peculiar noises, won't start, or has difficulty holding its direction down the road, you know that something is wrong. Similarly, you recognize a headache, fever, and loss of appetite as telltale evidences that all is not well in your body. In order to help you better understand the meaning of some of the signs and symptoms of illness, a few of the more common ones are discussed below.

Abdomen

Abdominal cramps. Cramping pain in the abdomen may be due to a number of disorders, and it may require extensive investigation on the part of your physician to determine the precise cause. Intestinal infections, such as those by salmonella or giardia ("traveler's diarrhea") may cause cramping (see "gastroenteritis," pages 461, 714). Other causes include appendicitis, intestinal obstruction, kidney stones, kidney infection, gallstones, inflammation of the gallbladder, disorders of the pan-

creas, certain cathartics, and food poisoning. "Indigestion," characterized by severe pain in the upper abdomen of an older adult, may signal a heart attack. Recurrent cramps may indicate a peptic ulcer, cancer of the stomach or bowel, diverticular disease, or ulcerative colitis (see also page 878).

Abdominal distension. Enlargement of the abdomen may result from the presence of either gas or fluid in the abdomen. Gastrointestinal gas has two main sources: swallowed air and gas produced by intestinal bacteria. Some people, without realizing it, develop the habit of swallowing air (aerophagia). Quantities of gas (air) are commonly generated within the digestive tract by bacterial activity on food and food residues. Gas in the stomach is usually released by belching, while that in the lower bowel by the passing of flatus (flatulence).

Nervousness, anxiety, and gum chewing tend to promote the swallowing of air. Certain foods are espe-

611

Important signs and symptoms

General

Change in weight; loss of appetite; weakness; fatigue; headaches; night sweats; fever; dizziness.

Heart, blood, and blood vessels

Heart: chest pain; shortness of breath, especially on exertion; irregular heartbeat; palpitations.

Blood: anemia; prolonged bleeding; easily bruising.

Blood vessels: swelling of ankles (edema); varicose veins; pain in legs on walking; inflammation of veins; legs cold or numb.

Respiratory system

Cough, dry or with sputum or with blood; shortness of breath; asthma or hay fever; wheezing; infections (colds, bronchitis, pneumonia).

Digestive system

Indigestion (heartburn); constipation; diarrhea; pain; loss of appetite; vomiting, especially with blood; blood in stools; jaundice; hemorrhoids; nausea; intolerance to foods; change in pattern of bowel movements.

Urinary system

Painful urination; frequency, especially at night; dribbling; blood in urine; infection; pain; inability to hold urine.

Genital system

Male: discharge, pain; sores; swelling; sexually transmitted disease.

Female: itching; discharge from vagina; painful intercourse; sexually transmitted disease. Menstrual period—irregular, intermittent, cramps, heavy or scant bleeding. Postmenopausal—bleeding, hot flashes, depression. Breasts—lumps, pain, nipple discharge, dimpling.

Nervous system

Weakness; paralysis; numbness or tingling; difficulty in walking; tremors; convulsions; dizziness; fainting spells; loss of feeling; loss of memory; difficulty speaking.

Muscles and bones

Muscular weakness or cramps; limitation of movement; pain or stiffness in joints; back pain.

Endocrine system

Excessive thirst, hunger, or urination; excessive sweating; feel too hot or too cold.

Skin

Dry; itching; rash; growths or masses; changes in color or texture of skin, hair, or nails.

Eyes

Changes in vision; double vision; sensitivity to light; blurring; itching; pain; infection.

Ears

Hearing loss; ringing in the ears; pain; infection; excess wax; dizziness.

Nose and sinuses

Discharge; nosebleeds; obstruction; hay fever; pain; frequent colds; loss of smell.

Mouth and throat

Sore throats; sore tongue; bleeding gums; lesions in mouth; difficulty swallowing; hoarseness; loss of taste.

Neck

Swollen glands; enlarged thyroid; pain; stiffness.

cially prone to cause flatulence, including cabbage, celery, cucumbers, onions, pears, peppers, beans, and broccoli. Carbonated drinks and alcohol may have the same effect. An inherited inability to digest milk sugar ("lactose intolerance," see page 858) or wheat gluten causes certain individuals to suffer from distension after eating these foods.

Stomach and intestinal gas may also occur in such illnesses as gastritis, intestinal obstruction, celiac disease, sprue, and ileus.

Distension due to the accumulation of fluid in the peritoneal cavity **(ascites)** may occur as a complication of such diseases as congestive heart failure, glomerulonephritis, cirrhosis of the liver, and abdominal or thoracic cancer.

Abdominal masses. Some masses felt within the abdomen are either normal or relatively harmless. In pregnancy, the uterus can be felt in the lower middle abdomen, and it becomes easily palpable as pregnancy advances. A bladder very full of urine may be detected as a soft mass above the pubic bone. In a thin person who is constipated, firm masses of fecal material may be felt in the lower colon on the left side.

Normal organs are generally difficult to feel. However, an enlarged liver, spleen, or kidney may be felt. Your physician will determine the cause. Enlarging cancers in the abdomen and upper pelvic area may be detected. These include cancer of the colon and, in women, tumors, cysts, and abscesses of the reproductive organs.

Abdominal rigidity. When the tissues inside the abdomen become inflamed, severe pain develops. The muscles overlying the inflamed area contract, making the abdominal wall rigid. This condition occurs in acute appendicitis (more apparent on the right side), perforated peptic ulcer, sometimes in acute inflammation of the gallbladder, in peritonitis from any cause, when there has been bleeding within the abdomen, and, strangely, in cases of black widow spider bites.

Abdominal tenderness. In acute abdominal inflammations, the abdominal wall overlying the inflamed area becomes sensitive, reinforcing, as it were, the protection afforded by the rigidity of the muscles mentioned above. In this way, the patient "guards" the internal area of inflammation.

Appetite

Loss of appetite. This may occur from emotional tensions, unappetizing food, unhappy circumstances during a meal, the use of tobacco, and the side effect of certain drugs. It is often the first symptom in many illnesses and is an important reason for weight loss in many chronic, wasting diseases. It is particularly noticeable in cancer of the stomach and infectious hepatitis.

Increase in appetite. Many people, unhappy with the circumstances of their life, find satisfaction in eating, and this, in turn, may result in obesity. Some people, during periods of strenuous physical activity or during pregnancy, become accustomed to eating heartily. When these situations change, their habit con-

613

tinues. A voracious appetite commonly occurs with an overactive thyroid gland (hyperthyroidism). The metabolic rate is elevated, and the person craves more food to provide the extra "fuel" used by the accelerated activities of the tissues. In certain tumors of the pancreas and diabetes, the appetite is increased because of excess insulin production. A vigorous appetite may accompany tapeworm infection.

Blisters

A blister is a small accumulation of fluid in the surface layer of the skin. Blood blisters, in which the fluid is bloody, are caused by bruising or pinching the skin. "Water blisters" are usually produced by continued localized friction against the skin. Blisters can result from a burn, from cold, and from certain chemicals. Certain skin allergies and some local and systemic infections may cause blisters. It is best not to puncture a blister. However, should a blister break, guard against infection. Blisters of unknown origin should be checked by your physician.

Blood loss (bleeding, hemorrhage)

Effects of bleeding. Blood accounts for 7 to 9 percent of the body's weight, or about 5 to 6 quarts (approximately 6 liters). A person can lose a pint of blood (half liter) with little or no adverse effect (this amount is commonly taken when blood is donated). When larger amounts are lost, symptoms develop that become increasingly severe as the loss continues. When the loss is

sudden and severe, the symptoms include pallor; thirst; cold sweating; buzzing in the ears; dizziness; light-headedness; blurred vision; restlessness; a rapid, faint pulse; rapid, shallow breathing; and, eventually, unconsciousness. The symptoms are the same whether the blood is lost to the outside of the body or into a body cavity (internal bleeding). **Severe blood loss, observed or suspected, should be reported to a physician.** For first-aid measures, see page 541.

From an injury. Blood loss from an injury may be of two types. The first, **external bleeding** from a crushing injury, tends to ooze, and is not as rapid as the bleeding from an injury inflicted with a sharp object. In a cleanly severed artery, the blood escapes in spurts, one spurt with each heartbeat. Severe blood loss must be controlled promptly. An injury may also cause **internal bleeding**. Internal bleeding may result from a hard blow, a fall, being thrown from a horse or vehicle, or from a crushing injury. Although no bleeding is apparent, watch for the symptoms of bleeding described above.

From the bladder. Blood in the urine (hematuria) may come from either the bladder or the kidneys. The common causes are cancer, kidney stones, acute nephritis, and infections causing hemorrhagic cystitis.

From the lungs. Blood from the lungs is expelled through the mouth and is usually "coughed up" or "spat up" rather than vomited. However, any lesion or injury in the mouth and nose cavities should be checked.

Causes for bleeding in the lungs include cancer and tuberculosis. Blood-streaked sputum is commonly seen in chronic bronchitis and bronchiectasis.

From the mouth. The most common cause of bleeding in the mouth is from the gums, due to poor oral hygiene and infection of the gum tissues (gingivitis). Injuries, ulcers, and tumors may also cause bleeding. Bleeding may occur from a defect in the clotting mechanism, deficiency of vitamin C (scurvy), and from certain drugs. If you have persistent bleeding in the mouth, see your dentist or physician.

From the nose. Nosebleeds result from the rupture of a small vein or veins in the lining of the nose. This can be due to "picking the nose," or it may develop spontaneously. For details, see page 907.

From the rectum. Bleeding from a lesion anywhere along the digestive tract will appear in the rectum. Bleeding from hemorrhoids or an anal fissure will be bright red. When the site of bleeding is distant, as from a peptic ulcer, the blood will be almost black, with a consistency like tar. Bleeding from intermediate points will be dark or light, depending on the distance the source is from the rectum. Bloody diarrhea is common in ulcerative colitis. Polyps (benign tumors) of the colon may bleed. Bleeding is an important symptom in cancer of the colon and rectum. Should you observe any bleeding from your rectum, see your physician.

From the skin. Cuts and abrasions of the skin will produce temporary superficial bleeding. Persistent bleeding and bleeding beneath the skin (purpura) suggest a defect in the blood-clotting mechanism and may occur in bleeding disorders (see page 819).

From the stomach. Blood in the stomach may be vomited or passed through the rectum. Its source may be a stomach ulcer, cancer, or bleeding veins in the lower esophagus (occurring in cirrhosis of the liver). The source may also be in the nose or pharynx. The color of the blood is a clue to how long it has been in the stomach. If it is bright red, the hemorrhage is recent. If the color is like "coffee grounds," it has been in the stomach long enough to be partially digested.

From the vagina. Periodic bleeding from the vagina occurs throughout a woman's reproductive period of life. This is normal during menstruation. Causes of abnormal vaginal bleeding include polyps of the lining of the uterus or cervix, fibroid tumors (myomas) in or near the lining of the uterus (mucosa), inflammation of the uterine mucosa, imbalance of the hormones controlling menstruation, and from cancer of the uterine tubes, uterus, or cervix. Certain serious complications of pregnancy can also cause abnormal vaginal bleeding.

The breast

The usual symptoms of breast disorders are a mass, pain or tenderness, and, less commonly, a discharge from the nipple.

Masses ("lumps"). During a woman's reproductive period, the glandular tissue in her breasts can produce milk. This tissue gives the breast a nodular consistency. On firm pressure, the finely alternating firm and soft areas can be felt. This normal nodularity undergoes cyclic changes each month, the nodules usually becoming firm and slightly tender just before menstruation.

Abnormal lumps may be benign or malignant. **Fibrocystic disease,** sometimes called **"lumpy breast,"** usually affects both breasts (although one side may predominate). The disorder tends to diminish after menopause. It may also be related to coffee drinking (see page 262).

Cancer of the breast is a most serious disease. Pain and tenderness are not common until the late stages. Often, but not always, a cancerous nodule tends to be fixed, and the overlying skin or nipple may be drawn in. It is wise for every woman to develop the technique of breast self-examination (see page 693).

Should you discover a lump in your breast, see your physician. A safe rule is to consider every lump a cancer until proved otherwise. The earlier the diagnosis, the better the prognosis.

Tenderness. As mentioned above, it is not uncommon for women, during their reproductive period, to have tender breasts just before they menstruate. The breasts also become tender during pregnancy, beginning about the third week after conception. Extreme tenderness during nursing (lactation) usually indicates an infection of the breast (mastitis) that may progress to abscess formation, so see your physi-cian. For additional information about the female breast and its problems, see pages 683, 697.

Male breast enlargement. Occasionally the breast of an adolescent boy may enlarge (gynecomastia), due to an imbalance in hormone production. It commonly affects one breast and usually disappears within a year, sometimes two.

In older men, one or both breasts may enlarge in response to hormone therapy for cancer of the prostate, from cirrhosis of the liver, and from a tumor of the testes. Breast enlargement may be a response to certain drugs or to the use of marijuana. Cancer of the male breast is very rare.

Breath: shortness of (dyspnea)

The rate and depth of breathing is automatically regulated by the body's need to receive oxygen and eliminate carbon dioxide. Breathing is stimulated any time more oxygen is required or excess carbon dioxide has accumulated in the tissues. "Shortness of breath," or dyspnea, is associated with more rapid and deeper breathing.

Shortness of breath normally occurs when a person exercises vigorously, since during this time the muscles need more oxygen and produce more carbon dioxide. Since these gases are carried in the blood to and from the muscles, the heart rate is also increased.

Obstructive dyspnea. Difficult breathing results any time there is an interference in the passage of air to and from the lungs. Such interference occurs when a person inhales a foreign body that blocks the air passages (choking). In children it may also be caused by croup, in which the tissues of the larynx become swollen and the laryngeal muscles go into spasm. Asthma is another cause of difficult breathing, in which exhaling is difficult because the smaller air passages have become narrowed.

Pulmonary dyspnea. When a disease interferes with the transfer of oxygen and carbon dioxide within the lungs, the body tissues need more oxygen than the lungs are able to supply, and carbon dioxide builds up. The brain stimulates the lungs to breathe, so the person breathes deeper and faster, even though the increase in depth and rate does not remove the basic cause of the problem. Shortness of breath from this cause may occur in pneumonia or in fibrosis of the lungs resulting from inhaling irritating dusts. Most importantly, difficulty in breathing is an outstanding symptom of chronic obstructive pulmonary disease (COPD) in which emphysema predominates.

Cardiac dyspnea. The blood carries oxygen from the lungs to the tissues of the body and carries carbon dioxide back to the lungs for elimination. When heart disease reduces the heart's capacity for pumping blood, the body experiences an oxygen shortage, and difficulty in breathing occurs. Thus, shortness of breath is a common and significant symptom of serious heart disease. In the early stages of heart disease, the dyspnea is noticed only at times of strenuous exertion. As the heart disease progresses, the dyspnea occurs with lesser degrees of exertion, until finally it occurs even when the person is resting.

Dyspnea of anemia. In anemia there is a deficiency in the blood's ability to carry sufficient oxygen for the body's needs, most noticeably when a person climbs stairs or engages in any form of vigorous physical activity. As in other conditions that cause an oxygen shortage, the person tries to breathe faster and more deeply.

Functional hyperventilation. People with this problem periodically breathe more deeply and rapidly, even though there is no lack of oxygen or excess of carbon dioxide in their body tissue, and their organs of circulation and respiration are perfectly normal. Such an attack typically occurs when the person is at rest and actually does not need additional oxygen. The hyperactive breathing is prompted by an unwarranted assumption that the person is "short of breath." Because of the excessive breathing, so much carbon dioxide is lost that a condition called **alkalosis** develops. The symptoms of hyperventilation syndrome include a feeling of lightheadedness, palpitation, tightness in the chest, tingling sensations around the mouth and in the hands, and a feeling of faintness.

Such attacks may be caused by bad breathing habits, but, more commonly, they result from anxiety.

Chills

A chill, with paleness of the skin, sense of coldness, and shivering, is one of the ways the body produces and conserves heat. Chills occur

617

when the environmental temperature is low or when the body temperature is rising suddenly. Chills typically occur in the early stages of pneumonia, when the body is reacting to a severe infection and fever develops.

The expression **"chills and fever"** describes a condition in which, even though the body's temperature is rising, the person feels chilly. Chills and fever occur in the early phase of many systemic infections. They are seen in each of the repeating episodes of malaria. When fever declines sharply, sweating occurs.

Complexion: ruddy

A conspicuous ruddiness is caused by dilatation of the capillaries, which increases the flow of blood through the skin. This condition occurs in fever, in alcoholic intoxication, in sunburn, when a person is angry, and when one blushes. Ruddiness is seen in certain forms of heart disease (mitral stenosis). A bluish redness of the skin occurs in polycythemia (excess of red blood cells). In carbon monoxide poisoning, the union of carbon monoxide to part of the hemoglobin imparts a cherry-red color to the skin.

Constipation

Constipation is a condition in which the bowel movements are poorly timed, infrequent, inadequate, and are hard and difficult to pass. There are many causes, the most common being inadequate drinking of water, lack of foods containing dietary fiber, and failure to exercise regularly. For a more detailed discussion, see page 877.

Cough

A cough is a sudden, noisy expulsion of air from the lungs. A person may restrain the urge to cough or, on the other extreme, may force a cough when it would not otherwise occur. Usually, however, coughing occurs automatically. A person in good health may cough in order to remove mucus and foreign materials such as dust that have accumulated in his upper air passages.

Coughing also occurs when fluid, food, or some foreign object accidentally finds its way into the air passages. A cough is provoked by inhaled smoke or gases, which irritate the lining of the air passages. This is the reason for smoker's cough. Another cause of coughing is a local inflammation of the air passages, as in laryngitis, tracheitis, and bronchitis. A tumor on the vocal cords will cause a dry, hacking cough. Coughing often accompanies such respiratory disorders as the common cold and influenza.

Coughing is usually a prominent symptom of diseases involving the tissues of the lungs, including pneumonia, pulmonary tuberculosis, emphysema, bronchiectasis, fungal infections of the lung, parasitic diseases of the lung, and lung abscess. Coughing also occurs in cancers of the lung, pleura, and mediastinum. Bronchiogenic carcinoma · (the lung cancer associated with cigarette smoking) usually becomes well established before it produces symptoms. But among its important symptoms, when they do occur, are coughing and spitting blood.

Strange as it may seem, heart failure can cause coughing. When the left side of the heart is unable to pump the blood out of its chambers, it backs up into the lungs, causing congestion. Fluid from the blood (plasma) seeps into the tiny air sacs and interferes with the normal exchange of oxygen. Coughing is a means of clearing out the air spaces.

Sometimes an aneurysm of the thoracic aorta (enlargement of the body's largest artery) and enlarging lymph nodes, due to leukemia, cause coughing by producing pressure against the trachea.

Certain contagious diseases inflame the lung tissues and produce coughing. Common among these are whooping cough, certain kinds of influenza, and measles.

Even wax in the ear canal can produce a cough! And sometimes coughing is caused by tricks of the mind. Called "psychogenic cough," this is an indication of a neurosis or just plain nervousness. It is often observed in speakers when they first get up to speak.

For treatment of cough, see page 453.

Cramps

Muscle cramps frequently occur at night, when the muscles in certain parts of the body go into violent spasm, especially those of the back of the thigh, calf of the leg, and feet. Although the precise cause is not known, cramps may occur from over-exercise, stretching the muscle too much, and dehydration. Relief may be obtained by gently massaging the cramping muscles, by applying heat, and by contracting the muscles that pull the limb in opposition to those that are in spasm. Drinking plenty of water will not bring immediate relief, but it can help to prevent future attacks. For further discussion of the causes and treatment of cramps, see page 963.

Cyanosis

Cyanosis is blueness of the skin and internal membranes, contrasting with their normal pink color. Cyanosis can be detected in a dark-skinned person by examining the lining of the eyelids or looking inside the mouth. The color of the skin and membranes varies from person to person and depends on the amount and quality of the pigment present in the tissues and on the color of the hemoglobin in the red blood cells. When hemoglobin, the protein pigment in red blood cells, combines with oxygen (as the blood passes through the lungs) it becomes bright red. Hemoglobin that has given up its oxygen (reduced hemoglobin) is a dark bluish red. When there is a marked increase in the amount of reduced hemoglobin for any reason, the skin and membranes appear bluish.

The skin of a "blue baby" appears blue. A congenital defect in the heart permits the blood coming from the lungs, filled with oxygen, to mix with blood that is on its way back to the lungs after having delivered its oxygen to the tissues. This mixture of oxygenated and unoxygenated blood gives the skin a bluish color.

At high altitudes, where the oxygen in the air is less concentrated, even normal people become somewhat cyanotic, particularly if they increase their need for oxygen by exercise. Exposure to cold may cause cyanosis in the exposed parts of the body (fingers, toes, nose, and ears) because, as a means of conserving heat, the blood to these structures is automatically curtailed by constriction of the blood vessels. Even nervous tension or intense emotion (fear, anger) can reduce the flow of blood to certain parts of the skin, producing cyanosis and cold, clammy skin.

Generalized cyanosis can be caused by pneumonia and certain chronic diseases that interfere with the oxygenation of blood in the lungs. In various forms of heart failure, because of sluggish circulation, more of the oxygen is withdrawn by the tissues. This lowers the oxygen concentration in the blood and imparts a blue color to the skin. Interference with the flow of blood to any part of the body by obstruction of either the arteries or the veins will slow down the circulation and cause cyanosis in that part.

Deafness

Deafness, which is the partial or complete loss of hearing, may result from disorders in the outer, middle, or inner ear; from disturbances in the conduction of impulses from the inner ear to the brain centers, where hearing is conceived; or from a lesion in the hearing center itself. For a full discussion of the types of hearing loss and methods available to correct many of their causes, see page 1152.

Diarrhea

Diarrhea is an increase in the number and looseness of the stool because of an excess of water in the intestines. The discharge of the stool may vary from mild to violent and may be accompanied by abdominal discomfort. Diarrhea can be caused by food sensitivities, infections, food poisonings, medications, emotional stress, and a number of diseases of the digestive tract. Diarrheas may be self-limited, but should they be violent and continuous, a physician should be consulted. Replacement of fluids (to prevent dehydration) and appropriate medications may be needed. For a more complete discussion, see page 877.

Discharge: mucus

A mucous discharge is an excess of mucus eliminated from some organ of the body. Mucus is a slippery, semifluid secretion produced by small glands located in the membranes that line many of the body's hollow organs and ducts (tubes). Mucus moistens and lubricates these membranes and protects them from injury. In response to the irritation of a membrane, mucus is produced in larger quantities than usual.

From the nose. A mucous discharge from the nose, often watery at first and becoming more viscid later, characterizes the early stages of the common cold and also an attack of hay fever. The nasal sinuses, opening as they do into the nasal cavities, are often involved, and add to the mucus already being produced by the membranes lining the nose.

From the trachea and bronchial tubes. Mucus is produced continuously by the membranes lining the air passages, but under usual circumstances, there is little or no excess to be eliminated. However, when the membranes are irritated or inflamed, as in bronchitis, an excess of mucus is produced, then is coughed up and expectorated (spat out). When the membrane is infected, pus cells will be present in the mucous discharge.

From the colon. When the lining membrane (mucosa) of the colon becomes irritated or involved in an inflammatory process, as in colitis, the excess mucus produced is eliminated with the stools at the time of defecation. In severe cases of mucous colitis, some of the stools are composed largely of mucus.

Discharge: purulent (containing pus)

When an infectious agent or a foreign body enters the tissues of the body, the body's defenses are aroused to rid it of the invader, and white blood cells are drawn to the site. In the process of doing their work, these white blood cells die, along with many of the tissues in the infected area. These dead cells, together with tissue debris and tissue fluid, constitute pus. If possible, the pus is expelled from the body and is called a **purulent discharge.** When the infection is localized, the area involved may form an ulcer or an abscess, which may drain to the outside.

A purulent discharge may escape from the bowel (through the anal opening), the ears, the eyes, the nose, the lungs (by coughing and expectorating), the urethra, the vagina, and from any part of the body where an abscess has ruptured. The presence of a purulent discharge is evidence of a serious infection that needs attention.

Dizziness

Dizziness describes a number of sensations in which a person feels lightheaded, unsteady, giddy, or faint. The problem may be due to a number of causes, including disturbances in the blood supply to the brain, disorders of the semicircular canals in the inner ear, anemia, allergies, and certain infections. The treatment, of course, depends on the underlying cause. For details as to cause and treatment, see page 1051.

Dyspepsia

Dyspepsia, or indigestion, covers a number of symptoms that are usually observed after eating or drinking. There is generally a sense of discomfort in the upper abdomen, belching, heartburn, and a feeling of fullness and bloating. The cause may be simply eating too much or too frequently, or it may be eating under emotional strain or eating foods to which one is unsuited. Sometimes it signals a more serious problem, such as peptic ulcer, gallbladder disease, or even cancer. For additional information about causes, prevention, and cure, see page 853.

Ears: symptoms

A wide variety of disorders may affect the ears, and many of these are discussed elsewhere (see page 1146).

621

Among the more common problems are discharge from the outer ear, dizziness, earache, ringing in the ear, impacted ear wax, infection in the ear canal, middle ear infection (otitis media), and deafness. The symptoms will differ according to the underlying problem, as will the treatment. See page 1146.

Edema

Edema is the accumulation of excess fluid in the tissues. Dependent areas of the body, such as the feet and ankles, show the puffiness first. Among the major causes of edema are heart failure, kidney failure, cirrhosis of the liver, malnutrition, allergies, local infection, local injury, obstruction of the veins (often seen in pregnancy), and sitting or standing for long periods of time. For additional discussion of the causes and treatment of edema, see page 809.

Energy loss

Loss of energy causes a feeling, or state, of exhaustion. It is a natural consequence of activity, mental or physical, that is continued too long. With it comes a reduction in the capacity to work. Loss of energy for muscular work may be due to a shortage or lack of oxygen, low blood sugar, an accumulation of body wastes, a rise in temperature (especially above 102° F), or a shortage of water (dehydration).

Disease states in which energy loss occurs include insufficient oxygen, as in anemia and certain diseases of the heart and lungs; inadequate glucose (food fuel) to meet tissue needs, as seen in severe malnutrition; a decrease in the rate of body metabolism, as in hypothyroidism; and in conditions of profound debility or severe systemic illnesses, as pneumonia.

Those who have experienced intolerable life situations or who are troubled by emotional tensions and conflicts may exhibit loss of energy. Although the symptom is functional, the victim sincerely feels physically handicapped. See also pages 639, 1057.

Eyes: symptoms

The eye is made up of many structures: the lids, conjunctiva, cornea, iris, lens, fluids within the eye chambers, retina, and the nerves connecting the eye to the vision centers of the brain. The external eye includes the muscles that move the eye and the nerves that activate them. More than one disorder may affect any one of these components of the eye, and the symptoms will vary according to the structure affected and the type of disorder. For an understanding of the problems that may be encountered and their diagnosis and treatment, see page 1125.

Fear

Fear is an emotion involving dread of unknown and possibly unpleasant consequences. Normally, it makes a person cautious and triggers the alarm reaction that prepares the body to protect itself, either by flight (leaving the scene) or fight (defense). For a discussion of childhood fears, see pages 448. For phobias in adults, see page 1055.

Fever

Fever is an abnormal or pathological elevation of body temperature above the normal. Vigorous exercise will physiologically raise the body temperature to approximately 100° F (38°C), but will not usually exceed this level if the intake of water has been adequate. This elevated temperature is not considered a fever. The *average* normal temperature is considered 98.6° or 37°C.

The body responds to infections, as well as to tissue destruction (as seen in extensive burns) with a fever. When the increase takes place rapidly, the patient may experience chills while the heat-regulating mechanism is accommodating its new, higher level. Sweating is common when fever is receding.

Fever occurs in heatstroke, in which there is a high external temperature coupled with a failure of the body's heat-dissipating mechanism. Certain drugs will cause a fever. Dehydration will also produce a fever in both children and adults.

Headache

Headache, as the term implies, is discomfort or pain in the head. About 25 percent of the time, headache is a symptom of some other disorder. In the majority of cases, a headache is not a serious problem and will disappear in a few minutes to a few hours. However, you should consult your physician about any headache that is different, that changes suddenly, and that persists. For a full discussion of headaches, including an outline of those that are serious and those that are not, see page 1050.

Heat cramps

Sudden spasm, or cramping, of the muscles of the lower limbs and abdomen may occur in persons who have been doing heavy physical work or vigorous activity in a temperature above 100°F (38°C) and who have been sweating profusely. These spasms are due primarily to an excessive loss of water (dehydration), rather than to a lack of salt (salt depletion), as formerly believed. For treatment and prevention, see page 556.

Heat exhaustion, or heat prostration

Heat exhaustion, due to prolonged exposure to excessive heat and high humidity, is often associated with vigorous exercise in a hot, humid environment. Heat exhaution may occur in persons exposed to hot, humid weather who have not become accustomed to such weather. There is only a moderate rise in temperature (up to 102°F), and the skin is damp and clammy.

The symptoms may include weakness, nausea, dizziness, headache, mental confusion, and stupor. There may also be heat cramps and a tendency to faint. Treatment consists of placing the individual in a cool place and administering lots of water. If salt is added to the water, it should be in small amounts (1/4 teaspoonful per glass). Elevating the feet is helpful. For additional discussion, see page 556.

Heatstroke or sunstroke

This is the result of prolonged exposure to excessive heat or to the sun, and is seen more commonly in the elderly or those who are debilitated. The most severe of the heat disorders, it is a medical emergency. The body's heat-control mechanisms are overwhelmed. Sweating ceases, and the skin becomes dry, hot, and flushed. The body temperature rises rapidly to as high as 105° F (40° C). The pulse rate may exceed 160 beats per minute.

Initially there may be weakness, nausea, headache, and a pain in the vicinity of the heart. This is followed by a rapid rise in body temperature and a loss of consciousness. In some, there may be convulsions, coma, and even death.

Treatment requires an all-out effort to lower the body temperature. Take the victim to a cool place indoors or to a shady spot outside. Fan him, or, if he is indoors, use an electric fan. Place cool, wet cloths on his forehead and over his body. If the victim is conscious, encourage him to drink cool water. Call for medical help, and take him to the nearest hospital.

Hemorrhage

Bleeding can be both external and internal. If severe, it can be life threatening and is a medical emergency. For a detailed discussion and emergency procedures, see page 541.

Hernia

A hernia is a protrusion of a portion of an organ or tissue through an abnormal opening in some body part. Examples include a loop of intestine passing through an opening in the abdominal wall into the region of the groin (inguinal hernial), or a portion of the stomach passing upward through an opening in the diaphragm into the lung area (hiatus hernia). For a more complete discussion of hernias and their treatment, see page 862.

Hiccup

A hiccup is a quick, involuntary intake of air that occurs spasmodically. It is brought about by the sudden contraction of the diaphragm and is abruptly checked by the closing of the larynx, often causing an audible sound. Hiccups occur at intervals of several seconds. Most attacks last a few minutes and subside spontaneously. Occasionally, however, usually during a serious illness or following surgery, an attack may last several hours or even days. At times, an attack of hiccups may even be life threatening. Further discussion and suggestions for treatment can be found on page 560.

Hoarseness

Hoarseness is a roughness of the voice and indicates a disorder of the larynx. It may be caused by misuse (shouting, singing too vigorously), overuse (speaking too long or when fatigued), irritation (dust), inflammation (infections), or from tumors (generally benign but sometimes cancerous, especially in smokers, tobacco chewers, and heavy drinkers). For a full discussion, see page 915.

Incontinence

Incontinence is the inability to control the passage of urine from the bladder or feces from the bowel. The problem is normal in infancy. It requires the maturing infant to gradually develop the ability to control when and where to pass urine and stool. In some children, nighttime bed-wetting continues into late childhood. For details, see page 445.

In adults, **urinary incontinence** may be due to an infection (cystitis), from injury (childbirth in a woman), from surgery (prostatic in a man), or from disorders in the spinal cord. Loss of control of the passage of feces or **fecal inconctinence** occurs commonly in severe diarrhea. Excessive use of cathartics (particularly mineral oil) often causes an involuntary loss of the watery or oily fecal material. Injury to the muscles that surround the anus, either by trauma or by tearing of these structures at the time of childbirth, can interfere with the normal control of fecal evacuation. Hemorrhoids and anal fissures can cause the passage of feces to be so painful that the rectal contents are retained until finally, the rectum is emptied involuntarily.

Certain injuries to the local nerves that supply the anal region or injury to the spinal cord can cause a permanent loss of control of the sphincter mechanisms that prevent the free passage of feces.

Indigestion

Indigestion and heartburn can be caused by a number of disorders of the upper digestive tract: the esophagus, stomach, duodenum, gallbladder, and pancreas. Feelings of fullness, gas, and burning in the lower esophagus (due to reflux of acid gastric contents), if continued, should be evaluated by your physician. For a full discussion of the problem, see page 853.

Intercourse: unsatisfactory

Sexual intercourse is a complex and very personal function, with physical, ethical, and moral components. When one or more of these are less than satisfying to the individual, the entire function becomes disappointing. The belief is fairly widespread that intercourse must always climax in ejaculation and orgasm. However, this is not necessarily true, and failure, because of this misconception, breeds failure. When the physical, ethical, and moral components of intercourse blend in a manner consistent with the individual's codes and personal expectations, the experience of sexual intercourse provides a gratifying reassurance of personal adequacy.

The sexual reflexes, which by their response to appropriate stimuli make intercourse possible, are powerful and compelling in comparison with other reflex mechanisms. But their activation rests on a delicate balance between affirmative desire and negative repulsion. Normally, the positive factors dominate. But minor rebuffs, incidental prejudices, and underlying emotional concerns and conflicts can easily tip the balance in the negative direction so that intercourse, if accomplished at all, is a disappointment. This background explains, in theory, why in most cases of unsatisfactory intercourse the basic causes are psychological, rather than physical.

The terms **frigidity** and **dyspareunia** refer to a wife's inability to

625

experience normal pleasure in sexual intercourse. **Impotence** refers to a man's inability to perform the sex act, a symptom that is less common in men than is frigidity in women. For a more complete discussion, see under "sexual problems of men," page 1111, and "sexual problems of women," page 1113.

Intoxication: alcohol

Alcohol intoxication is impairment of the physical and mental functions as a result of drinking beverage alcohol. The perceptual capacities are dulled, judgment is impaired, and reality is distorted. An intoxicated person's skin is flushed, his reflexes sluggish, and his muscular coordination poor. He may experience double vision, ringing in the ears, and numbness. His consciousness is impaired more or less in proportion to the amount of alcohol he has consumed, and in an extreme case, his condition may deteriorate to a state of coma.

Alcohol intoxication does not always follow the same pattern. It differs from one person to another, and even in the same person. Problems may arise when the intoxicated person becomes ill from some other cause, which may be overlooked because of the assumption that all his symptoms are caused by his alcohol.

The stupor of alcohol intoxication is easily confused with that caused by a serious head injury, especially if the injury is sustained while the person is intoxicated. The rupture or occlusion of a blood vessel in the brain ("stroke") may cause symptoms easily confused with alcoholic intoxication. The coma that occurs in diabetes, either from lack of insulin or from taking too much insulin, can be similarly confused.

Alcohol interacts in the body with many drugs, producing effects that greatly exceed the drug's usual actions, even to the extent of endangering the victim's life (see page 295).

Some persons react in an unusual manner when they take even a small amount of alcohol. They become mentally confused and disoriented; they experience delusions and hallucinations similar to those of a mentally ill person. The alcoholic who suddenly does not obtain his alcohol may develop symptoms of acute alcohol withdrawal (delirium tremens). An alcoholic may experience hallucinations of hearing "voices" accusing him of unmentionable conduct. The mental deterioration of a chronic alcoholic must be treated in the same way psychoses characterized by the loss of intellectual capacity are treated. For further discussion, see page 289.

Itching

Itching is an uncomfortable sensation in the skin that creates the urge to rub or scratch the affected area. It may be limited to a small area, or it may be generalized. It is quite normal for various areas of the skin to itch mildly at times. Dryness of the skin caused by low humidity in the air or removal of the skin's oil by the excessive use of soap may cause itching. Itching commonly occurs in the latter part of pregnancy and at menopause.

Itching is the most frequent symptom of diseases of the skin, such as in certain allergies, in response to irritants (chemicals and drugs), and in emotional states, such as anxiety.

Itching may occur in certain systemic diseases, such as those affecting the liver or the bile passages (associated with jaundice), in diabetes, in some forms of kidney disease, and in certain cancers.

Itching is especially troublesome when it occurs in the region of the anus (pruritus ani). In addition to the general causes for itching elsewhere in the skin, itching at or near the anus may be caused by lack of cleanliness, by local infections, or by the presence of pinworms.

Jaundice

Jaundice occurs when bilirubin, a bile pigment, is deposited in certain tissues of the body, giving the skin, the mucous membranes, and the whites of the eyes a yellow color.

Bilirubin is a normal product released by the breakdown of hemoglobin, the protein pigment present in red blood cells. The average life of a red blood cell is about 120 days. As red blood cells reach this approximate age, they wear out and are destroyed by macrophages (large cells occurring in various tissues of the body, including the spleen). As the red blood cells are broken apart, the iron present in the hemoglobin molecules is salvaged and used again to manufacture new hemoglobin. Another part of the hemoglobin molecule is altered to form biliverdin and bilirubin, both of which happen to be colored substances.

An example of what happens to old red blood cells is seen on a small

scale when a person bruises himself. Immediately after the injury, the area turns "black and blue." The bruise fades to produce shades of green and yellow, resulting from the decomposition of hemoglobin to biliverdin and bilirubin.

Normally the bilirubin produced by the destruction of aging red blood cells is transported in the blood to the liver, where it becomes part of the bile. However, when bilirubin in the blood builds beyond normal levels, some of the pigment is deposited in the skin, and the person becomes yellow, or jaundiced. There are three common causes of jaundice.

Increased destruction of red blood cells. As already mentioned, when red blood cells break down so rapidly that the amount of bilirubin released exceeds the capacity of the liver to handle it, part of the pigment seeps into the spaces between the cells, causing the tissues to look yellow, or jaundiced. Examples include certain anemias (hemolytic), pneumococcal pneumonia, and, occasionally, malaria.

Liver disease. In certain liver diseases, the liver cannot dispose of the usual amount of bilirubin brought to it by the blood. As a result, the concentration of this pigment increases in the blood, causing jaundice. Viral hepatitis will cause this type of jaundice, as does cirrhosis of the liver.

Obstruction to the flow of bile. Possible causes for this type of jaundice are: (1) the occasional effect of certain drugs or hormones (including contraceptive pills) in constricting the small bile ducts within the liver; (2) a gallstone blocking the common bile duct (the duct leading from the liver to the intestine); and (3) a cancer in the head of the pancreas that obstructs the outflow of bile from the common bile duct into the duodenum. For further study of jaundice, see page 869.

Lump in the throat

This symptom is usually not the result of an actual disease, but the result of anxiety. The individual faces some unsolved problem, and the pent-up emotional tension causes him to be apprehensive about his health. He may be afraid that he will contract cancer of the throat or some other life-threatening disease. A lump in the throat may also follow the loss of a loved one or unresolved grief.

Nausea

Nausea is an unpleasant, uneasy sensation in the area of the stomach that often terminates in vomiting. It can be triggered by disorders of the middle ear, the digestive tract, and certain areas of the brain. For a detailed discussion, see under "vomiting," pages 419, 561.

Neck: stiffness

The common stiff neck occurs from sleeping in an awkward position or from exposure to cold. It is probably due to persistent muscular tension that reduces the blood supply to the involved muscles. An inflammation of the muscles (fibromyositis) may cause muscle pain in the neck, shoulder, and lower back. A more chronic form is torticollis (wryneck),

which may last more or less throughout life (see page 964).

Pain in the neck that interferes with the usual motions may occur when the lymph nodes become enlarged (lymphadenopathy). Stiffness and pain may be the result of arthritis or an injury involving the neck.

Extreme pain in the neck when the head is bent (flexed) forward may indicate an infection (meningitis) of the membranes covering the brain and spinal cord (meninges).

Neck: swellings

Swellings in the neck are commonly due to an enlargement of the lymph nodes, the thyroid gland, or the salivary glands. Congenital cysts and benign fatty tumors can also produce local enlargements.

Enlargement of the lymph nodes (lymphadenopathy) is often caused by infections in the mouth (tooth abscess), throat, and ear. A cancer in this area will also cause the nodes to enlarge. The thyroid gland may enlarge from an infection, certain types of goiter, or from a cancer of the gland itself. The salivary glands enlarge in mumps and in tumors of these glands.

Nervousness

Nervousness is an unpleasant feeling of restlessness, often coupled with anxiety, that distracts the attention and makes concentration difficult.

The causes of nervousness may be either psychological or physical. Psychological causes include emotional conflicts, lack of a goal in life, lack of a sense of belonging, thwarted ambition, and mental depression.

Nervousness may also be due to an overactive thyroid gland. It may accompany chronic systemic diseases such as tuberculosis, and it commonly occurs in dietary insufficiencies. Nervousness often occurs when the brain is damaged, as by encephalitis, brain tumor, or head injury. Heavy use of coffee and other caffeine-containing beverages, and other central nervous system stimulants (such as amphetamines) may cause nervousness.

Nose: obstruction by polyps and deviated septum

The passage of air through the nose is sometimes hindered by a benign tumor called a polyp—an overgrowth of the tissue of the lining membrane. It can be removed by a simple surgical procedure.

The septum, made partly of cartilage and partly of bone structure covered by mucous membrane, separates the nasal cavity into its right and left halves. When this septum is displaced to one side or the other, generally due to an injury (fracture), it may interfere with the passage of air. For further discussion, see page 908.

Offensive odors

Odors from the skin. Odor from a person's skin or clothing may result from lack of cleanliness, or it may be caused by a skin disease. Sweat—the fluid produced by the sweat glands—is normally odorless. Glands associated with the hair follicles in the skin produce oil. These two products, sweat and oil, particularly when produced in excess, undergo chemical changes as a result of bacterial action, and this mixture of decomposed sweat and oil produces the objectionable body odor.

A simple way to prevent this odor is to bathe frequently and change underclothing after each bath or shower. Antiperspirants, properly used, help to control excess sweating in the armpits. Deodorants serve only to cover up offensive odors and do not attack the problem at its source.

When diseases of the skin cause body odor, it is usually because the skin lesions have become secondarily infected. Obviously, removal of the odor requires proper treatment of the skin disease and infection.

Odors from the mouth and nose (bad breath—halitosis). The usual cause of "bad breath" is poor oral hygiene. When the mouth is not rinsed after each meal or the teeth brushed regularly, food fragments and tissue debris accumulate between the teeth and the crevices of the membrane that lines the mouth and covers the tongue. Bacterial action causes these particles to decompose, giving rise to an offensive odor. This situation also favors diseases of the gums and teeth, which are an added cause of bad breath. Unhealthy conditions in the nose and pharynx, such as sinusitis and tonsillitis, are yet other causes of bad breath.

The use of tobacco may taint the breath for many hours after the last cigar or cigarette, particularly when the smoker inhales.

An unpleasant odor originating in the lungs may be exhaled as "bad breath." This occurs in such diseases as bronchiectasis, lung abscess, or lung cancer, particularly when there is cough or expectoration. Volatile substances liberated into the lungs can produce characteristic odors, such as the odor of alcohol from liquor and the odor of onions and garlic from food. In certain systemic diseases, volatile substances may be eliminated through the lungs, as in one of the complications of diabetes (sweet, fruity odor of acetone), uremia (odor of urine), or in liver failure (musty odor).

Certain forms of indigestion can also cause "bad breath," especially when there is eructation (belching) or regurgitating of stomach contents.

Emotional states, such as anxiety, nervousness, or irritation, may aggravate the problem of "bad breath," presumably by reflex interference with the flow of saliva or by producing indigestion.

Odors from incontinence. The person who loses control of his bladder or rectum requires diligent nursing care to prevent offensive odors. This is often a problem with patients who have surgery involving the lower bowel.

Pain

Pain is doubtless the most common symptom that brings a patient to his physician or dentist. The type of pain, its location, whether the pain is continuous or intermittent, its time of onset, and its duration are all important indicators that your physician must evaluate in attempting to determine the cause and its subsequent treatment. A detailed discussion is found on page 1157.

Pallor

Paleness of the skin and membranes occurs whenever the blood fails to move briskly enough or when it carries less hemoglobin than normal. Blood with a low oxygen content permits the skin and membranes to appear pale, in contrast to bright red blood that has just picked up a fresh supply of oxygen from the lungs.

Because complexions vary, it is not always possible to judge whether a person is pale by merely looking at his skin. The membrane lining the eyelid (observed by pulling down the lower eyelid) serves as a better index of the true color of the blood than does the skin.

Temporary pallor may occur in intense emotional states (fear or anger) or when a person faints.

Pallor occurs in the various forms of anemia, as when blood is lost through hemorrhage, when the body is deficient in iron, when the production of red blood cells falls below normal, or when red blood cells are destroyed at an abnormally high rate. The type of anemia causing the pallor can only be determined by an examination of the patient's blood in a laboratory.

Pallor occurs in those heart and lung diseases in which there is an inadequate circulation of blood through the tissues. It occurs commonly in cancer and in certain systemic diseases, as scurvy and AIDS.

Palpitation

The heart is an active organ and dilates and constricts with each heartbeat. Normally a person is unaware that his heart is beating, much less that it is pumping vigorously within his chest.

Palpitation is awareness of the unduly rapid beating of the heart. This awareness of the heart's contraction is common among persons nervously inclined or those who are anxious about their health. People become aware that their heart is beating when it is irregular, unusually rapid, or extremely forceful. The diseases with which palpitation may be associated include anemia, disease of the thyroid gland, and certain disorders of the heart.

Of itself, palpitation is not an alarming symptom, but when it occurs other than during extreme exercise or intense emotion, the cause should be determined by a physician.

Paralysis

Paralysis is a condition in which a muscle or muscles do not respond to the nerve signal for contraction. The usual cause is damage to the nerve or nerve tract that normally activates the muscle or muscle group. The situation can be compared to an electric motor that no longer functions because the wire connecting it to the power source has been severed. Common instances of paralysis are as follows:

Paralysis from stroke (cerebrovascular accident). When the part of the brain that supplies a group of muscles is deprived of its blood supply, the muscles become paralyzed. Brain damage occurs when the artery supplying that area becomes obstructed (stroke) or ruptures (hemorrhage). The obstruction results either from a thrombus (local blood clot) or from an embolus (fragment of a blood clot carried in the blood). See also page 808.

Paralysis from injury. When the nerve impulses carried from the brain along the nerve pathways of the spinal cord are obstructed or when the nerves conveying these impulses to muscles are damaged or severed, the muscles thus supplied are paralyzed. See also pages 549, 1036.

Paralysis from cerebral palsy. This disorder stems from damage to the brain tissue at or before the time of birth and produces a weakness of the muscles in one or more parts of the body. Coupled with this weakness is spasticity (stiffness) and, often, involuntary jerking movements. The extent and severity of the body's involvement varies from case to case. The legs are usually more severely involved than the arms. Birth injury, prematurity, or congenital developmental defects are usually responsible. For further details, see page 427.

Paralysis in neuritis. There are many kinds of neuritis (inflammation of the nerves). Most nerves carry fibers that control muscle action as well as those that carry sensory impulses. Hence, when a nerve becomes inflamed, there will be a loss of control, or at least a weakness of the muscles that nerve supplies. In some cases of polyneuritis (inflammation of many nerves), the loss of muscle function may be so general

631

that the patient's life can be saved only by means of a mechanical respirator (to compensate for the paralysis of the breathing muscles). For further discussion, see page 1041.

Facial paralysis. This paralysis involves the nerve that supplies the muscles of facial expression. It occurs on just one side, permitting the mouth to be drawn and the eye to be opened on the good side, and making it difficult to draw the mouth or close the eye on the affected side. The onset is usually sudden, and generally there is improvement within two weeks. For further details, see page 1045.

Paralysis in hysteria. Paralysis of certain parts of the body is one of the common, though mysterious, manifestations of hysteria. The paralysis usually involves one whole arm and hand or one whole leg and foot, but does not correspond to the exact anatomical pattern of distribution of the nerves. For further information, see page 1055.

Rash (skin eruption)

A rash is a temporary eruption on the skin, a visible lesion characterized by redness or prominence, or both. Careful observation of the characteristics of a rash and the circumstances under which it appears will help to determine its cause (see also page 971).

Rashes from infectious diseases. The common communicable and infectious diseases in which rashes appear are chickenpox (varicella), German measles (rubella), measles (rubeola), Rocky Mountain spotted fever, scarlet fever, syphilis, typhoid fever, and typhus fever.

Rash of pellagra. Pellagra, a disease caused by a deficiency of niacin (vitamin B3), is common in some of the developing areas of the world. The rash resembles sunburn, appears in those areas exposed to light and sun, and, interestingly, is aggravated by exposure to sunlight.

Rash in diseases of the skin. As might be expected, many skin diseases are associated with some form of rash. For a discussion of their diagnosis and treatment, see page 972.

Rash from drugs. Redness (erythema) or itching (urticaria) may develop from sensitivity to a drug. Some drugs are more likely to cause an allergic response than others. There is also a great difference in the way different people react to a drug. One person will be sensitive to one drug and another person to an entirely different drug. Some reactions develop promptly, while others occur days later.

Urticarial reactions. Hives (urticaria) may be caused by many conditions: allergy to certain foods and to substances contacting the skin; sensitivity to injections containing protein; reaction to infection by parasitic worms and bites by lice, mosquitoes, or bedbugs; hormonal imbalances (as during menstruation or at the time of menopause); and instances of psychic stress or emotional unrest. For more a detailed discussion, see pages 471, 989.

Rash in infants. An infant's skin is tender and subject to rash from a variety of causes, among the more common being diaper rash, heat rash, infantile eczema, seborrheic eczema, rashes from contact with certain substances, and from infections to which infants are prone (measles, German measles, etc.). For further details, see pages 723-728.

Rectum: prolapse

Protrusion of the rectum lining occurs chiefly in infants or in elderly persons. The immediate cause is straining at stool, or, in the more serious cases, merely coughing or engaging in muscular exertion such as lifting. The condition becomes serious if the tissue is allowed to remain prolapsed long enough to be damaged because of inadequate blood supply.

The immediate remedy consists of returning the tissue to its normal internal location. It should first be lubricated thoroughly with mineral oil, vaseline, or mild soap, and then, using gradual pressure through a clean towel, the tissue should be pushed into the anus. The easiest way to do this with an infant is to lift the baby by its heels while making the replacement. In an adult, the replacement is best done with the person in the knee-chest position. If the replacement is not successful, consult a physician immediately.

Sleeplessness (insomnia)

Many people suffer from inability to sleep at appointed times or from a tendency to awaken before the desired number of hours of sleep have been obtained. In some, it is simply an inability to put aside the activities, and especially the concerns, of life, to allow body and mind to sink into deep, refreshing sleep. In others, the problem may stem from a more serious cause.

Sleep is an essential component of life, and physicians today are much more concerned with sleep loss than in previous years. Sleep-disturbance laboratories are now part of most large medical institutions, with the result that sleep disorders are much better understood. Medication to induce sleep is, at best, only of short-term benefit, and for most sufferers of insomnia, there are better and more physiological ways of handling the problem. For a full discussion, see page 57.

Sneezing

Sneezing is a natural reflex action designed to aid in expelling an irritant from the nasal passages. These irritants commonly consist of dust or powders. The membranes lining the nasal passages can also be irritated by anything that causes them to swell. The two most common causes of such sneezing are infection (such as the common cold) and allergy (sensitivity to certain foreign materials that enter the nostrils along with the air, as in hay fever). Chilling of the skin, especially of the lower extremities, can cause reflex congestion in the membranes of the nose and thus induce sneezing. For further information, see page 911.

Sore throat

Sore throat, an inflammation of the mucous membrane that lines the pharynx (back of the mouth), is a common disorder resulting from many causes. The throat may become sore from simply breathing

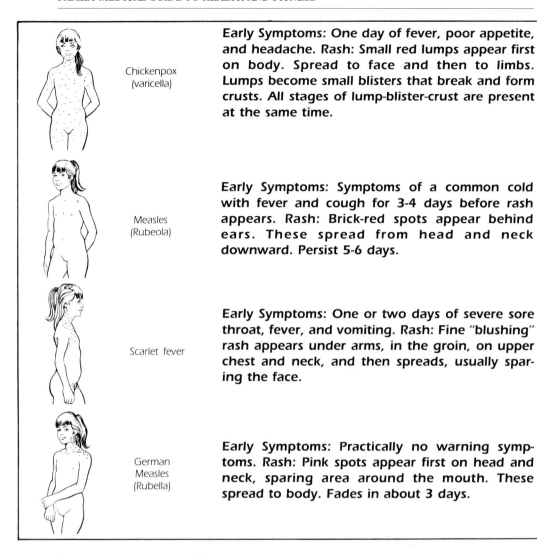

Chickenpox (varicella)

Early Symptoms: One day of fever, poor appetite, and headache. Rash: Small red lumps appear first on body. Spread to face and then to limbs. Lumps become small blisters that break and form crusts. All stages of lump-blister-crust are present at the same time.

Measles (Rubeola)

Early Symptoms: Symptoms of a common cold with fever and cough for 3-4 days before rash appears. Rash: Brick-red spots appear behind ears. These spread from head and neck downward. Persist 5-6 days.

Scarlet fever

Early Symptoms: One or two days of severe sore throat, fever, and vomiting. Rash: Fine "blushing" rash appears under arms, in the groin, on upper chest and neck, and then spreads, usually sparing the face.

German Measles (Rubella)

Early Symptoms: Practically no warning symptoms. Rash: Pink spots appear first on head and neck, sparing area around the mouth. These spread to body. Fades in about 3 days.

hot, dry air; from drinking irritating or excessively hot drinks; or from being exposed to tobacco smoke. However, infections, commonly from the streptococcus organism **(strep throat)** or a viral infection, such as the common cold, will produce the inflammation. For a full discussion, see page 912.

Speech disturbances

The use of language for transmitting ideas is one of the highest intellectual accomplishments of human beings. Understanding speech involves the ability to attach significance to symbols and to select the right symbols to express thoughts. This function, whether performed by speaking or writing, requires the integrated activity of many brain areas, as well as a high degree of muscle coordination.

Speech disturbances may result from disturbances of the speech area of the brain, faulty control of the speech organs, disorders of the larynx, and defects in the auxiliary organs of speech such as the lips and palate. For further details, see page 451.

Stupor

In stupor there is a reduction of alertness, a semiconsciousness from which the person can be partially aroused. Stupor can progress to coma, shock, or unconsciousness. It can be caused by drugs or epilepsy. In cases of mental illness, the term *stupor* describes a condition of reduced responsiveness, as in depression or dementia.

Swallowing difficulty (dysphagia)

Swallowing is a complicated function involving a complex coordination of muscles in the face, tongue, pharynx, and esophagus. These muscles are under the control of five pairs of nerves and the corresponding integration centers of the brain. Thus, a number of disorders can cause difficulty in swallowing. These include:

Foreign body within the esophagus. Large, irregular-shaped objects, if swallowed, may lodge in the back of the pharynx. Objects of the right shape and size to enter the upper part of the esophagus usually pass through its entire length. Those that become lodged usually do so in the upper part of the esophagus, which interferes with swallowing. An object with sharp edges is likely to injure the lining of the esophagus, causing symptoms that persist even after the object is removed. The re-moval of such a foreign object requires special equipment and the services of a specialist.

Corrosive injury and stricture of the esophagus. Swallowing a strong acid or alkali will cause serious injury to the lining of the esophagus. In the acute phase, the patient may have to be fed by vein or into the stomach by a tube passed through the abdominal wall. As the injury heals, there is gradual shrinking of the tissues, with scar formation and narrowing of the lumen of the esophagus. Thus, swallowing food, or even liquid, may become difficult or impossible. Special procedures are used to enlarge the esophagus, or surgical repair may be required.

Cancer of the esophagus. Cancer of the esophagus occurs most commonly in the lower third (nearer to the stomach than to the throat). Difficulty in swallowing is usually the first symptom to develop. The sooner this is reported to a physician, the better.

Paralysis of the swallowing muscles. This disorder takes one of two forms:

1. Cardiospasm, or achalasia. In this condition, the waves of contraction that normally push the food or drink through the esophagus stop short of the stomach, and the food or drink accumulates in the lower part of the esophagus, causing it to stretch. Besides difficulty in swallowing, there may be pain behind the breastbone after eating. Emotional stress often aggravates the problem.

2. Bulbar palsy. In bulbar palsy the nerve cells in the brain stem that normally control swallowing are damaged. This condition can be

635

caused by an inadequate blood supply (atherosclerosis) or by toxins, such as those produced in diphtheria.

Pressure against the esophagus. Pressure on the esophagus can be produced by an aneurysm of the aorta, a tumor, or a diaphragmatic hernia.

Esophagitis. Inflammation of the tissues of the esophagus may make swallowing painful.

Lesions of related structures. Conditions in the mouth, pharynx, or larynx may interfere with swallowing, either because they are painful or because they interfere in a mechanical way. These include cancer of the tongue, cleft palate, inflammation of the lining of the mouth or pharynx (stomatitis or pharyngitis), and cancer of the larynx.

Emotional conditions. Fear or acute anxiety may cause a person to "feel" a lump in the throat that makes swallowing difficult. A related condition, called globus hystericus, occurs under conditions of emotional conflict and makes it difficult for a person to initiate swallowing.

Tensions: emotional

Emotional tensions occur in persons who feel ill at ease or baffled by problems that seem too difficult to solve. In some cases the person knows, on the intellectual level, what to do, but is deterred by his emotions (fear, love, hate) from doing anything about it. Sometimes, moving in the sensible direction would require the individual to forfeit some cherished desire, so emotional pressures build up while the solution to the problem is delayed. Emotional tensions cause many functional symptoms.

The tongue: its appearance

One symptom of illness is a white coating on the tongue. The generally accepted view is that this coat is formed from dying cells on the tongue's surface that have dehydrated and turned white. The thickness of the coat depends on the rate at which new cells are produced and dead ones are worn off. Talking and eating erode these superficial cells. Conditions that slow the production of cells leave the tongue looking clean. If talking and eating are reduced, as happens when a person is sick, the coat will be thick.

Thus, the appearance of the tongue may vary according to the condition of a person's general health. In simple anemia, the tongue appears pale and small; in pernicious anemia, it appears beefy red, sore, and smooth. With a niacin (vitamin B3) deficiency (pellagra) the tongue looks black, while in riboflavin deficiency it has a magenta cast. Generally, in multiple vitamin deficiencies (from a poor diet), the tongue is beefy red, sore, and without a coat. In chronic vitamin deficiencies and in chronic iron deficiency, the tongue may appear smooth. When certain anticancer agents (including vitamin antagonists) are being administered, the tongue will appear small and smooth. People who use alcohol often have a heavily coated tongue.

Tremors

A tremor is a repetitious, involuntary shaking movement produced by the alternate contraction of opposing groups of muscles. Characteristic tremors, which occur in several forms of disease, usually disappear during sleep.

Parkinsonism (paralysis agitans) is a slow-motion tremor, most noticeable when the muscles are otherwise at rest. This condition involves the fingers (with a "pill-rolling" gesture), the forearms, the head, and the tongue. Multiple sclerosis is characterized by a tremor that increases in the part of the body under immediate use. Tremor appears in many cases of advanced atherosclerosis of the brain vessels, as well as in some brain tumors and brain abscesses.

A fine, rapid tremor of the fingers is present in many cases of overactivity of the thyroid gland. Tremor is also common in alcoholics and is sometimes seen in the hands of those who use large quantities of caffeine (from coffee, tea, cola drinks, and mate [mah-teh]). An overdose of certain drugs may cause tremor. Tremor ("the shakes") is also a typical response to extremely low blood sugar (hypoglycemia), as when a diabetic has taken more insulin than needed. Tremor may develop in certain functional disorders, as in anxiety states and hysteria.

Elderly persons sometimes develop a mild tremor, often involving just the head, which persists during most of their waking hours. This tremor has no particular significance except that it is a nuisance.

Ulcers

An ulcer is an open lesion in which there is a gradual loss of substance due to the disintegration and death of the skin tissue or mucous membrane. The types and forms of ulcers are many. For details, see under "ulcer," pages 855, 975, 986.

Unconsciousness

Unconsciousness, a state in which the mind is unresponsive to the impressions made by the senses, has many causes. Some are serious ailments that require proper treatment if the person's life is to be saved.

Unconsciousness from taking alcohol, drugs, or poisons. Intoxication by alcohol is the most common cause of unconsciousness among patients admitted to the hospital.

Overdose of a number of drugs will also cause unconsciousness. These include sedatives, tranquilizers, barbiturates, and narcotics (such as heroin and morphine).

Among the poisons that produce unconsciousness, carbon monoxide gas (from automobile exhaust, and fumes from improperly ventilated heating stoves) is probably the most common.

If an unconscious person has been working with an insecticide or a weed killer, poisoning by such chemicals should be suspected. For first-aid treatment of various kinds of poisoning, see page 520.

Unconsciousness due to head injury. Unconsciousness is common among victims of severe head injury, such as from a blow, a fall, or an automobile accident. The unconsciousness that immediately follows a head injury results from damage to the brain tissue. The extent of the damage can be measured, roughly, by the length of time the victim remains unconscious.

In some cases of severe head injury with damage to the blood vessels and the membranes surrounding the brain, the person may regain consciousness after the injury, only to become unconscious again several hours later. This lapse of consciousness after a lucid interval indicates increasing pressure within the skull, caused by an expanding blood clot. It threatens the victim's life and requires prompt treatment by surgical intervention.

Unconsciousness caused by diseased blood vessels. The blood vessels that supply the brain may become weakened because of atherosclerosis. These weakened vessels may rupture, producing a hemorrhage in the brain, or they may become plugged by a thrombus (clot) forming at the site where the vessel is diseased. A piece of blood clot carried by the blood may also block one of the vessels supplying the brain. An individual so injured suffers a stroke.

Unconsciousness in epilepsy. Unconsciousness occurs as a part of the usual seizure ("fit") of epilepsy. The duration of the unconsciousness varies from a few seconds, in milder cases, to a few hours.

Unconsciousness in diabetes and other metabolic disorders. A number of metabolic disorders can result in unconsciousness. Among these are diabetic coma, hypoglycemic coma, uremic coma, and hepatic coma.

1. In so-called "diabetic coma" the body's system for regulating sugar in the blood malfunctions, causing an overabundant supply. Toxic products build up in the blood, causing unconsciousness. The breath of a diabetic-coma victim has a "fruity" odor (acetone breath).

2. Hypoglycemic coma may occur when the blood sugar falls below the level necessary to maintain the brain's normal activity. This may happen when a diabetic receives too much insulin or too large a dose of an oral antibiotic agent.

Diabetic coma and hypoglycemic coma in a diabetic must be differentiated, as the emergency treatment in the two situations is different: administration of insulin in diabetic coma and administration of sugar (or intravenous glucose) in hypoglycemic coma. For details, see page 1017.

3. Uremic coma develops when the diseased kidneys are unable to eliminate waste products from the blood. As their concentration rises, unconsciousness ensues.

4. Hepatic coma may develop in a person with liver disease (cirrhosis or hepatitis) as a result of the accumulation in the blood of ammonia and related substances normally detoxified by the liver.

Unconsciousness associated with brain tumor or abscess. The onset of unconsciousness with brain tumor or brain abscess is usually gradual, but may be sudden when complications develop. The unconsciousness may not be associated with paralysis.

Unconsciousness in meningitis and encephalitis. The usual symptoms and signs in meningitis are severe headache and rigidity of the neck, followed by unconsciousness. Loss of consciousness is particularly characteristic of the "lethargic" type of encephalitis.

Unconsciousness caused by reduced blood supply to the brain (fainting). Many circumstances, some emotional and some physical, can deprive the brain of sufficient blood, causing unconsciousness. For more information, see page 803.

Unconsciousness in hysteria. Persons with hysteria may lose consciousness as a functional response to some emotional stress.

For treatment of the various forms of unconsciousness, consult the general index.

Vomiting

Vomiting is usually preceded by nausea. Vomiting is controlled by a nerve center in the brain stem. Nerve impulses from the center cause a vigorous contraction of the abdominal muscles and the diaphragm, with a relaxation of the muscle fibers at the junction of the esophagus and stomach. This allows the stomach contents to be ejected through the esophagus and mouth. There are many causes for nausea and vomiting.

1. Psychic reactions. Emotional shock (as sudden bad news), pain, fright, grief, unpleasant tastes, and offensive smells may trigger the vomiting mechanism.

2. Drugs. Some drugs produce vomiting by irritating the lining of the digestive tract. Others directly stimulate the vomiting center of the brain stem.

3. Poisons. Nausea and vomiting are prominent symptoms in most cases of poisoning, either in food poisoning or in poisoning by chemical substances (other than those in offensive food).

4. Disturbances of the abdominal organs. Irritation of the digestive organs, intestinal infections, intestinal obstruction, cancer of the digestive organs, inflammation of the appendix or gallbladder, and gallstones commonly cause nausea and vomiting.

5. Toxicity. Nausea and vomiting occur in uremia, severe liver disease, and some types of cancer, presumably because of the toxicity these conditions produce.

6. Increased intracranial pressure. Increased pressure within the skull resulting from brain injury, brain tumor, brain abscess, and hemorrhage in or around the brain may cause nausea or vomiting, or vomiting without nausea, probably because of interference with the blood supply to the vomiting center.

7. Excessive stimulation of the semicircular canals. Dizziness or excess stimulation of the sense organs for equilibrium (as in motion sickness) typically cause nausea and vomiting by reflex influence on the vomiting center.

8. Pregnancy. It is typical for an expectant mother, in the early weeks of her pregnancy, to experience nausea and vomiting.

For details on the various causes of vomiting, see the general index under specific items.

Weakness

Weakness involves an actual loss (complete or partial) of the ability to

639

perform in a normal manner.

Gradually progressive weakness may occur in the declining years of old age, particularly when the elderly person has some chronic illness. It occurs to persons of any age who have been long confined to bed. Even after recovery from an illness, the person will go through a period of getting his strength back, during which he must increase his activities gradually.

General weakness typically occurs in illnesses associated with fever, and in systemic diseases such as AIDS, tuberculosis, and malaria.

Weakness is common in disorders in which there is insufficient oxygen available to the tissues, as in anemia and certain forms of congenital heart disease. It is seen in starvation, when insufficient food energy is available to nourish the body and provide energy. In anorexia nervosa, a disease in which the person has a compulsion to avoid gaining weight, there is weakness because of inadequate food intake.

Weakness accompanies such disorders of the endocrine organs as adrenal insufficiency, pituitary insufficiency, thyroid disease in which there is either hypo- or hyperfunction of the thyroid gland, diabetes, and hyperparathyroidism.

Weakness is common in viral hepatitis and certain other liver disorders. It occurs in chronic kidney failure, in which the kidneys can no longer eliminate the accumulating metabolic wastes.

Weakness occurs in those diseases of the nervous system in which the nerve centers controlling the actions of the muscles or of the nerve fibers leading to these muscles are injured or destroyed. Such conditions as stroke, tumors of the brain and other nerve tissues, and poliomyelitis cause weakness and even paralysis of the muscles that would normally be controlled by the affected nerve structures. Weakness occurs in such muscular disorders as myasthenia gravis, myotonia, and progressive muscular dystrophy.

Weakness even occurs in cases of chronic alcoholism or in persons who use certain drugs for long periods of time (such as bromides and barbiturates).

See also "energy, loss of," page 622.

Weight: sudden change

A sudden change in weight, either a loss or gain, is a warning that a physician should investigate.

Weight loss. Loss of weight, other than when a person is attempting to lose weight, is cause for alarm. Loss of weight occurs in acute diseases with fever or in any illness in which food intake is sharply curtailed. Unexpected weight loss is one of the signs of a possible cancer.

Loss of weight in newborn babies may be due to pyloric obstruction, in which little or no food enters the small intestine. Weight loss is seen in hyperthyroidism, in diabetes if poorly controlled, in Hodgkin's disease, and in infection with hookworm.

Weight gain. A sudden gain in weight is usually due to a rapid accumulation of water in the body tissues and may occur with congestive heart failure, cirrhosis of the liver, acute kidney failure, and certain malignancies.

Ready diagnosis of common problems

The flowcharts on the pages that follow will help you to quickly diagnose some of the more common symptoms that people complain about. All of the questions can be answered by Yes or No. After you have answered a question, follow its answer to the next question and the next, till you reach the "end of the line," at which point recommendations will be made for treatment. You will be advised if you should consult a physician. Where the symptom suggests a medical emergency if it is not treated immediately, the box around the recommendation will be red.

The following example shows how to use these flowcharts. If your back pain is severe, you would answer Yes and follow the line to the box that asks, "Did it come on suddenly?" The green lines are one possible series of answers that might be given, ending in the recommendation to "consult your physician immediately." Since this is a medical emergency, the box around this recommendation is printed in red.

Back pain

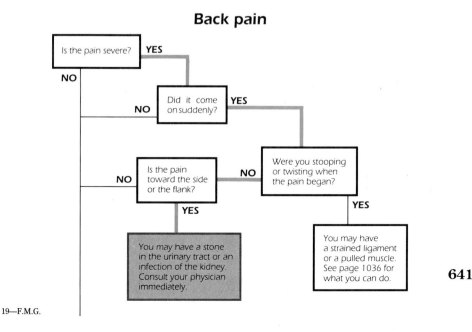

641

Back pain

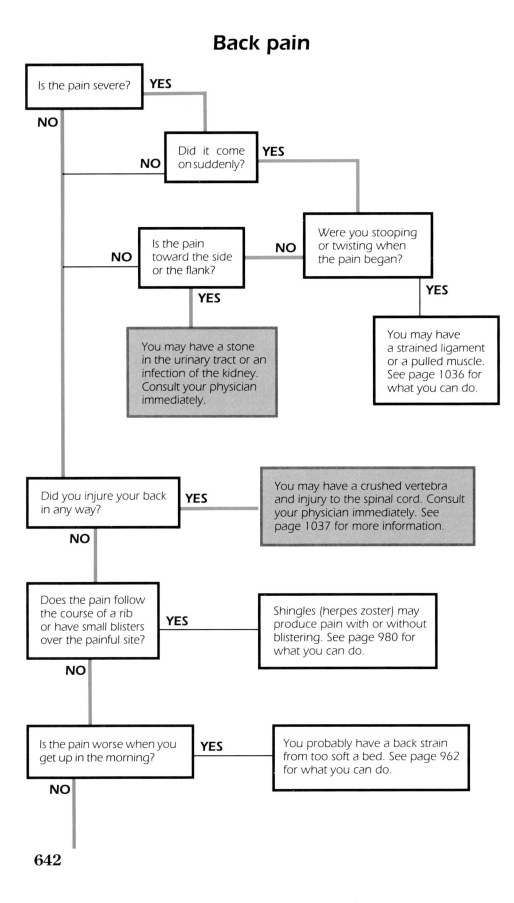

Is the pain severe?

YES → Did it come on suddenly?

NO →

Did it come on suddenly?

NO → Is the pain toward the side or the flank?

YES → Were you stooping or twisting when the pain began?

Is the pain toward the side or the flank?

NO → Were you stooping or twisting when the pain began?

YES →

You may have a stone in the urinary tract or an infection of the kidney. Consult your physician immediately.

Were you stooping or twisting when the pain began?

YES →

You may have a strained ligament or a pulled muscle. See page 1036 for what you can do.

Did you injure your back in any way?

YES →

You may have a crushed vertebra and injury to the spinal cord. Consult your physician immediately. See page 1037 for more information.

NO →

Does the pain follow the course of a rib or have small blisters over the painful site?

YES →

Shingles (herpes zoster) may produce pain with or without blistering. See page 980 for what you can do.

NO →

Is the pain worse when you get up in the morning?

YES →

You probably have a back strain from too soft a bed. See page 962 for what you can do.

NO

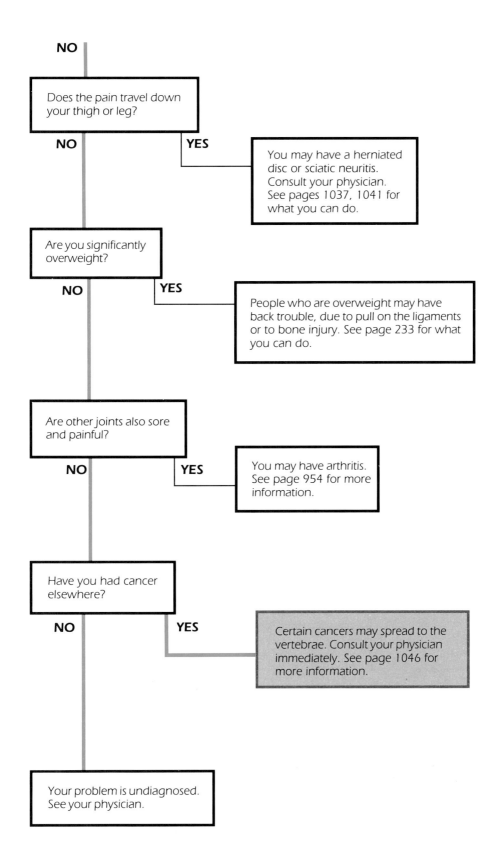

NO

Does the pain travel down your thigh or leg?

NO   **YES**

You may have a herniated disc or sciatic neuritis. Consult your physician. See pages 1037, 1041 for what you can do.

Are you significantly overweight?

NO   **YES**

People who are overweight may have back trouble, due to pull on the ligaments or to bone injury. See page 233 for what you can do.

Are other joints also sore and painful?

NO   **YES**

You may have arthritis. See page 954 for more information.

Have you had cancer elsewhere?

NO   **YES**

Certain cancers may spread to the vertebrae. Consult your physician immediately. See page 1046 for more information.

Your problem is undiagnosed. See your physician.

Breathing difficulty

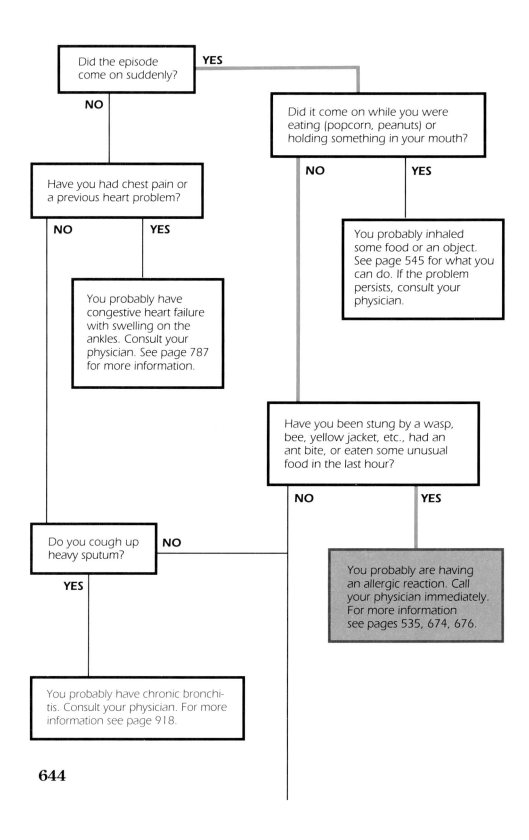

Did the episode come on suddenly?

YES

NO

Did it come on while you were eating (popcorn, peanuts) or holding something in your mouth?

NO

YES

Have you had chest pain or a previous heart problem?

NO

YES

You probably inhaled some food or an object. See page 545 for what you can do. If the problem persists, consult your physician.

You probably have congestive heart failure with swelling on the ankles. Consult your physician. See page 787 for more information.

Have you been stung by a wasp, bee, yellow jacket, etc., had an ant bite, or eaten some unusual food in the last hour?

NO

YES

Do you cough up heavy sputum?

NO

YES

You probably are having an allergic reaction. Call your physician immediately. For more information see pages 535, 674, 676.

You probably have chronic bronchitis. Consult your physician. For more information see page 918.

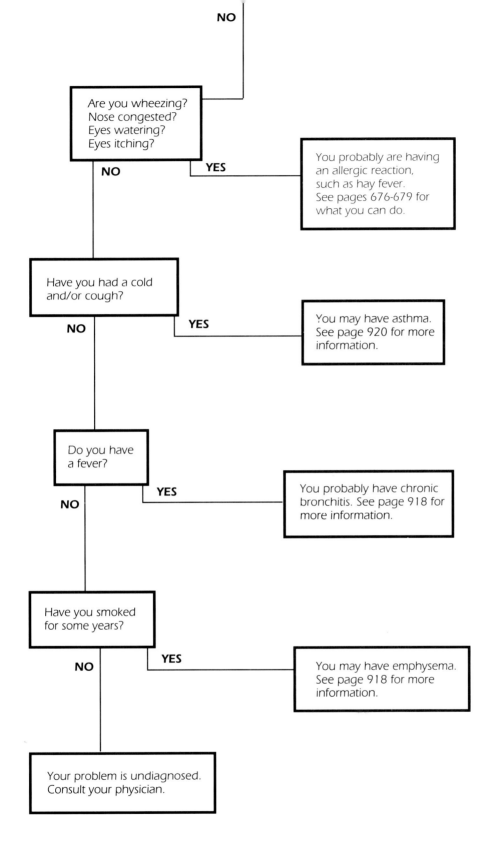

NO

Are you wheezing?
Nose congested?
Eyes watering?
Eyes itching?

NO   **YES**

You probably are having
an allergic reaction,
such as hay fever.
See pages 676-679 for
what you can do.

Have you had a cold
and/or cough?

NO   **YES**

You may have asthma.
See page 920 for more
information.

Do you have
a fever?

NO   **YES**

You probably have chronic
bronchitis. See page 918 for
more information.

Have you smoked
for some years?

NO   **YES**

You may have emphysema.
See page 918 for more
information.

Your problem is undiagnosed.
Consult your physician.

Chest pain

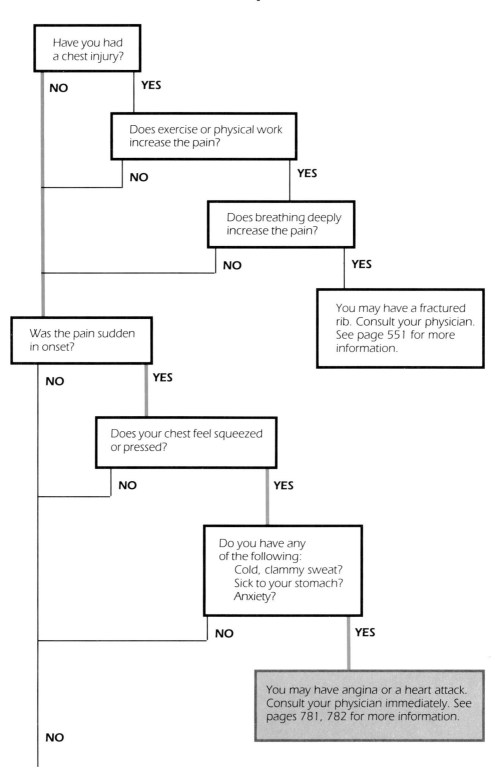

Have you had a chest injury?

NO / **YES**

Does exercise or physical work increase the pain?

NO / **YES**

Does breathing deeply increase the pain?

NO / **YES**

You may have a fractured rib. Consult your physician. See page 551 for more information.

Was the pain sudden in onset?

NO / **YES**

Does your chest feel squeezed or pressed?

NO / **YES**

Do you have any of the following:
Cold, clammy sweat?
Sick to your stomach?
Anxiety?

NO / **YES**

You may have angina or a heart attack. Consult your physician immediately. See pages 781, 782 for more information.

NO

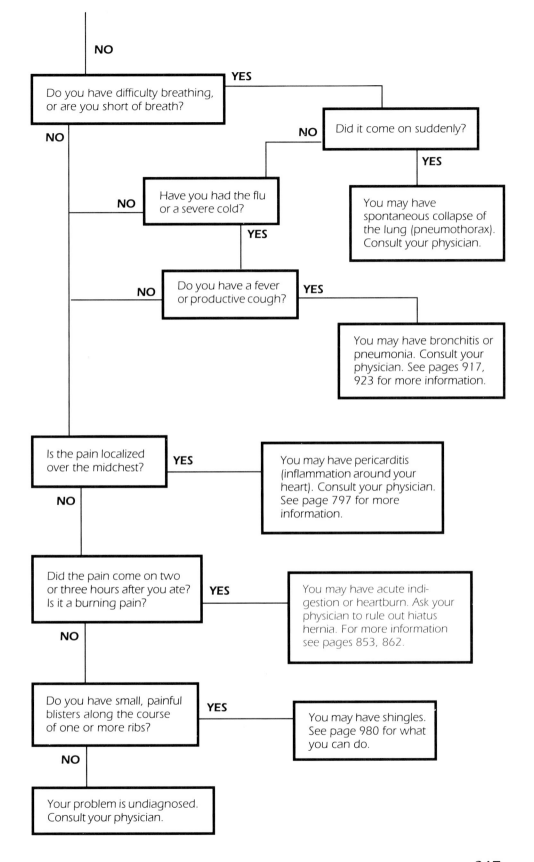

NO

Do you have difficulty breathing, or are you short of breath?

YES

NO

Did it come on suddenly?

YES

You may have spontaneous collapse of the lung (pneumothorax). Consult your physician.

NO

Have you had the flu or a severe cold?

YES

NO

Do you have a fever or productive cough?

YES

You may have bronchitis or pneumonia. Consult your physician. See pages 917, 923 for more information.

Is the pain localized over the midchest?

YES

You may have pericarditis (inflammation around your heart). Consult your physician. See page 797 for more information.

NO

Did the pain come on two or three hours after you ate? Is it a burning pain?

YES

You may have acute indigestion or heartburn. Ask your physician to rule out hiatus hernia. For more information see pages 853, 862.

NO

Do you have small, painful blisters along the course of one or more ribs?

YES

You may have shingles. See page 980 for what you can do.

NO

Your problem is undiagnosed. Consult your physician.

647

Cough

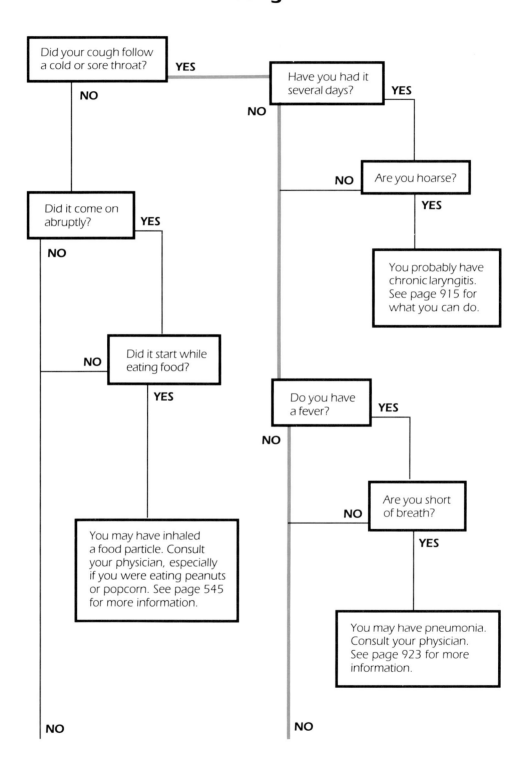

Did your cough follow a cold or sore throat?

YES → Have you had it several days?

NO ↓

Did it come on abruptly?

Have you had it several days?

YES → Are you hoarse?

NO ↓

Are you hoarse?

NO →

YES ↓

You probably have chronic laryngitis. See page 915 for what you can do.

Did it come on abruptly?

YES → Did it start while eating food?

NO ↓

Did it start while eating food?

NO →

YES ↓

You may have inhaled a food particle. Consult your physician, especially if you were eating peanuts or popcorn. See page 545 for more information.

Do you have a fever?

YES → Are you short of breath?

NO ↓

Are you short of breath?

NO →

YES ↓

You may have pneumonia. Consult your physician. See page 923 for more information.

NO

NO

648

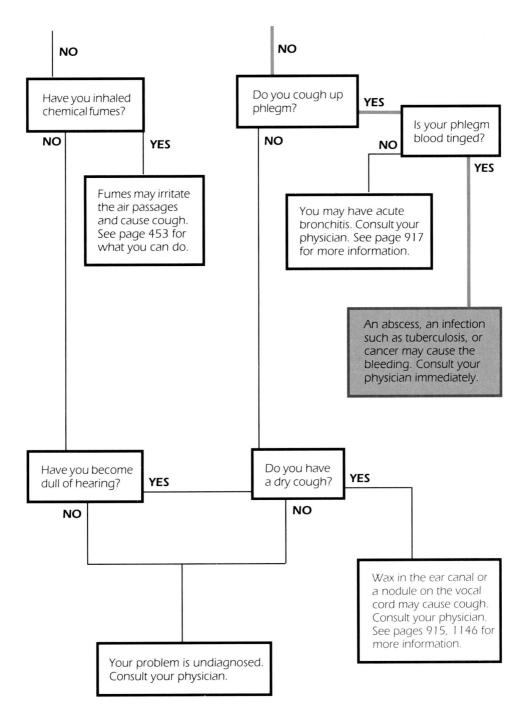

NO

Have you inhaled chemical fumes?

NO   YES

Fumes may irritate the air passages and cause cough. See page 453 for what you can do.

NO

Do you cough up phlegm?   YES

Is your phlegm blood tinged?

NO   NO

YES

You may have acute bronchitis. Consult your physician. See page 917 for more information.

An abscess, an infection such as tuberculosis, or cancer may cause the bleeding. Consult your physician immediately.

Have you become dull of hearing?   YES

NO

Do you have a dry cough?   YES

NO

Wax in the ear canal or a nodule on the vocal cord may cause cough. Consult your physician. See pages 915, 1146 for more information.

Your problem is undiagnosed. Consult your physician.

649

Earache

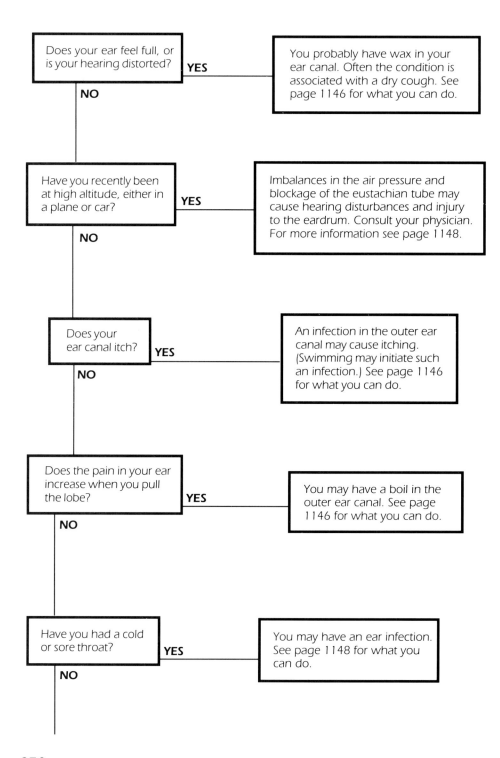

Does your ear feel full, or is your hearing distorted?

YES → You probably have wax in your ear canal. Often the condition is associated with a dry cough. See page 1146 for what you can do.

NO

Have you recently been at high altitude, either in a plane or car?

YES → Imbalances in the air pressure and blockage of the eustachian tube may cause hearing disturbances and injury to the eardrum. Consult your physician. For more information see page 1148.

NO

Does your ear canal itch?

YES → An infection in the outer ear canal may cause itching. (Swimming may initiate such an infection.) See page 1146 for what you can do.

NO

Does the pain in your ear increase when you pull the lobe?

YES → You may have a boil in the outer ear canal. See page 1146 for what you can do.

NO

Have you had a cold or sore throat?

YES → You may have an ear infection. See page 1148 for what you can do.

NO

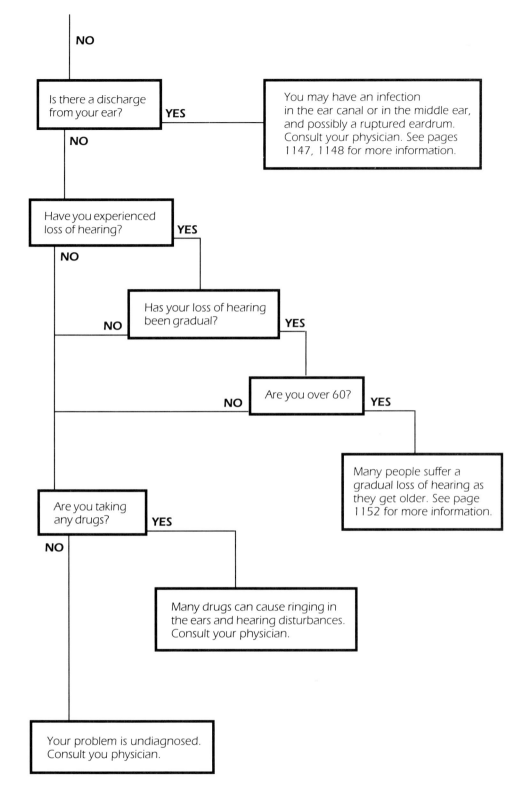

NO

Is there a discharge from your ear?

YES — You may have an infection in the ear canal or in the middle ear, and possibly a ruptured eardrum. Consult your physician. See pages 1147, 1148 for more information.

NO

Have you experienced loss of hearing?

YES

NO

Has your loss of hearing been gradual?

YES

Are you over 60?

NO

YES — Many people suffer a gradual loss of hearing as they get older. See page 1152 for more information.

Are you taking any drugs?

YES — Many drugs can cause ringing in the ears and hearing disturbances. Consult your physician.

NO

Your problem is undiagnosed. Consult you physician.

Eye problems

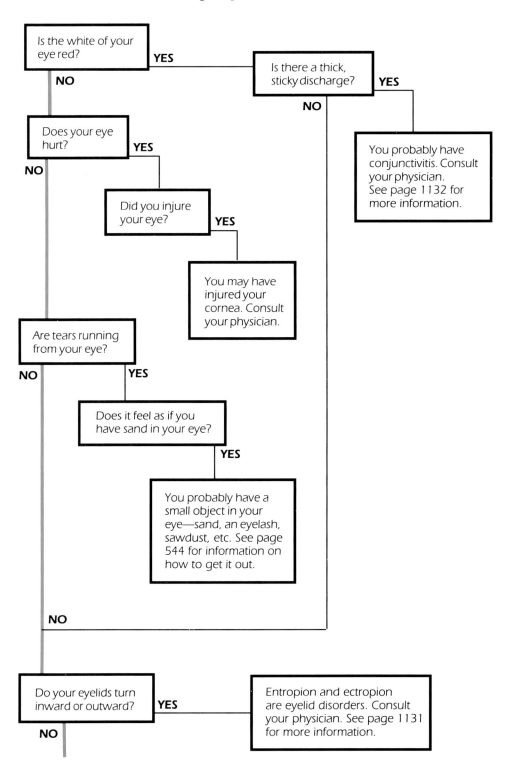

Is the white of your eye red?

YES → Is there a thick, sticky discharge?

YES → You probably have conjunctivitis. Consult your physician. See page 1132 for more information.

NO

NO ↓

Does your eye hurt?

YES → Did you injure your eye?

YES → You may have injured your cornea. Consult your physician.

NO

Are tears running from your eye?

YES → Does it feel as if you have sand in your eye?

YES → You probably have a small object in your eye—sand, an eyelash, sawdust, etc. See page 544 for information on how to get it out.

NO

Do your eyelids turn inward or outward?

YES → Entropion and ectropion are eyelid disorders. Consult your physician. See page 1131 for more information.

NO

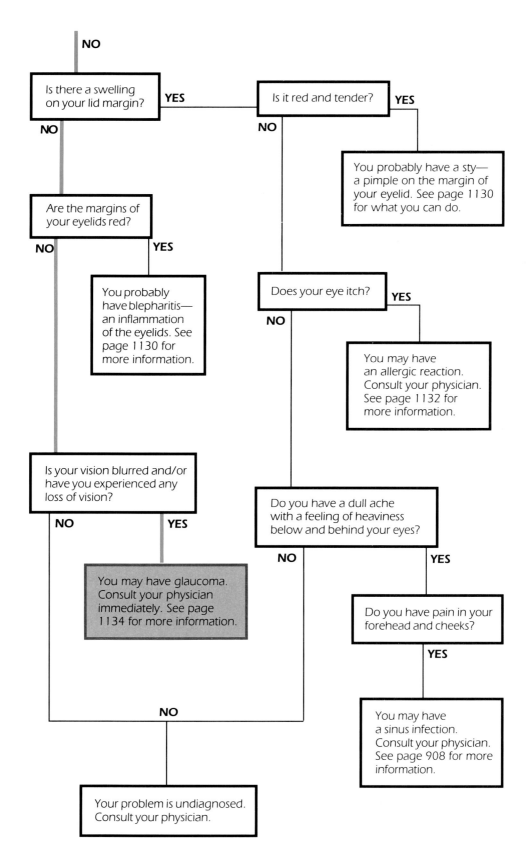

NO

Is there a swelling on your lid margin?

YES → Is it red and tender?

YES

You probably have a sty—a pimple on the margin of your eyelid. See page 1130 for what you can do.

NO

Are the margins of your eyelids red?

NO

YES

You probably have blepharitis—an inflammation of the eyelids. See page 1130 for more information.

NO

Does your eye itch?

YES

You may have an allergic reaction. Consult your physician. See page 1132 for more information.

NO

Is your vision blurred and/or have you experienced any loss of vision?

NO

YES

You may have glaucoma. Consult your physician immediately. See page 1134 for more information.

Do you have a dull ache with a feeling of heaviness below and behind your eyes?

NO

YES

Do you have pain in your forehead and cheeks?

YES

You may have a sinus infection. Consult your physician. See page 908 for more information.

NO

Your problem is undiagnosed. Consult your physician.

Fever (Adult)

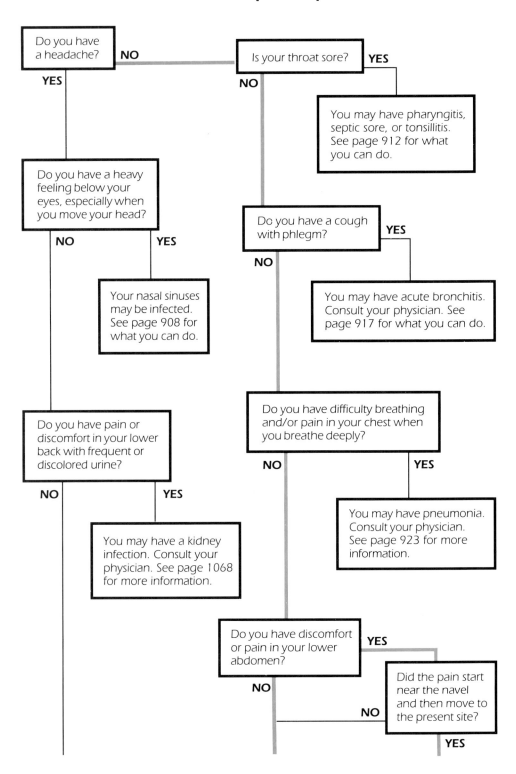

Do you have a headache?

NO — Is your throat sore? **YES**

YES

NO

You may have pharyngitis, septic sore, or tonsillitis. See page 912 for what you can do.

Do you have a heavy feeling below your eyes, especially when you move your head?

NO   **YES**

Your nasal sinuses may be infected. See page 908 for what you can do.

Do you have a cough with phlegm? **YES**

NO

You may have acute bronchitis. Consult your physician. See page 917 for what you can do.

Do you have pain or discomfort in your lower back with frequent or discolored urine?

NO   **YES**

You may have a kidney infection. Consult your physician. See page 1068 for more information.

Do you have difficulty breathing and/or pain in your chest when you breathe deeply?

NO   **YES**

You may have pneumonia. Consult your physician. See page 923 for more information.

Do you have discomfort or pain in your lower abdomen? **YES**

NO

Did the pain start near the navel and then move to the present site?

NO

YES

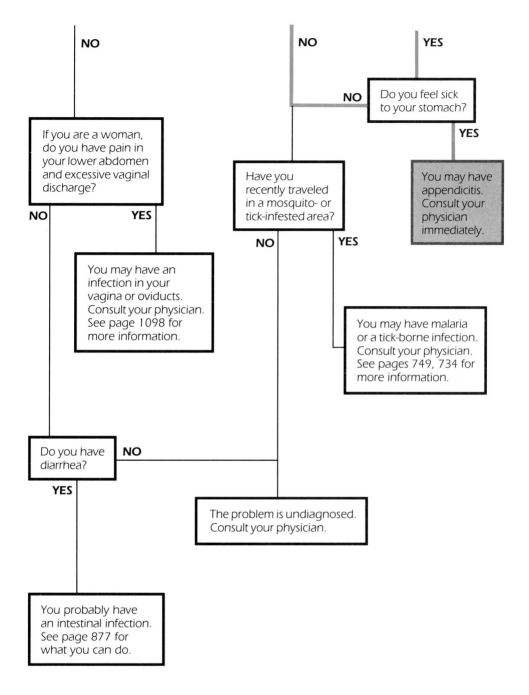

NO

NO   **YES**

If you are a woman, do you have pain in your lower abdomen and excessive vaginal discharge?

NO   Do you feel sick to your stomach?

NO   **YES**   **YES**

Have you recently traveled in a mosquito- or tick-infested area?

NO   **YES**

You may have appendicitis. Consult your physician immediately.

You may have an infection in your vagina or oviducts. Consult your physician. See page 1098 for more information.

You may have malaria or a tick-borne infection. Consult your physician. See pages 749, 734 for more information.

Do you have diarrhea?   **NO**

YES

The problem is undiagnosed. Consult your physician.

You probably have an intestinal infection. See page 877 for what you can do.

Fever (Infant or child)

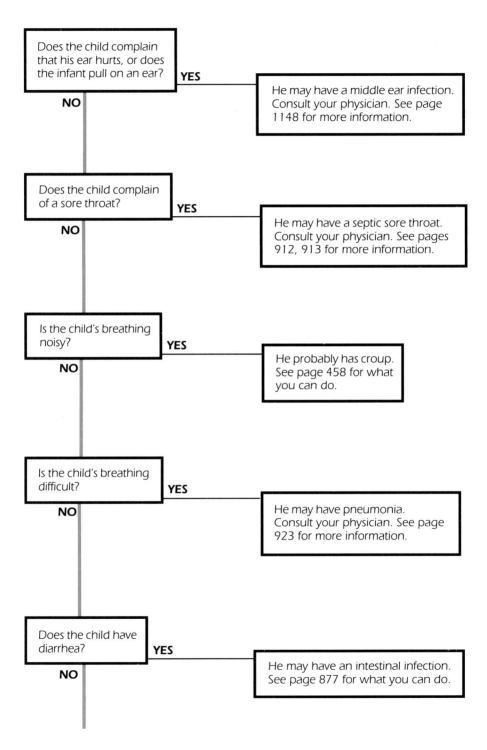

Does the child complain that his ear hurts, or does the infant pull on an ear?

YES — He may have a middle ear infection. Consult your physician. See page 1148 for more information.

NO

Does the child complain of a sore throat?

YES — He may have a septic sore throat. Consult your physician. See pages 912, 913 for more information.

NO

Is the child's breathing noisy?

YES — He probably has croup. See page 458 for what you can do.

NO

Is the child's breathing difficult?

YES — He may have pneumonia. Consult your physician. See page 923 for more information.

NO

Does the child have diarrhea?

YES — He may have an intestinal infection. See page 877 for what you can do.

NO

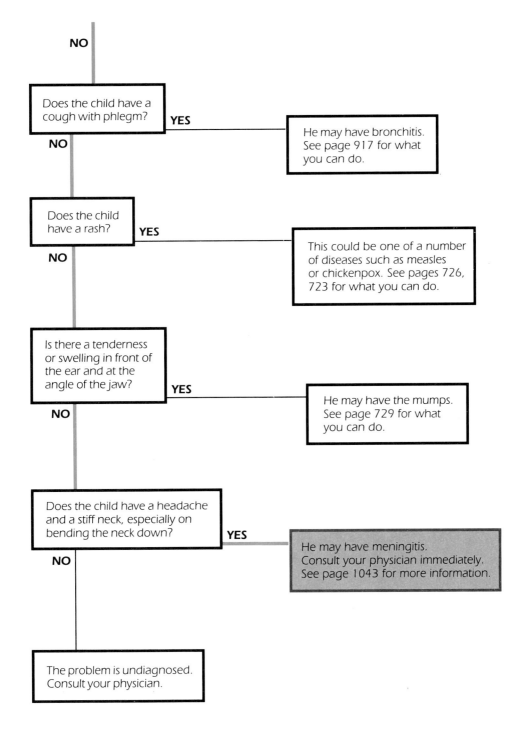

NO

Does the child have a cough with phlegm?

YES

He may have bronchitis. See page 917 for what you can do.

NO

Does the child have a rash?

YES

This could be one of a number of diseases such as measles or chickenpox. See pages 726, 723 for what you can do.

NO

Is there a tenderness or swelling in front of the ear and at the angle of the jaw?

YES

He may have the mumps. See page 729 for what you can do.

NO

Does the child have a headache and a stiff neck, especially on bending the neck down?

YES

He may have meningitis. Consult your physician immediately. See page 1043 for more information.

NO

The problem is undiagnosed. Consult your physician.

20—F.M.G.

Headache

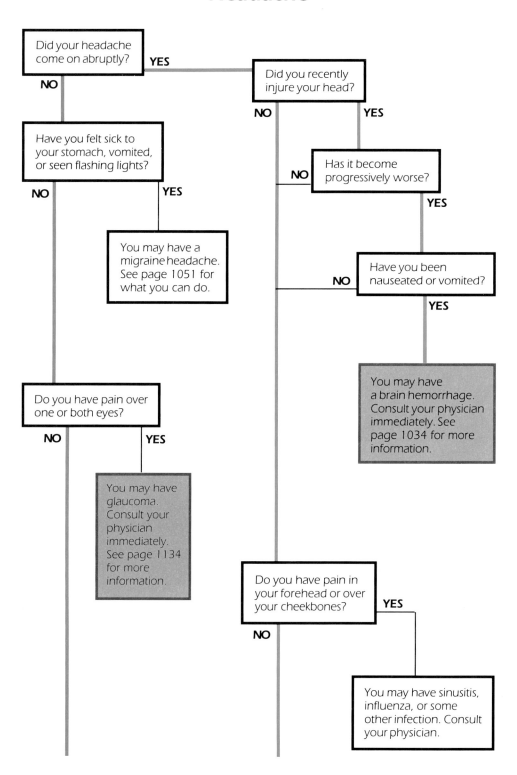

Did your headache come on abruptly?

NO / **YES**

Did you recently injure your head?

NO / **YES**

Have you felt sick to your stomach, vomited, or seen flashing lights?

NO / **YES**

Has it become progressively worse?

NO / **YES**

You may have a migraine headache. See page 1051 for what you can do.

Have you been nauseated or vomited?

NO / **YES**

You may have a brain hemorrhage. Consult your physician immediately. See page 1034 for more information.

Do you have pain over one or both eyes?

NO / **YES**

You may have glaucoma. Consult your physician immediately. See page 1134 for more information.

Do you have pain in your forehead or over your cheekbones?

NO / **YES**

You may have sinusitis, influenza, or some other infection. Consult your physician.

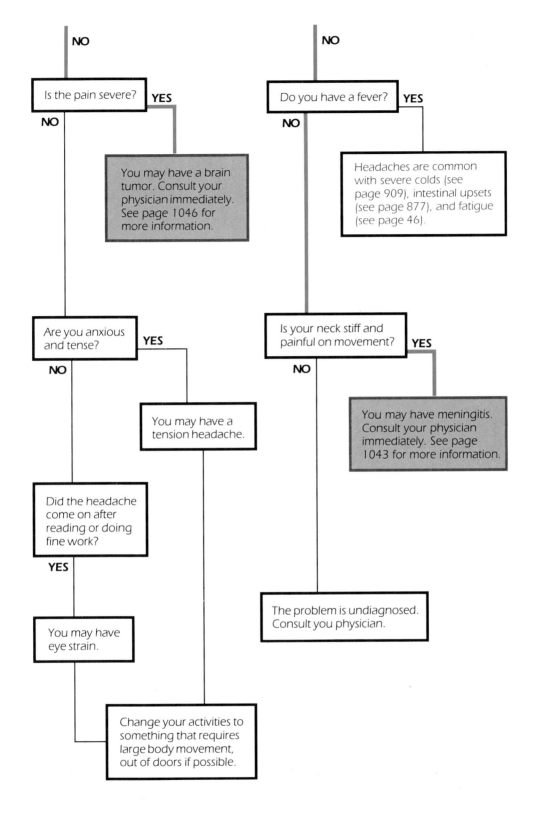

NO

Is the pain severe? **YES**

NO

You may have a brain tumor. Consult your physician immediately. See page 1046 for more information.

Are you anxious and tense? **YES**

NO

You may have a tension headache.

Did the headache come on after reading or doing fine work?

YES

You may have eye strain.

Change your activities to something that requires large body movement, out of doors if possible.

NO

Do you have a fever? **YES**

NO

Headaches are common with severe colds (see page 909), intestinal upsets (see page 877), and fatigue (see page 46).

Is your neck stiff and painful on movement? **YES**

NO

You may have meningitis. Consult your physician immediately. See page 1043 for more information.

The problem is undiagnosed. Consult you physician.

Itching

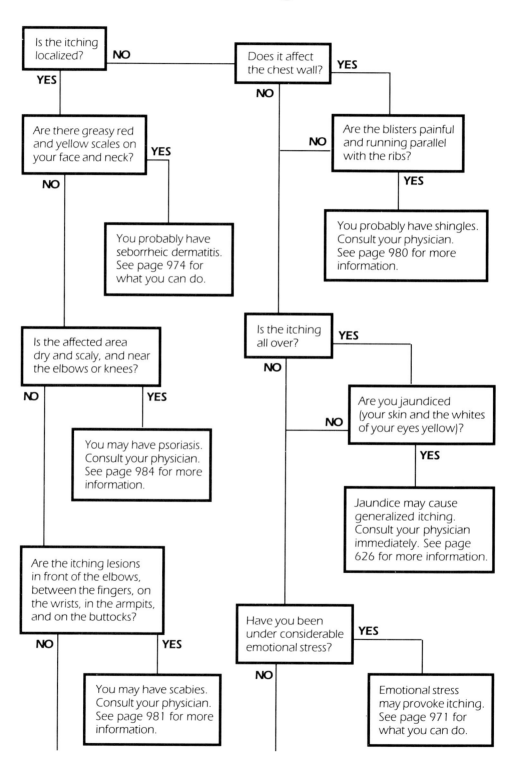

Is the itching localized?

NO → Does it affect the chest wall?

YES (localized) ↓

Are there greasy red and yellow scales on your face and neck?

YES → You probably have seborrheic dermatitis. See page 974 for what you can do.

NO ↓

Is the affected area dry and scaly, and near the elbows or knees?

YES → You may have psoriasis. Consult your physician. See page 984 for more information.

NO ↓

Are the itching lesions in front of the elbows, between the fingers, on the wrists, in the armpits, and on the buttocks?

YES → You may have scabies. Consult your physician. See page 981 for more information.

NO ↓

Does it affect the chest wall?

YES ↓

Are the blisters painful and running parallel with the ribs?

YES → You probably have shingles. Consult your physician. See page 980 for more information.

NO ↓

Is the itching all over?

YES ↓

Are you jaundiced (your skin and the whites of your eyes yellow)?

YES → Jaundice may cause generalized itching. Consult your physician immediately. See page 626 for more information.

NO ↓

Have you been under considerable emotional stress?

YES → Emotional stress may provoke itching. See page 971 for what you can do.

NO ↓

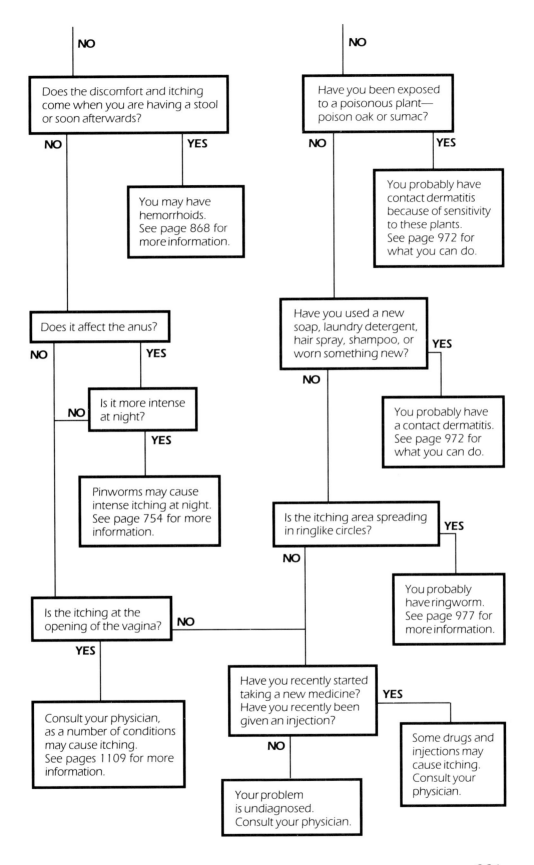

NO

Does the discomfort and itching come when you are having a stool or soon afterwards?

NO   YES

You may have hemorrhoids. See page 868 for more information.

Does it affect the anus?

NO   YES

Is it more intense at night?

NO

YES

Pinworms may cause intense itching at night. See page 754 for more information.

Is the itching at the opening of the vagina?   NO

YES

Consult your physician, as a number of conditions may cause itching. See pages 1109 for more information.

NO

Have you been exposed to a poisonous plant— poison oak or sumac?

NO   YES

You probably have contact dermatitis because of sensitivity to these plants. See page 972 for what you can do.

Have you used a new soap, laundry detergent, hair spray, shampoo, or worn something new?   YES

NO

You probably have a contact dermatitis. See page 972 for what you can do.

Is the itching area spreading in ringlike circles?   YES

NO

You probably have ringworm. See page 977 for more information.

Have you recently started taking a new medicine? Have you recently been given an injection?   YES

NO

Some drugs and injections may cause itching. Consult your physician.

Your problem is undiagnosed. Consult your physician.

Joint pain

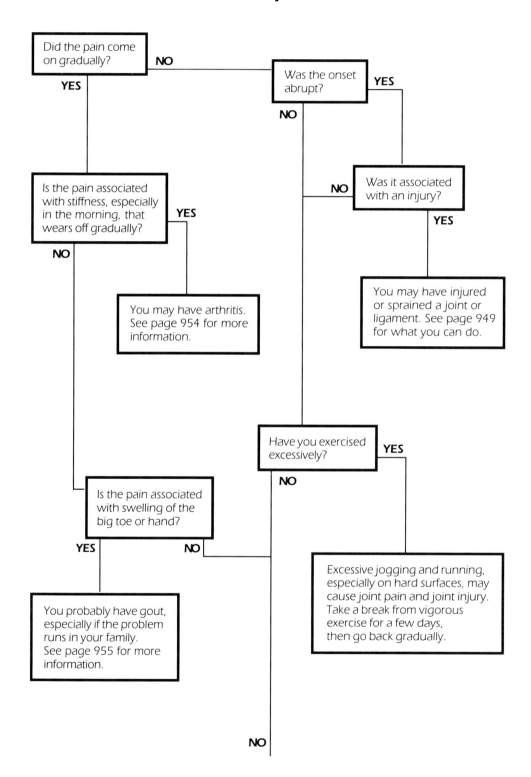

Did the pain come on gradually?

NO → Was the onset abrupt?

YES ↓

Is the pain associated with stiffness, especially in the morning, that wears off gradually?

YES → You may have arthritis. See page 954 for more information.

NO ↓

Is the pain associated with swelling of the big toe or hand?

YES → You probably have gout, especially if the problem runs in your family. See page 955 for more information.

NO

Was the onset abrupt?

YES ↓

Was it associated with an injury?

NO

YES → You may have injured or sprained a joint or ligament. See page 949 for what you can do.

Have you exercised excessively?

YES → Excessive jogging and running, especially on hard surfaces, may cause joint pain and joint injury. Take a break from vigorous exercise for a few days, then go back gradually.

NO

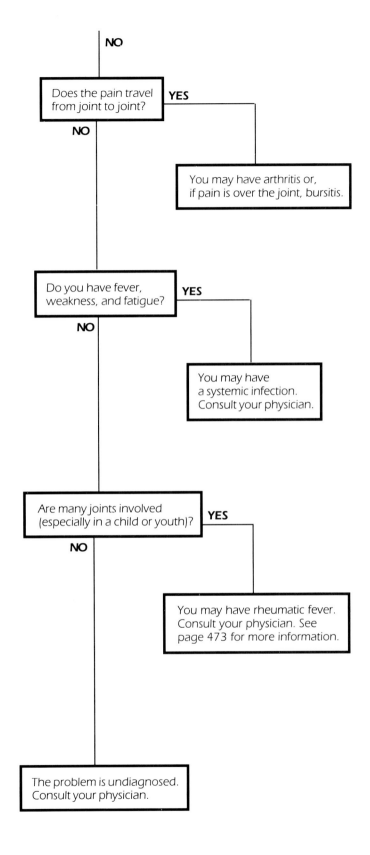

NO

Does the pain travel
from joint to joint?

YES

NO

You may have arthritis or,
if pain is over the joint, bursitis.

Do you have fever,
weakness, and fatigue?

YES

NO

You may have
a systemic infection.
Consult your physician.

Are many joints involved
(especially in a child or youth)?

YES

NO

You may have rheumatic fever.
Consult your physician. See
page 473 for more information.

The problem is undiagnosed.
Consult your physician.

Neck pain

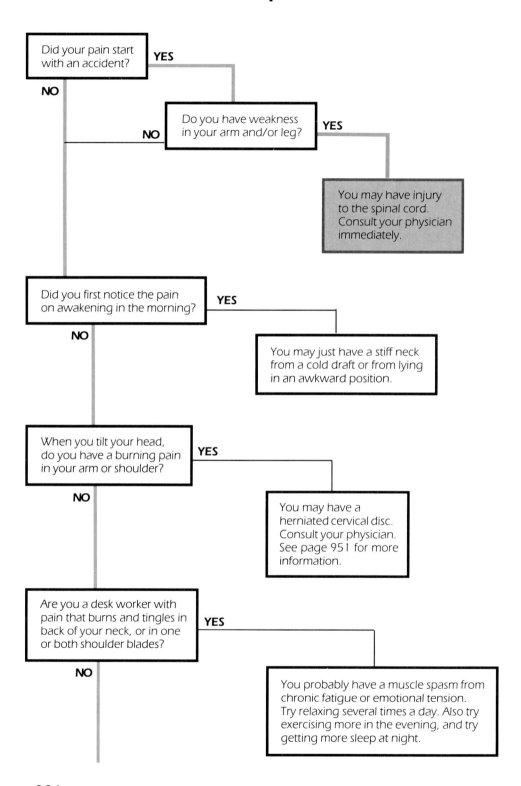

Did your pain start with an accident?

YES → Do you have weakness in your arm and/or leg?

NO

Do you have weakness in your arm and/or leg?

YES → You may have injury to the spinal cord. Consult your physician immediately.

NO →

Did you first notice the pain on awakening in the morning?

YES → You may just have a stiff neck from a cold draft or from lying in an awkward position.

NO

When you tilt your head, do you have a burning pain in your arm or shoulder?

YES → You may have a herniated cervical disc. Consult your physician. See page 951 for more information.

NO

Are you a desk worker with pain that burns and tingles in back of your neck, or in one or both shoulder blades?

YES → You probably have a muscle spasm from chronic fatigue or emotional tension. Try relaxing several times a day. Also try exercising more in the evening, and try getting more sleep at night.

NO

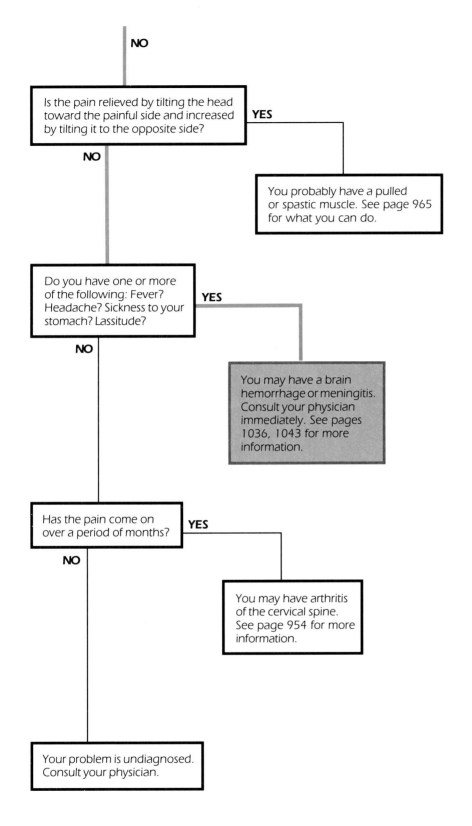

NO

Is the pain relieved by tilting the head toward the painful side and increased by tilting it to the opposite side?

YES

NO

You probably have a pulled or spastic muscle. See page 965 for what you can do.

Do you have one or more of the following: Fever? Headache? Sickness to your stomach? Lassitude?

YES

NO

You may have a brain hemorrhage or meningitis. Consult your physician immediately. See pages 1036, 1043 for more information.

Has the pain come on over a period of months?

YES

NO

You may have arthritis of the cervical spine. See page 954 for more information.

Your problem is undiagnosed. Consult your physician.

665

Sick feeling (malaise)

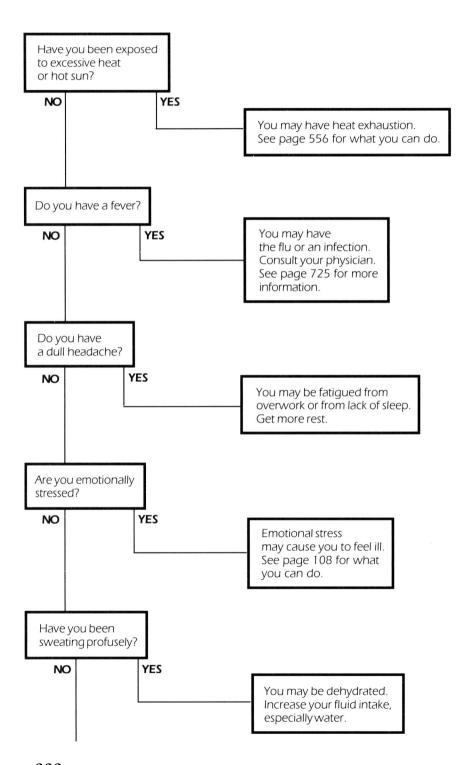

Have you been exposed
to excessive heat
or hot sun?

NO   **YES**

You may have heat exhaustion.
See page 556 for what you can do.

Do you have a fever?

NO   **YES**

You may have
the flu or an infection.
Consult your physician.
See page 725 for more
information.

Do you have
a dull headache?

NO   **YES**

You may be fatigued from
overwork or from lack of sleep.
Get more rest.

Are you emotionally
stressed?

NO   **YES**

Emotional stress
may cause you to feel ill.
See page 108 for what
you can do.

Have you been
sweating profusely?

NO   **YES**

You may be dehydrated.
Increase your fluid intake,
especially water.

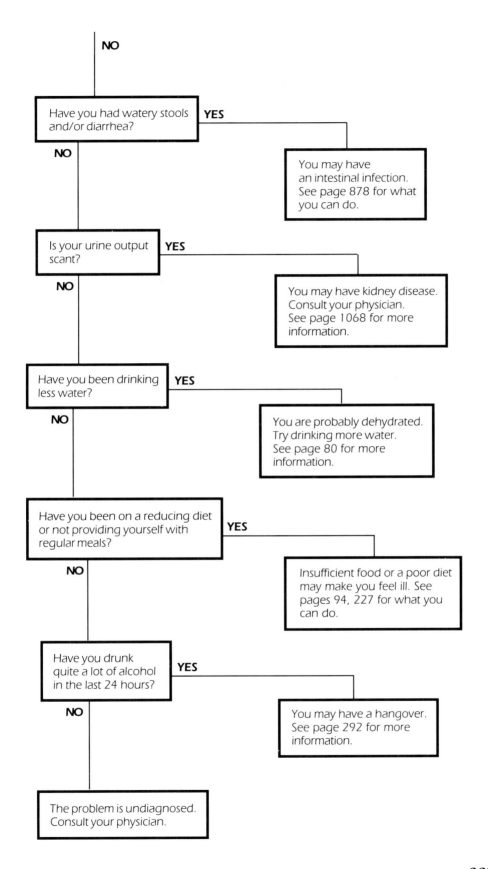

NO

Have you had watery stools and/or diarrhea?

YES

NO

You may have an intestinal infection. See page 878 for what you can do.

Is your urine output scant?

YES

NO

You may have kidney disease. Consult your physician. See page 1068 for more information.

Have you been drinking less water?

YES

NO

You are probably dehydrated. Try drinking more water. See page 80 for more information.

Have you been on a reducing diet or not providing yourself with regular meals?

YES

NO

Insufficient food or a poor diet may make you feel ill. See pages 94, 227 for what you can do.

Have you drunk quite a lot of alcohol in the last 24 hours?

YES

NO

You may have a hangover. See page 292 for more information.

The problem is undiagnosed. Consult your physician.

667

Periods, missed

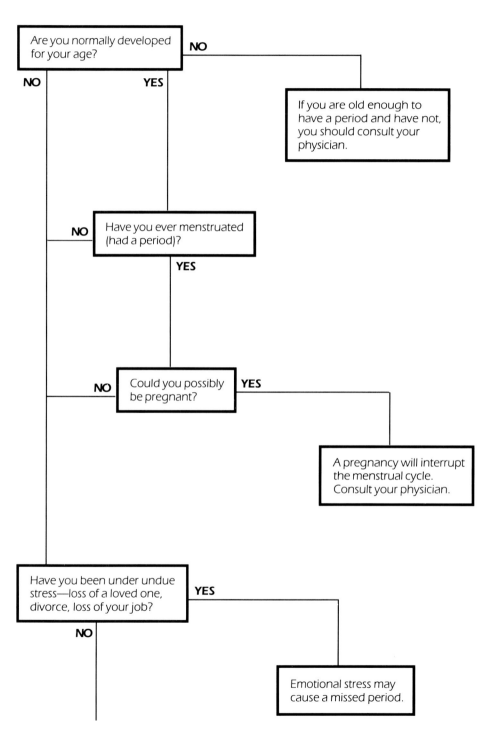

Are you normally developed for your age?

NO → If you are old enough to have a period and have not, you should consult your physician.

NO · **YES**

Have you ever menstruated (had a period)?

NO

YES

Could you possibly be pregnant?

NO · **YES** → A pregnancy will interrupt the menstrual cycle. Consult your physician.

Have you been under undue stress—loss of a loved one, divorce, loss of your job?

YES → Emotional stress may cause a missed period.

NO

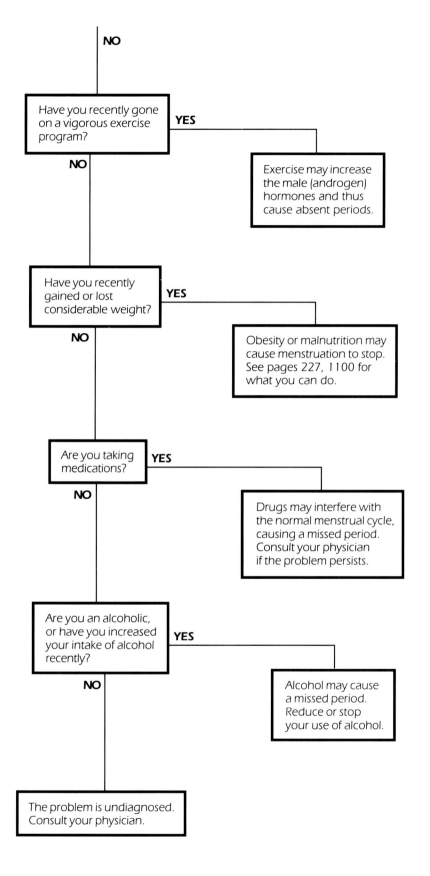

NO

Have you recently gone
on a vigorous exercise
program?

YES

Exercise may increase
the male (androgen)
hormones and thus
cause absent periods.

NO

Have you recently
gained or lost
considerable weight?

YES

Obesity or malnutrition may
cause menstruation to stop.
See pages 227, 1100 for
what you can do.

NO

Are you taking
medications?

YES

Drugs may interfere with
the normal menstrual cycle,
causing a missed period.
Consult your physician
if the problem persists.

NO

Are you an alcoholic,
or have you increased
your intake of alcohol
recently?

YES

Alcohol may cause
a missed period.
Reduce or stop
your use of alcohol.

NO

The problem is undiagnosed.
Consult your physician.

Throat, sore

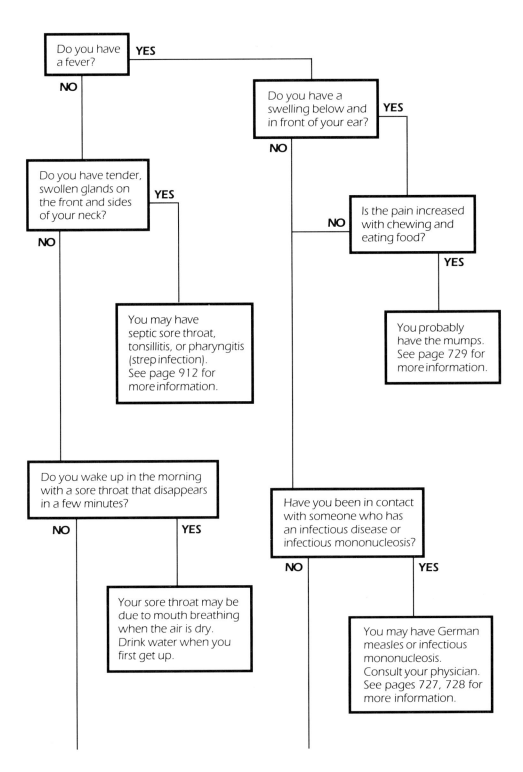

Do you have a fever?

YES

NO

Do you have a swelling below and in front of your ear?

YES

NO

Do you have tender, swollen glands on the front and sides of your neck?

YES

NO

Is the pain increased with chewing and eating food?

NO

YES

You may have septic sore throat, tonsillitis, or pharyngitis (strep infection). See page 912 for more information.

You probably have the mumps. See page 729 for more information.

Do you wake up in the morning with a sore throat that disappears in a few minutes?

NO

YES

Have you been in contact with someone who has an infectious disease or infectious mononucleosis?

NO

YES

Your sore throat may be due to mouth breathing when the air is dry. Drink water when you first get up.

You may have German measles or infectious mononucleosis. Consult your physician. See pages 727, 728 for more information.

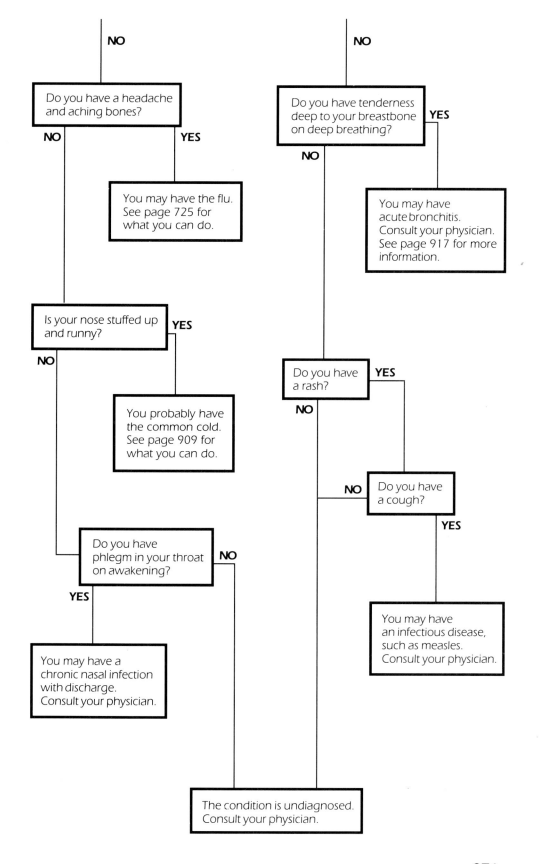

NO

Do you have a headache and aching bones?

NO **YES**

You may have the flu. See page 725 for what you can do.

Is your nose stuffed up and runny?

YES

NO

You probably have the common cold. See page 909 for what you can do.

Do you have phlegm in your throat on awakening?

NO

YES

You may have a chronic nasal infection with discharge. Consult your physician.

NO

Do you have tenderness deep to your breastbone on deep breathing?

YES

NO

You may have acute bronchitis. Consult your physician. See page 917 for more information.

Do you have a rash?

YES

NO

NO Do you have a cough?

YES

You may have an infectious disease, such as measles. Consult your physician.

The condition is undiagnosed. Consult your physician.

CHAPTER **22**

Allergy

You live in a hostile environment, with enemies all around. These enemies are generally microbes or germs (bacteria, viruses, fungi, and others). They are ever on the offensive, awaiting an opportunity to invade your body—through your skin, your lungs, or your intestinal wall. Your major defense forces are organized under your immune system (see page 827), an arrangement of organs, glands, cells, and chemicals.

When enemy forces attempt to enter your body, skin cells block their pathway. Should this first line of defense be breached, sentry cells in the tissues called T lymphocytes or T cells sound an alarm. While killer cells (macrophages) are being mobilized, the T cells provide detailed information regarding the enemy to B lymphocytes. The B lymphocytes prepare chemicals specifically designed to inactivate or destroy the enemy forces. It's a very real form of chemical warfare. Enemy forces exposed to these special chemicals are more easily de-

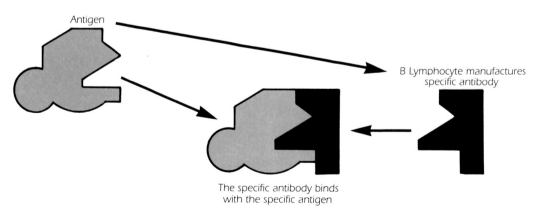

Antigen

B Lymphocyte manufactures specific antibody

The specific antibody binds with the specific antigen

How a specific antibody is designed for and binds with a specific antigen.

stroyed by the defense forces, the phagocytes or macrophages.

Another name for the enemy or invader is **allergen,** while the chemical weapon designed to attack and destroy the allergen is called an **antibody.** For each allergen there is a custom-made molecule or antibody that will only attack that specific allergen.

Besides microbes, you are constantly being exposed to countless chemicals in the air, on the objects you touch, and in the food and water you eat and drink. Some people inherit an immune system that fails to

distinguish between these "harmless" substances and those that are real enemies (see diagram below). The immune systems of these people are overly sensitive to these substances and react to them as if they were enemies. If your body overreacts to one or more otherwise harmless substances, you are said to have a **hypersensitivity** or **allergy.** You are **allergic** to these substances.

Kinds of allergens

Allergies can be caused by a wide variety of substances. Those listed in the categories below are merely sug-

Antigen (A substance; usually protein, pollen, milk, feathers, etc.)	
Person A	Person B
Antibody formed	Antibody not formed
The immunity protects the person.	No immunity, with tissue damage.
An antigen in Person A stimulates the body to form a protective antibody. It is called an immunogen.	The antigen in Person B fails to provoke antibody formation. It is called an allergen.
Individuals differ in their ability to handle antigens. Person A is protected, while Person B is not.	

673

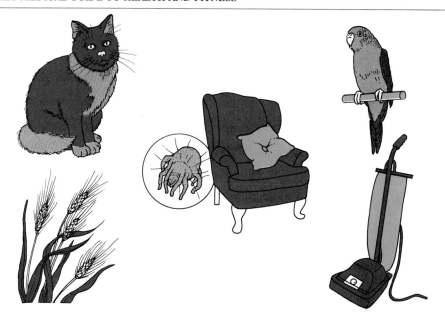

Allergens are of many types, such as feathers, hair, dandruff, house dust, pollens, and certain foods.

gestive of the many allergens commonly known to cause problems.

- **Skin allergens.** Chemicals (mercury, wood alcohol, grease, solvents, detergents), plants (poison ivy, poison oak, poison sumac), dyes (as in leather, shoe polish), furs, feathers, cosmetics, fingernail polish, metals (nickel, jewelry), and insecticides.
- **Inhaled allergens.** Causing conjunctivitis, hay fever, and asthma. Pollens (Bermuda grass, ragweed, flowers of trees), animal dandruff (cats, dogs), feathers, molds, dust, mites, tobacco smoke; and perfumes.
- **Food allergens.** Present in wheat, corn, peas, beans, strawberries, nuts, sesame seed, milk, eggs, pork, fish, shellfish, chocolate, and certain food dyes and vegetable gum thickeners.

- **Additives and preservatives** have been implicated as allergens. Among them are sodium and potassium metabisulfite, used to preserve dried fruits, some canned items, and fresh vegetables. BHA, BHT, and tartrazine (FD&C yellow dye no. 5), and butylated hydroxytoluene may also provoke allergic reactions.
- **"Injected" allergens.** Insect bites, such as from bees, wasps, yellow jackets, hornets, and the bites of ants. Injection of certain drugs, especially penicillin, and hormones, such as insulin, may provoke a reaction.
- **Drug allergens**—antibiotics (penicillin, streptomycin), sulfa drugs, local anesthetics, hormones (as insulin), and certain vitamins may cause allergic reactions. Morphine, codeine, and aspirin may mimic allergic-type re-

actions but do not work through an allergic mechanism.

- **"Germ" allergens.** Bacteria, viruses, fungi, and certain parasites may at times provoke allergic reactions.
- **"Physical allergens."** Heat, cold, pressure, and light may provoke allergiclike symptoms. Whether the response is a true allergic reaction in all cases is not clear.
- **"Emotional allergens."** Strong emotions of any type, including anxiety, laughter, or depression, may, in some people, provoke an allergic type of response, such as hives and asthma, but this does not appear to be due to an allergic mechanism.

The body's response to allergens

In response to allergens, your immune system produces several types of antibodies. The most common one causing allergic reactions is immunoglobulin E, or IgE. As mentioned above, every allergen has its own specific IgE. When an antibody attacks an allergen, the allergic response is caused by the release of a variety of chemicals, often called mediators. These mediators are released from mast cells—tiny chemical factories that line the tissues of the nose, nasal sinuses, lungs, skin, and intestinal tract. Thus, when an antibody attaches itself to an allergen on the membrane of these mast cells, the mediators released include histamine, serotonin, leukotrienes, prostaglandins, and various others that are known as chemotactic factors.

The action of these mediators can be divided into three broad classes: (1) Those that allow fluid to leak through the small blood vessels and contract smooth or involuntary muscles. (2) Those that attract other inflammatory cells into the area of reaction that, in turn, may cause allergic symptoms. (3) Those that modulate the release of other mediators. The net effect of these chemicals depends on the sensitivity of the tissue in which they collect.

Histamine is probably the best-studied chemical to date. Histamine contracts some smooth muscles, but relaxes others. Those of the bronchi and gut contract, while those of the small blood vessels relax. Histamine stimulates many glands to secrete, such as the hydrochloric acid secreting glands in the stomach wall, and mucus and other glands in the lining of the eyes, nose, throat, and bronchi. Histamine allows fluid to seep out of the small blood vessels. This is the cause of runny eyes and nose. It also stimulates nerve endings, which causes itching and pain. A knowledge of the effects of histamine and other mediators provides some understanding of an allergic reaction.

Allergic reactions

Allergic reactions differ, depending on the area of the body in which the allergen and antibody have their disagreement. Following are some examples:

- **Skin allergens.** Allergens affecting the skin cause itching, swelling, redness, and blistering.

- **Inhaled allergens.** Allergens that are inhaled affect the respiratory tract, causing sneezing and runny nose. In the lungs these allergens cause difficulty in breathing (asthma).
- **Food allergens.** The allergens in food may cause local reactions, such as itching and swelling of the lips and lining of the mouth, or, after being swallowed, they may cause nausea, cramps, and diarrhea. A food allergen may also be absorbed into the bloodstream.
- **Blood allergens.** Allergens that enter the bloodstream from food or from an injection (such as an insect sting) may cause generalized hives and an itching, runny nose, or asthma. Some people may experience swelling within the larynx, constriction (narrowing) of the smaller airways, and a drop in blood pressure. A severe response may end in collapse, unconsciousness, and death. This type of reaction is termed **anaphylactic shock.**

Allergic symptoms

Anaphylaxis. When a specific allergen enters the circulation, the reactions are widespread. Histamine entering the circulation causes the small blood vessels to dilate and fluid and protein to seep from the blood into the tissues. In a severe case, circulation will collapse, causing the victim to die. However, chemicals or mediators other than histamine (which are less well understood) are also probably involved in anaphylaxis, especially when the lungs are affected. They cause the air passage-ways (bronchi) in the lungs to constrict, producing "asthma." A severe case of asthma will result in death from suffocation.

Rhinitis (hay fever). When the allergen-antibody reaction takes place in the nose, histamine causes the blood vessels to dilate, which allows fluid to leave the blood. The glands in the lining of the nose pour out their secretions, causing the nose to become runny and congested; sneezing is common.

Hives. An allergic reaction in the skin causes the release of histamine. The blood vessels dilate, and fluid flows out of the capillaries. The result is a red flare and local swelling with itching, which is typically called hives.

Conjunctivitis. The allergic response seen in the eyes is due to a reaction similar to that which occurs in the nose. Dilation of the blood vessels causes redness, and stimulation of the nerves provokes itching. Fluid entering the tissues causes swelling, which stimulates the lachrymal glands, causing tears to flow.

Wheezing, coughing, and tightness in the chest. These symptoms are often produced when an allergen-antibody reaction takes place in the bronchioles (small air passages). Many chemicals are released from mast cells that line the tissue of the breathing passages. Other white blood cells are attracted to the lung and also release chemicals. This results in a spasm of the muscles that surround the breathing tubes (bronchioles). It also causes the secretion of a very thick, tenacious mucus into the opening of the bronchioles and swelling of the lining of these air passageways. The combined effect is a narrowing of the breathing passageways with symptoms of wheezing, coughing, and tightness of the chest.

Diagnosing allergies

To diagnose an allergic condition, or sensitivity to allergens, a doctor must first obtain a very thorough history of the patient, give him or her a physical examination, and carry out certain laboratory procedures. Once the results of these studies are correlated, the doctor will try to discover the particular allergen that is triggering the allergic response. Allergen skin testing (scratch testing) is the method most often used. The doctor places drops from extracts of common allergens (grasses, weeds, molds, animal danders, etc.) on the skin, and then punctures the skin. After several minutes the drop is blotted off. A person is allergic to a particular allergen if, within fifteen minutes of puncturing the skin, a red, raised, itchy bump appears, similar to a hive.

Where skin testing is not feasible, a blood test can detect allergies. The RAST test measures specific IgE antibodies directed against particular antigens. Unfortunately, it is not as sensitive as skin testing and is considerably more expensive.

Testing for food allergies is somewhat more difficult and is not as accurate as skin testing. The suspected food is completely eliminated from the patient's diet for two to three weeks, and is then reintroduced. If the symptoms decrease or disappear during the diet, then resume after the special diet is terminated, the doctor will suspect a food allergy as the cause of the problem.

Preventing the allergic reaction

Since an allergy is an inherited sensitivity to one or more allergens, or an inherited capability of developing such a sensitivity, there is no real cure. However, there are five ways to prevent or modify the allergic response.

● **Avoid the allergen.** This is not always possible, but once an allergic person has learned what allergens trigger his attacks of allergy, avoiding the allergens makes common sense. Stay indoors at certain times of the year when plants are blooming and producing pollens to which you are sensitive. If the pollens are confined to a certain locality, then stay away from that area. If animal dander is the problem, avoid contact with animals to which you are sensitive. You may use a mask when house cleaning to protect yourself against a dust allergy. Some people find that air-conditioning units with good filters bring relief. However, if molds get into the filters, they may cause trouble.

● **Use antihistamines.** As discussed above under "Allergic reactions," when the allergen to which you are sensitive causes the release of histamine, an antihistamine may relieve the attack. Histamine attaches itself to specific receptors (or sites), which then brings about the allergic re-

677

sponse—the allergic symptom. Antihistamines are molecules that attach themselves to the same receptors that histamines attach to, but they do not bring about the allergic response. Flooding the bloodstream with antihistamine molecules prevents most of the histamine molecules from attaching to their receptors. Thus the allergic reaction is averted.

Unfortunately, many antihistamines cause drowsiness, making it unwise to drive an automobile or work around machinery when taking this type of medication. Certain relatively new antihistamines that do not cause sedation are, for most people, a good alternative to conventional antihistamines. Your physician can advise you which antihistamine would be best for you.

- **Topical sprays and inhalers.** These are available by prescription only for allergic rhinitis and asthma, and should be used under the direct supervision of a physician. They prevent allergic reactions from developing. These agents, which include corticosteroids, cromolyn sodium, and beta-adrenergic compounds, are not to be confused with over-the-counter decongestants.
- **Desensitization.** This procedure requires a series of injections, in gradually increasing doses, of the allergen to which you are sensitive. This allows your body to build up neutralizing antibodies, which may help to prevent the allergen from producing the allergic

response. It will also make available less of the IgE antibodies that provoke the allergic response. While desensitization will not cure your hypersensitivity, it will allow you to be free of your allergy for reasonable lengths of time. Large numbers of desensitizing allergens are available. If you are troubled with allergies, you should seek the advice of a physician who specializes in handling these disorders.

- **Hormone therapy.** Oral and injectable corticosteroids are available for serious allergic reactions that cannot be controlled by the use of antihistamines, topical sprays, or inhalers. They should be used under the direct supervision of a physician.

Allergic disorders

The various allergic disorders are discussed under the systems of the body in which they occur. To avoid repetition, and for the convenience of the reader, the reference is given to where the common disorder is described, together with its suggested treatment.

Atopic dermatitis (eczema). Atopic dermatitis is an inherited disorder that, in most cases, affects the skin. It causes itching, burning, and a red, blistering rash, possibly accompanied by hives, hay fever, and asthma. It is likely to occur during three age periods: infancy, childhood, and adulthood. It may appear for the first time during any one of these periods. For a more complete discussion and suggested treatment, see page 971.

Allergic dermatitis (contact dermatitis). Allergic dermatitis occurs when a person touches something to which he has developed a sensitivity from a previous exporsure. The two most common examples are poison ivy and poison oak. Sensitivity may be acquired to a wide variety of substances. For a more complete discussion, see page 972.

Hay fever (allergic rhinitis). Hay fever is an allergic response to substances carried in the air that are breathed into the lungs. It is often associated with allergic conjunctivitis. The nose is congested and runny, and there is frequent sneezing. For details, see page 910.

Asthma (bronchial asthma). Doubtless half or more of the episodes of asthma are due to an allergic response. The smaller air passageways are narrowed by contraction of the bronchial muscles, swelling of the lining membrane, and an outpouring of mucus that narrows the bronchial tubes. Breathing becomes extremely difficult. For a full discussion, see page 920, and for emergency treatment, see page 529.

Drug allergy. An allergic reaction may occur in sensitive individuals after the taking of certain drugs. Many drugs can cause a reaction, although there are a few in which an adverse response is more frequently seen (see page 674 for examples). A rash is the usual manifestation. Fever and symptoms of shock may occur in more extreme cases. Treatment will depend on the severity of the reaction. The drug must, of course, be promptly discontinued. If you know that you are sensitive to a particular drug, report this to your physician. For details about causes and treatment, see page 326.

Serum sickness. Serum sickness may result from the injection of animal serum into a human (horse, bovine, rabbit), or from the use of a number of drugs (penicillin, streptomycin, sulfonamides). The adverse reaction may come on immediately, or it may be delayed for two to three weeks. It generally starts with hives, accompanied by fever, nausea, pain in the abdomen, swelling of the lymph nodes, and joint pains. Emergency treatment requires the use of epinephrine. See your physician immediately or go to an emergency room. For additional discussion, see page 471.

Anaphylactic shock. In some persons an allergic reaction to an insect sting or to a drug such as penicillin is so sudden and so intense that it is called "anaphylactic shock." The symptoms include skin rash (hives), swelling of the lining of the air passages, difficult breathing, a drop in blood pressure, collapse, unconsciousness, and, if not treated immediately, possible death. For further details, see page 676, and for emergency treatment, see page 535.

CHAPTER 23

Cancer

Cancer is doubtless the most dreaded disease afflicting the human race today. Although deaths from cancer, the second most common killer in the United States, are exceeded only by those from heart disease, cancer creates far greater fear in the sufferer than do coronary heart disease, stroke, diabetes, or chronic kidney failure—diseases that also take a heavy toll on life. Every two years cancer kills more Americans than the total number killed in the four most recent wars: World War I, World War II, Korea, and Vietnam. And every year cancer kills seven times the number of Americans killed in automobile accidents!

More than 1.3 million new cases of cancer occur every year in the United States. Of these, 400,000 are skin cancers with a relatively low mortality, but for the remaining 900,000, the annual death rate is about 50 percent! Cancer of the lung accounts for the largest number of these deaths, among both men and women. For those who receive treatment, the results are often given in terms of five-year survival rates. Un-fortunately, this often causes the victims to be haunted by fear that the cancer will recur.

In spite of these somber facts, though, the outlook for cancer victims has been steadily improving. The five-year survival rate has doubled in the last fifty years, and of those who do die, one-third could be saved by early diagnosis and prompt treatment. If one adds to this the fact that almost all lung cancers could be eliminated if tobacco smoking were abolished, the outlook for anyone dying from this disease is far less discouraging than it was just a few years ago.

What is a cancer?

Cancer is not a single disease, but takes more than 100 forms, all of which are characterized by a multiplication of cells that threaten life. In this sense, the term **neoplasm,** or new growth, is most fitting. In most types, a **tumor,** or enlarging mass, develops as a result of a steady and abnormal multiplication of cells. Cell multiplication that is restricted to a single site is called a **benign tumor.**

When the multiplying cells invade adjoining tissues, or when they are carried in body fluids (blood, lymph) to other parts of the body, the mass is called a **malignant** tumor, or **carcinoma.** Thus, the most common medical terms used to designate a cancer are *malignant* tumor, *malignant growth, neoplasm,* or *carcinoma.*

All but the most highly specialized cells of the body can replace themselves when worn out, injured, or aged. The superficial cells of the skin, and those lining the intestinal tract and the uterus, are constantly being rubbed or sloughed off. New cells forming in the deeper layers replace those that are lost, thus maintaining a constant balance between loss and renewal.

This is also true of blood cells. Red blood cells live for about 120 days. Each second some two to three million worn-out red corpuscles are taken out of circulation by the spleen. At the same time, a similar number of new red blood cells enter the circulatory system from the bone marrow, where they are manufactured. White blood cells always increase in number under the stimulus of an infection, but the body will return to a normal production level when the infection is over.

Normally, the human body maintains a precise control over the number of cells that make up its tissues, so that it produces only the cells that it needs. When the required number is reached, cell production stops. This control over cell production resides in the genes that are found in the nucleus of each cell. The DNA molecules in the genes are "coded" to regulate how each cell grows and the work it does, thus enabling every cell in the body to work in cooperation with all other cells. As the body grows, beginning at conception and continuing to adulthood, the number of cells increases enormously, but the rate of increase is always controlled very carefully so that only the proper number of each cell is produced.

In a cancer cell, though, the DNA molecules have been altered or rearranged in subtle ways that change them into what we call "oncogenes," or cancer genes. The oncogene cells in a developing neoplasm or cancer multiply in spite of the body's normal checks and balances. The body loses control of its cell growth, and the cancer cells no longer obey the signal to stop growing.

Types of cancer

Cancers are subdivided into two large classes: benign and malignant. **Benign tumors,** as already mentioned, remain isolated from the surrounding tissues and grow within their own capsule. Although *benign* means harmless, the increasing size of these tumors may displace adjoining structures, and by placing pressure on adjacent tissues may sometimes cause damage. A fatty tumor called *lipoma*, which develops

Characteristics of benign and malignant tumors		
	Benign	**Malignant**
Structure	Normal	Abnormal
Spread	Limited	Widespread
Growth	Slow	Usually rapid
Outlook	Excellent	Serious to fatal
Treatment	Cautery, surgery	Radiation, Chemotherapy

under the skin, causing a bump on the body's surface, belongs to this benign class.

Malignant tumors

Malignant tumors are composed of cells whose multiplication is out of control, and as they continue to multiply they send out tentaclelike projections called *processes* that invade surrounding tissues. The invading growth often destroys these structures, usually by interfering with and appropriating their supply of blood. This may lead to bleeding and ulceration.

Often these wildly-growing cells break away in small groups and, carried in the blood or lymph, travel to distant organs. Here they set up a beach-head, and, once established, develop into secondary tumors similar to the original one. This process of migration is called **metastasis.** Metastatic tumors may endanger the victim's life even more than the original tumor.

As a cancer develops in a particular part of the body, its cells more or less partake of the nature of the nor-

mal cells of the tissue or organ in which it originates. For this reason, the various kinds of cancer roughly parallel the various kinds of normal tissue in which a malignant tumor may grow. While there are numerous classes and subclasses of cancers, we will mention only four major types:

Carcinomas. The largest group of cancers, known as carcinomas, originate from epithelial cells. Some of these cover the body's surfaces, such as the skin. Others line its tubes and cavities, such as the mucous membranes of the air passageways, intestines, bladder, and uterus. Still others compose the functioning cells of its glands, as in the salivary glands, the liver, pancreas, and prostate.

Leukemias develop in the tissues that produce blood cells, such as the bone marrow and lymph nodes.

Lymphomas develop from the cells of the lymph glands, as for example, the spleen and lymph nodes.

Sarcomas arise in the body's supporting tissues—bone, blood vessels, muscle, and fibrous tissue.

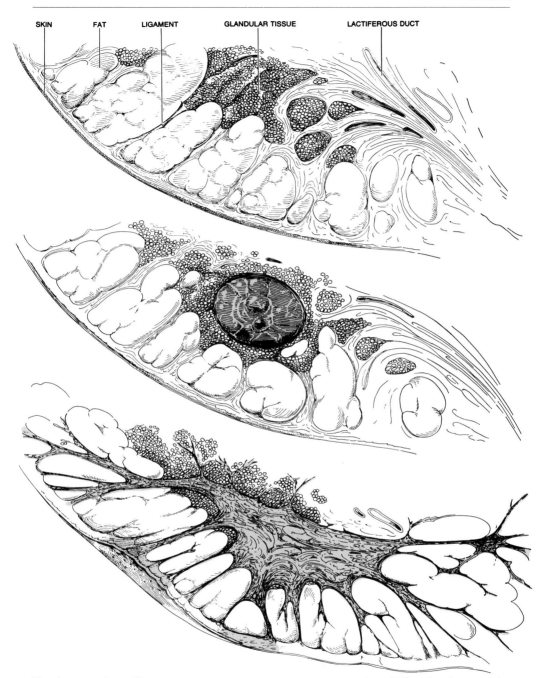

SKIN   FAT   LIGAMENT   GLANDULAR TISSUE   LACTIFEROUS DUCT

Benign and malignant tumors may develop in the breast. Top: the structures of the normal breast. Middle: a benign tumor has developed in the glandular tissue. It is circumscribed and remains within the breast. Bottom: a cancerous tumor spreads within the breast tissues. It may invade adjoining structures (muscle and chest wall), or it may be carried by the blood and lymph to distant parts of the body (metastasis).

683

What causes cancer?

The precise cause of cancer is not known. However, a vast amount of research over the past half century has helped us to make large strides in our understanding of this very complex and difficult disease. It now appears that most cancers develop because of a series of events that take place in a single cell of the body over a period of years. These events convert this once normal cell into an abnormal cancer cell.

Two types of factors contribute to this change: those that start the process of change, and those that continue the process once it has started. The first group of agents are called **initiators,** while the second group are called **promoters.** An initiator may be a chemical, radiation, or virus. A promoter may be a different agent in one of the same three groups.

Research has revealed that certain oncogenes produce a protein that establishes itself in the nucleus, or command post, of the cell. Other oncogenes produce a different protein found in the edges of the cell. It is possible that one of these proteins is produced by the initiator and the other by the promoter. Working hand in hand, these agents cause the cell to multiply and spread without control.

Chemicals that can produce a first or subsequent event in the transformation of a normal cell to a cancerous cell are called **carcinogens.** Carcinogens often require some other agent to work with them. These agents are called **co-carcinogens.** Over time, the action of one or

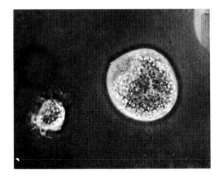

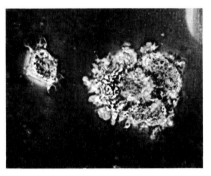

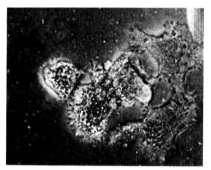

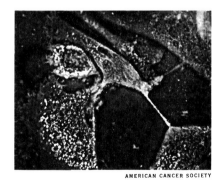

AMERICAN CANCER SOCIETY

A time-lapse study of the division of a malignant cell, showing four stages of development and growth.

684

several carcinogens (or co-carcinogens) alters the DNA in the chromosomes that are in the nucleus of a cell, especially those that control the multiplication of cells. When the genes that control cell reproduction finally change into an oncogene (or cancer gene), the body's normal control over the growth and multiplication of cells is lost, and a wild-growing cancer starts on its fateful course.

Predisposing factors

Heredity, environment, and lifestyle all play important roles, either singly or in combination, in the development of cancer. Many experts believe that as many as 90 percent of human cancers result from exposure to carcinogens that could be avoided.

Heredity. There appears to be a strong hereditary tendency for the development of certain types of cancer. A woman whose female relatives have had breast cancer carries a three- to five-times greater risk of developing breast cancer than does the woman without such a family history. Again, two individuals may smoke the same number of cigarettes a day and inhale just as deeply, yet twenty years later one will develop a lung cancer and the other continue in apparently perfect health. Heredity may be one reason for this. However, the conclusion that heredity caused the difference must be tempered by the fact that other important lifestyle differences between the two individuals may have caused one to contract cancer and the other to remain free, even though their smoking habits were identical.

Environment. It is now recognized that modern man's environment is filled with opportunities for coming in contact with agents that, over the longterm, can initiate a malignant growth. We can mention several.

Physical agents. Excessive exposure to **sunlight** is an important predisposing factor to cancers of the skin. The solar keratoses (thickening of epidermal cells) that occur on those portions of the body exposed to the sun are the intermediate stage between normal skin and skin cancer. These develop more frequently in farmers, sailors, and other workmen whose activities expose them to large amounts of ultraviolet radiation from sunlight. Sunbathing with prolonged and unnecessary exposure to the sun is unwise. Because of the high level of pigment in their skin, dark people are less susceptible to skin cancer than are those with a fair complexion. For details, see page 73.

Exposure to **radiation** in X-rays or atomic radiation increases a person's susceptibility to cancer. When X-ray equipment was first introduced, the precautions required today were not used, with the result that those working in this field were needlessly exposed to radiation. For example, radiologists had ten times the incidence of leukemia as did physicians in general. Because of improved technology, the X-rays used today expose both radiologist and patient to a minimal amount of radiation, thus drastically reducing the risk of adverse effects.

685

Excessive **temperature** appears to make tissues vulnerable. Cancer of the lip is quite common among pipe smokers. The heat from the pipe stem is thought to be an important factor (a promoter) in causing cancer of the lip. A testicle that has not descended into the scrotum is more likely to develop a malignant change because the body temperature inside the body is higher than in the scrotal sack (see page 1092).

Chemical agents. The number of chemicals to which a person living in today's society is exposed staggers the imagination. The industrial revolution started more than 100 years ago, but the chemical revolution came into full bloom during World War II. Thousands of new chemicals enter the marketplace every year.

Stop and think about it for a moment. Your clothes are made of chemicals and dyed with chemicals. The walls in your home are painted with chemicals, your drapes, carpets, and upholstered chairs are made from chemicals. The food you eat is colored, flavored, preserved, and packaged in chemicals. Whether you are at home, driving a car, or at work, you are constantly exposed to chemicals. Indeed, the very air you breathe is all too often filled with chemicals!

We know beyond a reasonable doubt that certain chemicals increase the risk of contracting cancer. Arsenic preparations, even when taken internally, cause skin cancer in humans. Workers exposed to aniline dyes are particularly susceptible to cancer of the urinary bladder. Those exposed to asbestos, especially if they smoke tobacco, are much more prone to contract cancer of the lung.

The United States Food and Drug Administration and similar organizations in other countries attempt to protect their citizens from exposure to chemicals that might put them at risk to develop cancer. Carefully controlled laboratory tests are conducted, and any substance that shows a potential for causing cancer is banned. Thus, the use of the artificial sweetener cyclamate, and the dye formerly used to color butter and margarine yellow, have been banned.

However, as can well be imagined, it takes years—often as much as twenty or thirty years—to test for the long term effects of a single chemical, let alone combinations of chemicals. Thus, extensive testing of all chemicals and chemical combinations is not feasible. It behooves each individual to take those precautions that are practical to avoid all unnecessary exposure to substances that might place him or her at risk. The first and foremost of these precautions is to avoid the use of tobacco, especially smoking.

Cigarette smoking is now responsible for one in every four cancer deaths in the United States, making it the greatest single cause of cancer in this country. Smoking is the culprit in over 90 percent of the cases of lung cancer, and it is increasingly being implicated as a precipitating cause of cancer in other parts of the body. The prospect of developing lung cancer is ten times greater for the cigarette smoker than for the nonsmoker, and forty times greater if he has smoked forty cigarettes a day for twenty years or more.

Tobacco smoke taken into the lungs contains carcinogens that both initiate and promote the transformation of lung cells into cancer cells. Many of these cancer producing agents enter the bloodstream, circulate throughout the body, and are eventually eliminated by the kidneys and concentrated in the urine. It is not surprising to find that cancer of the bladder is significantly more common among smokers than among nonsmokers. For details, see page 273.

Users of alcohol have a higher incidence of cancer of the liver, larynx, and esophagus than do nondrinkers. Some authorities class alcohol as a co-carcinogen, meaning that it augments the influence of other conditions that predispose to cancer. Those who use alcohol often smoke, and the alcohol user and smoker commonly drinks coffee, which contains caffeine—a chemical that may damage the chromosomes. Thus, singly and in combination, those who use alcohol, nicotine, and caffeine constantly expose themselves to conditions that increase their risk of developing cancer.

Biological agents. The precise role of viruses in causing cancer is not yet understood. Viruses are minute infectious agents that live and multiply within the cells that support them. They are so small that they can only be seen under an electron microscope. They are formed of protein and a nucleic acid, either DNA or RNA. Occasionally, the DNA or RNA of a certain virus will become integrated with the DNA or RNA in the chromosomes of the cells that it infects. On a rare occasion a portion of the virus's DNA or RNA may act as an initiator or promoter. A number of DNA and RNA viruses are known to be associated with human cancers.

There are many predisposing factors to cancer, and it appears that at least two of these must be present and working side by side in order to produce a cancer. The mere presence of a cancer-related virus in a person's body will not, of itself, produce cancer. It takes some additional factor, in the presence of a virus, to either lower the body's resistance or to weaken the body's tissues, in order to trigger the transformation of normal cells to cancer cells.

Lifestyle factors

The term lifestyle is used here in a rather broad sense and includes both habits of life and certain times of life.

Age. Cancer is responsible for more deaths in children one to fourteen years of age than from any other cause except accidents. More deaths occur from cancer during the first five years of life than during the next ten years combined. Many of these cancers occur in parts of the body where cell development has not yet reached full maturity. They are, in a way, carry-overs from embryonic life. The organs most commonly affected are the blood-producing tissues (with resulting leukemia), the brain and other parts of the nervous system, the eye, the adrenal glands, muscle tissue, bone tissue, and the kidneys. Because the tissues in children's bodies are in a state of transition, with rapid changes in growth and

687

development, their cancers appear to grow more rapidly.

The likelihood of cancer increases year by year throughout adulthood. Many predisposing factors require long periods of time to bring about a malignant change in normal cells. Exposure to cancer-producing chemicals in the home or on the job often require a lag period of twenty or more years before the cancer occurs, as is the case with people who smoke. Again, some malignancies are slow-growing. For example, cancer of the prostate is infrequent in men in their forties, but common in those eighty or ninety years of age.

Sex. The incidence of cancer among men is different from what it is among women, as can be seen in the charts on pages 688 and 689. Habits of life as well as biological differences contribute to this situation.

Deaths from cancer of the lung remain the most frequent cause of death among men. Cigarette smoking became particularly common among men during and after World War I, and deaths from lung cancer increased far more rapidly among men after that time. Following World War II, women also took up smoking in large numbers, and since that time deaths from lung cancer among women have also risen steadily, after a lag period of twenty to twenty-five years. In 1986 lung cancer surpassed breast cancer as the number one killer among women.

Marital status. There seems to be no doubt that hormones play an important role in the development or prevention of certain cancers. Cancer of the breast is less common among married than among unmarried women. Also, the woman who has

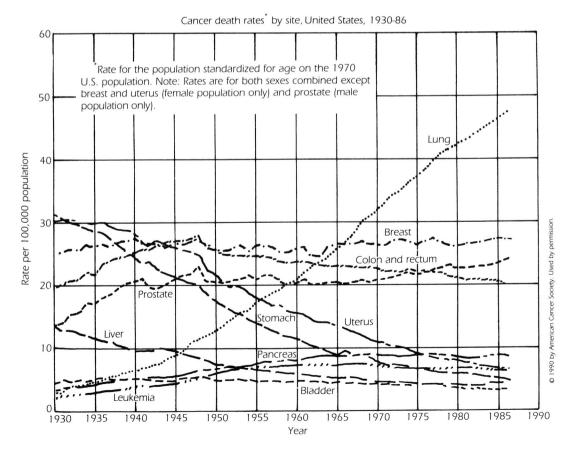

Cancer death rates* by site, United States, 1930-86

*Rate for the population standardized for age on the 1970 U.S. population. Note: Rates are for both sexes combined except breast and uterus (female population only) and prostate (male population only).

Rate per 100,000 population

Lung

Breast

Colon and rectum

Prostate

Stomach

Uterus

Liver

Pancreas

Leukemia

Bladder

Year

© 1990 by American Cancer Society. Used by permission.

her first child before age twenty-five has a lower risk of breast cancer than does the woman who has her first child after age thirty-five.

However, marriage seems to have just the opposite effect in cancer of the cervix. Among girls married in their teens, or who first experience sexual intercourse in their early

they are at increased risk (see predisposing factors and lifestyle factors on the preceding pages) should be alert to the telltale signs and symptoms that indicate the possible presence of a cancer. For example, smokers are in a high risk category, not only for cancer of the lung (90 percent of all lung cancers), but for

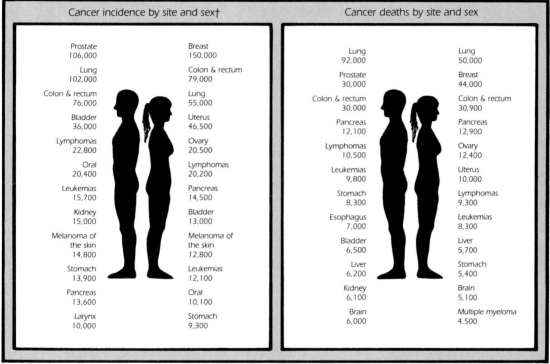

Cancer incidence by site and sex†		Cancer deaths by site and sex	
Prostate 106,000	Breast 150,000	Lung 92,000	Lung 50,000
Lung 102,000	Colon & rectum 79,000	Prostate 30,000	Breast 44,000
Colon & rectum 76,000	Lung 55,000	Colon & rectum 30,000	Colon & rectum 30,900
Bladder 36,000	Uterus 46,500	Pancreas 12,100	Pancreas 12,900
Lymphomas 22,800	Ovary 20,500	Lymphomas 10,500	Ovary 12,400
Oral 20,400	Lymphomas 20,200	Leukemias 9,800	Uterus 10,000
Leukemias 15,700	Pancreas 14,500	Stomach 8,300	Lymphomas 9,300
Kidney 15,000	Bladder 13,000	Esophagus 7,000	Leukemias 8,300
Melanoma of the skin 14,800	Melanoma of the skin 12,800	Bladder 6,500	Liver 5,700
Stomach 13,900	Leukemias 12,100	Liver 6,200	Stomach 5,400
Pancreas 13,600	Oral 10,100	Kidney 6,100	Brain 5,100
Larynx 10,000	Stomach 9,300	Brain 6,000	Multiple myeloma 4,500

† Excluding non-melanoma skin cancer and carcinoma in situ.

© 1990 by American Cancer Society. Used by permission.

teens, cancer of the cervix is far more frequent than among girls who marry in their twenties or who never marry.

Cancer detection

The earlier a cancer can be detected, the better are the prospects for its cure. Once the growth has spread to adjacent tissues or metastasized to distant organs, eradication or control of the malignancy is much more difficult. Those who know that

cancers in general (30 percent of all cancers). Another group who should be careful is persons with a family history of cancer. A third group is people who have already had a cancer.

The chart on page 690 points out the early signals of a developing malignancy in the various tissues and organs of the body.

There are also a number of symptoms of cancer of a more general na-

689

Cancer danger signals

The telltale symptoms listed in the right-hand column suggest the possibility of cancer in the organs named on the left. Any time these symptoms appear, you should immediately arrange for an examination by your doctor.

Bladder	Blood in the urine; increase in the frequency of urination.
Bone	Local pain, tenderness; unusual thickening of bone; walking with an unexplained limp.
Blood (leukemia)	Vague symptoms: fever, pallor, blood spreading into the tissues.
Breast	Lump or deformity in the breast or nipple.
Cervix	Abnormal bleeding, spotting with blood, or abnormal discharge.
Colon and rectum	Bleeding from the rectum, change in bowel habits.
Esophagus	Difficulty in swallowing.
Kidney (in adult)	Blood in urine (usually without pain); loss of appetite, fatigue, and loss of weight.
Kidney (in three-year-olds or younger)	Firm, painless mass in one side of abdomen.
Larynx	Sudden, unexplained, progressive hoarseness; later, difficult breathing.
Lip	Warty growth; crusting ulcer or fissure (resting in a disklike, firm area).
Lung	Cough (particularly different from the usual smoker's cough); transient sneezing. Later, spitting blood.

(continued on the next page)

Mouth and tongue	An area of roughening; mild burning when eating highly seasoned foods. Later, ulceration.
Skin	A pimple or small sore fails to heal and gradually enlarges; an old skin lesion now begins to grow; a persistent lesion crusts but bleeds when the crust is removed; an old wart or mole changes size or color.
Stomach	Persistent distress in upper abdomen, loss of appetite, loss of weight.
Uterus	Episodes of vaginal bleeding unrelated to menstruation.

NOTE: Most cancers are not painful, at least in their early stages. Thousands of cancer victims have lost their lives needlessly because they waited too long before seeing their doctor, thinking that their lesion could not be cancer because it was not painful.

Some cancers do not give a warning signal; they develop "silently," and the best prospects of cure have passed by the time the symptoms appear. Hence the advice: *See your physician for a periodic cancer checkup.*

ture. While not specific for cancer alone, they certainly should be considered and immediately reported to your physician. These include:

- Loss of appetite
- Loss of weight—for no apparent reason
- Tiredness—more than expected
- Headaches—out of the ordinary, and recurring
- Vomiting—sudden attacks without feeling sick
- Pain—steady, in the bones or deeply placed
- Fever—low grade, continual
- Weakness and pallor

The American Cancer Society points out seven warning signs:

- Change in bowel or bladder habits
- A sore that does not heal
- Unusual bleeding or discharge
- Thickening or lump in the breast, or elsewhere
- Indigestion or difficulty in swallowing
- Obvious change in a wart or mole
- Nagging cough or hoarseness

Diagnostic procedures

Should you suspect that you have cancer, immediately see your physician. He will give you a thorough medical checkup. Denial of facts is a serious mistake. If you have a family background of cancer, discuss this with your doctor. Have you been exposed to a known cancer-producing agent, such as tobacco

691

smoke? Do you smoke, have you ever smoked, or have you lived in a smoke-filled environment at home or at work?

Your physician will carefully examine the suspected site of the lesion. A number of diagnostic procedures are available today, including X-rays, ultrasound, radioisotope scanning, CT scans, and laboratory analysis of specimens of blood, urine, and other body discharges. Depending on the possible site of the cancer, a **mammogram** of the breasts or a **Pap smear** of vaginal discharge is appropriate in women. Medical Resonance Imaging (MRI) is particularly helpful in the diagnosis of brain tumors. Instruments are also available to visually examine the colon, the bladder, the bronchial tree, and the esophagus and stomach. The conclusive test, of course, is a biopsy of the lesion that has been examined by a pathologist. Your physician may wish to consult with a specialist himself, or he may refer you to one.

If you have cancer

Many people's first reaction to a cancer diagnosis is consternation or even panic. Fortunately, modern methods of treatment have greatly changed the picture, and many forms of cancer respond to appropriate therapy. If you are diagnosed with cancer, the following steps will help you relate to the problem intelligently in spite of how you feel.

Face the facts

Face the reality of the situation and get council from your physician and friends. If you have any doubt as to the diagnosis, request a second opinion. You may wish a diagnostic study at a reputable medical center. But **do not waste time.**

Plan realistically

Become well informed about the particular kind of cancer you have. Contact the American Cancer Society, 777 Third Avenue, New York, NY 10017, or the society's office nearest your home. They will provide you with literature that discusses cancer in general and your particular type of cancer in detail. Make two plans for the immediate future: one in case the treatment is successful, and the other in case it is not. Arrange your personal affairs and your commitments accordingly.

Beware of nostrums

Because of the dread that attends the discovery that a person has cancer, the disease lends itself to exploitation by unscrupulous persons who claim to have access to a "cure" for malignancy. "Cancer cures" have come and gone for as long as the disease has been recognized. Cancer still persists, but the promoters and their cures have run their courses and disappeared.

Quackery in the field of cancer therapy is a multibillion dollar busi-

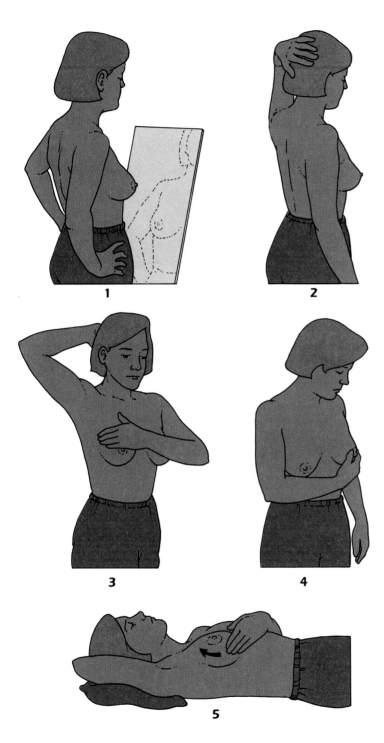

You should examine your breasts once a month after your period. Check each breast in the following manner:

1. Stand in front of a mirror and drop your arms. Become familiar with the appearance of your breasts, the texture of the surface, and their size and shape. You should especially watch for changes. A rough texture may indicate a lump underneath.

2. Raise each arm above your head, and, turning from side to side, again watch for changes.

3. With your arm still raised above your head, press the flat of your hand against the surface of your breast. Check for changes in what you feel, especially lumps. Work your way around the entire breast.

4. Squeeze the nipple to see if there is a discharge.

5. Because the pressure of the tendons holding up your breasts when you stand may "hide" a lump, you should lie on your back with a pillow under your shoulders and check each breast again, following the instructions in number 3.

Self-examination of the breast.

How to select your physician

Questionable therapy	Standard therapy
1. Practitioner is warm, friendly, and exudes confidence, but is not qualified by well-established specialty boards.	1. Practioner is qualified by well-established specialty boards.
2. Claims are carefully phrased and supported by testimonials, not by scientific research.	2. Claims are guarded and the treatment offered is supported by wide experience and research.
3. Diagnosis is made by unconventional methods. The results are not shared with other physicians.	3. Diagnosis is made by established procedures including biopsy. The results are gladly shared with other physicians.
4. The treatment is unique, and the practitioner claims regular physicians do not wish to use it because the cures would lose them money.	4. The therapy is not confined to a single individual or institution. The therapy is available at many medical centers.
5. The cost of therapy is high.	5. Costs are well established.
6. The surroundings are often exotic, as are the regime and diet.	6. The surroundings are not exotic, nor are the diet and procedures.
7. The practitioner claims that the government bans the therapy because of "big business."	7. The government and professional agencies cooperate to make the treatments available.
8. The practitioner and his support group exhibit a martyr or persecution complex.	8. There is an openness about all activities.

ness. Its promoters nearly always appear to be solicitous, warm, and caring. This, together with carefully-worded claims and voluminous support by testimonials (not research), often leads sufferers and their loved ones into spending precious time and large sums of money on questionable and unproven treatments. However, over and over again, this "can't lose" or "last resort" mentality has proven fatal to cancer victims.

Quacks frequently accuse the medical profession of refusing to use their particular therapy because of selfish reasons, and they indict the government for banning it out of support for "big business." They pay little attention to the fact that the American Cancer Society, the National Cancer Institute, and similar organizations in the United States and other countries are constantly evaluating every possible agent claimed to be effective in the treatment of cancer.

It would be bad enough if the loss of the sufferer's finances and those of his family were the only consideration. Unfortunately, all too often these irregular cures cause the cancer victim to neglect tried methods of treatment. Meanwhile, the cancer steadily progresses, reaching a stage where any treatment becomes hopeless. Thus many lives have been needlessly sacrificed.

While it is sometimes difficult for a professional, let alone a lay person, to evaluate the claims for a particular cancer cure, there are some serious questions you can ask regarding any purported remedy for cancer.

- Does the effectiveness of the remedy rest on testimonials of those supposedly cured, and on statements released to the news media by its promoters? If so, it should raise a serious doubt in your mind.
- Check to see whether the academic degrees the promoter claims to have are real. Is he a graduate of a bona fide academic institution? If he gives you the name of such an institution, call the university's public relations officer and ask whether he is really an alumnus. (The title "Doctor" applies to a number of degrees. Even the use of "M.D." is no assurance of valid qualifications, since this degree can be "bought" in certain countries.) Also call your local medical society and the American Cancer Society and ask about that person's professional standing among his peers. Another source of valuable information is the local office of the federal government's Food and Drug Administration. Their people can tell you the status of the remedy that is being recommended to you.
- What experience has this health practitioner had in diagnosing and treating malignancies? If he says you have a cancer, what tests did he employ, and how willing is he to share his findings with your physician? If he is, ask him to send your physician or pathologist a report for evaluation.
- Has this person published his findings in a reputable scientific journal, or is his literature in the form of *self-published* books, pamphlets, and papers?

- Is the treatment you are being offered found only in a distant geographical location (some other country) where surveillance by reputable professionals and government agencies does not exist?
- Does the promoter of this cure have a "secret formula" that he has promised some now deceased researcher to not disclose?
- Does he have a "martyr complex"? That is, did he have to leave the United States, or some other country with high medical standards, because his "remedy" would put regular medical practitioners out of business?
- Does he claim that he is being persecuted, and forced to "practice" where he is, because of his desire to help humanity?

Some years ago, a substance called *laetrile,* derived from apricot seeds, was widely promoted for its ability to cure cancer. It was heralded as a "natural remedy" and given the designation of a "missing vitamin" (vitamin B_{17}). Laetrile is amygdalin, a chemical that contains 6 percent cyanide by weight. A single 500 mg dose contains enough cyanide to kill a person if the cyanide were released from its chemical combination. Fortunately, most of a dose of laetrile is excreted without being broken into its constituent chemicals.

A study of nearly 200 laetrile treated cancer patients by independent researchers failed to show a single case in which there was a clear-cut anticancer benefit. Since laetrile costs very little to produce, the promoters did very well financially. During a twenty-seven month period, the documented bank deposits of one promoter totaled $2.5 million!

Cooperate in your treatment plan

Different types of cancer have differing treatment programs. Place yourself in the hands of a specialist in the treatment of your particular cancer. Your family physician can recommend the right person for you, as can the local medical society or the American Cancer Society.

Treatment of cancer

Your treatment may involve surgery, radiation, or chemotherapy, or a combination of these procedures. Depending on the malignancy, a hormonal therapy may be used.

When **surgery** is employed, the cancerous lesion and the surrounding tissues are removed. This is especially true if the cancer is discovered early, and while it is still localized. On occasion, surgery is preceded by radiation or chemotherapy—treatments used to reduce the size of the malignancy.

Irradiation therapy consists of exposing the tumor to X-rays or other forms of radiation. Modern techniques carefully direct the rays, concentrating them almost exclusively on the cancer, so that far less normal tissue adjacent to the cancer is destroyed. As a result, radiation sickness is now much less severe than in the past.

Chemotherapy employs chemical agents that destroy rapidly multiplying cells. These agents are used when the cancer is not localized, such as in leukemia. It is also used in cases when the cancer has been surgically removed but the possibility exists that some spread may have occurred, and when the cancer has already spread to so many areas of the body that the use of irradiation and surgery are not feasible. And, as already mentioned, chemotherapy may be used as a pretreatment to surgery.

In **hormonal therapy,** hormones or their synthetic counterparts are used to suppress the growth of cancers whose cells arose from endocrine organs, and are thus susceptible to the influence of these substances.

Medical specialists have long looked forward to the development of **immunotherapy**—treatment in which a person is protected from developing cancer by activating his own immune defenses. Newer immunotherapy techniques are proving to be effective in the treatment of certain animal tumors, and there is considerable optimism that similar approaches will soon be available in the fight against human cancer.

Below are a few examples of treatments directed against particular types of cancer that illustrate how the various therapeutic measures are used.

Lung cancer. No uniformly effective treatment for lung cancer exists, though early surgical removal of the affected portion of the lung, sometimes supplemented by irradiation therapy and/or chemotherapy, saves up to about 10 percent of cases.

Breast cancer. For cancer of the breast, the current trend is to use surgery conservatively, followed by irradiation to kill cancer cells that may remain in the region of the breast, and chemotherapy to suppress or prevent the growth of cancer cells that may have migrated to other parts of the body.

Leukemia. With leukemias (cancer of the blood-forming tissues) chemotherapy, sometimes supplemented by irradiation therapy, gives the best results.

Prostate cancer. Hormone therapy is especially useful in treating this cancer.

Preventing cancer—what you can do

The best "treatment" for cancer is to avoid it in the first place. Many experts believe that up to 90 percent of all cancer is due at least in part to environmental or lifestyle exposures, and that most, if not all, of these could be avoided.

One of your best precautions is a complete medical checkup by your physician on a regular basis, especially as you get older. Women should request a Pap smear at least as often as they have a regular checkup, and occasionally a mammogram.

We have already mentioned tobacco, alcohol, and caffeine (the chemical found in coffee, tea, many soft drinks, and mate [mah-teh]—a popular South American drink) as potential cancer producers. Cigarette smoke is the single greatest culprit in many of today's societies. Unfortunately, cigarette smoke is intimately associated with the use of alcohol and coffee drinking, and these in turn may all be linked directly or indirectly to dietary factors.

Some researchers maintain that approximately two-thirds of all cancer deaths can be ascribed to tobacco and diet. They believe that in the United States diet plays the major role in female cancer, while tobacco is the primary cause of cancer in men. Dietary fats, especially those derived from animal sources (fatty steaks, lard, butter) may promote cancerous growths in the tissues of the breast and the lining of the colon. It also appears that animal protein may increase the risk of cancers of the prostate, colon, and kidneys.

Cancer of the colon is rare in people with a diet that is high in fiber and low in animal protein, fat, and refined sugar. In such diets, the passage of waste through the intestinal tract (called transit time) is significantly shorter than it is for people who eat the typical Western diet. A high-fiber diet also changes the mix of intestinal organisms, and it ap-

pears that the extra bulk provided by the fiber may dilute carcinogens and co-carcinogens, making them less effective. In these and other ways, high dietary fiber reduces the risk of colon and rectal cancer (see also page 92).

For these reasons it would seem wise, as you plan your diet, to avoid refined foods from which much of the fiber has been removed. Choose foods that are low in fat (especially fat of animal origin) and that have low to moderate amounts of protein. Plant proteins are best. Obese women have a higher incidence of breast cancer than women of normal weight, so you should plan on just enough calories to avoid becoming overweight (see page 231).

Use common-sense measures to avoid or minimize exposure to chemicals in your home, garage, garden, and workplace. For example, avoid inhaling aerosol sprays such as hair spray, insect repellent, lubricant, and home cleaner. Also, avoid all unnecessary contact with laundry detergents, polishes, gasoline, oils, and chemicals at large. Be sure to wear a mask any time you must use pesticides and other sprays, and thoroughly wash your skin when you are through to remove contaminants.

Recent research indicates that a healthy body has several methods of blocking certain cancer-causing events. Your body has a mechanism that prevents the transformation of a normal cell into a cancer cell, and even when such a transformation has occurred, the newly formed cancer cell and its offspring may be destroyed. Thus a healthy lifestyle (see page 117) is a preventive not only for cancer, but also for many of the other killer diseases so common in our society.

Here is a summary of things that you can do to lower your risk of getting cancer:

- **Avoid exposure to known cancer-producing agents.** These include tobacco smoke, beverage alcohol, caffeine-containing drinks, aerosols, paints and solvents, poison sprays, excessive sunshine, and unnecessary X-ray radiation.
- **Dietary cautions.** Eat plenty of fruits and vegetables, especially broccoli, cabbage, brussels sprouts, and other green leafy vegetables. Eat whole grain cereals and some legumes (beans) to ensure a generous intake of fiber.

    Do not overeat, and if you are overweight, regain your normal weight. Reduce your intake of fat to 15 to 20 percent of your total calories. If you are an average American, this means cutting your fat intake to a little less than half what it now is. Where possible, replace red meat with fish, or, even better, with milk and vegetable proteins. Most cheeses are high in fat.

- **Maintain physical well-being.** These are discussed under a healthful lifestyle.
- **Maintain mental well-being.** Studies have shown that happy people—especially those who are very happy—live much longer than those who are unhappy. "Laughter wards" have actually been established in many hospitals today, because of the healing benefit of cheerfulness. The Good Book says, "A merry heart doeth good like a medicine" (Proverbs 17:22). Trust God. Try to help someone who has greater needs than you do, and be grateful for the blessings you do have.

Cancers at large

The cancers that occur in the various tissues and organs of the body are described in detail under the diseases of each organ or system. They are also listed in the general index.

699

CHAPTER 24

General infections

The human body is veritably bathed in an ocean of germs: bacteria, viruses, and fungi. While most are friendly or harmless, some are hostile and dangerous. A newborn baby is sterile, but immediately upon birth it is invaded by countless microorganisms. Fungal spores in the air and the touch of helping hands and loving lips soon blanket the infant in germs. On the skin, in the hair follicles, up the nose, down the throat, in the intestinal tract, and on and in the external sex organs, microscopic and submicroscopic invaders establish residence.

Infection refers to the entrance into the body's tissues of disease-producing organisms. To gain this entrance they must cross one of two barriers: the skin or the mucous membranes. The skin is covered by an acid coat that hampers the growth of microbes, both bacteria and fungi, while the normal inhabitants of the skin are also hostile to any newcomers. The mucous membranes are no less defensive, as their fluid secretions are toxic to numerous germs. Mucus and other watery secretions pour from countless glands embedded in the membranes of the respiratory, digestive, and genito-urinary tracts.

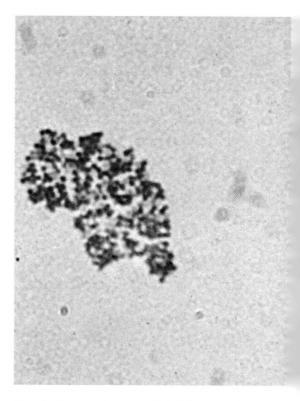

Staphylococcal germs (highly magnified).

The respiratory tract filters the air you breathe. The tortuous path that air must follow after it is breathed traps dust and associated germs. The mucus that lines the bronchial passages traps additional germs, and by means of the mucus elevator (see page 902) expels it into the mouth, where it is either spat out or swallowed. Coughing clears the respiratory tree of large accumulations of mucus and debris.

The digestive tract provides an inhospitable environment to germs. The highly acid secretions of the stomach act as a chlorinating plant that kills many organisms. The contents of the stomach, including germs, move into the highly alkaline small intestine, where concentrated bile and digestive enzymes destroy additional germs. Mucus also flows from the intestinal walls, and the wavelike contractions of the walls sweep the contents of the intestine downward into the colon, where all newcomers in the germ population must defend themselves against es-

tablished residents or be carried out in the stool. The urinary and genital tracts of both men and women are also designed to resist the inroads of germs. Many of their secretions contain anti-infective constituents.

Should the skin break or a mucous membrane be breached, the microbes face another formidable line of defense in the tissues and the circulating blood that is designed to combat any invasion by disease-producing organisms. Phagocytic cells (cells that surround germs and foreign particles) can engulf invading germs like giant vacuum sweepers, and even destroy them. Any microbe that escapes the phagocytic cells must still face chemical warfare as the body's immune mechanisms (see page 827) come into play. Each unfriendly germ stimulates the production of specific antibodies and other lethal chemicals that have been custom-made to combat it. The body makes every possible effort to expel or destroy every foreign invader.

As the invaders and the defense

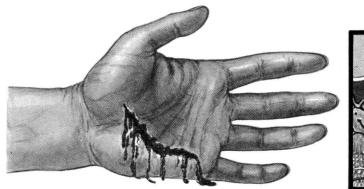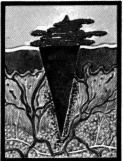

Injuries may introduce disease-producing organisms into the body.

701

forces lock in mortal combat, certain factors tend to swing the outcome in either a favorable or unfavorable direction. Sometimes the enemy's superior numbers overwhelm the body's defenses. At other times the defense forces are more deadly in their attack.

The individual's relative susceptibility is another variable. Immunity is one of the body's strongest defenses against invading microbes. For example, anyone who has recovered from rubella has antibodies within his system that protect him for the remainder of his life from any future illness caused by this particular virus, but the person whose tissues do not contain these antibodies may become an easy victim once the virus has breached his defenses.

On the other hand, fatigue, malnourishment, or other illnesses reduce the efficiency of the body's defense system, making the person more susceptible to infections. Even mental attitudes can affect the defense system. Immunity is enhanced in people who are happy and contented while anger and resentment diminish resistance. The old saying has been proved true today: "A merry heart doeth good like a medicine, but a broken spirit drieth the bones" (Proverbs 17:22).

Local infections

Should infective organisms break through the defenses at some particular site, every effort is made to limit, or localize, the spread of the infection. Soldier cells called phagocytes (white blood cells) pour into the infected area, "closing ranks" to

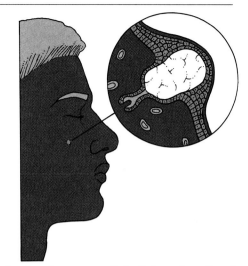

A pimple or small boil is a localized infection in the skin.

literally wall off the zone of conflict. When this occurs in tissue that is near the surface of the body, the resulting local infection is called a **boil,** or on a smaller scale, a **pimple.** Virulent germs may destroy some of the tissue. This tissue debris, together with dead germs, active germs, and phagocytes, fills the center of the mass, forming what we call **pus.**

A similar scenario occurs when a local infection develops deeper inside the body, but the localized infection is called an **abscess.** In both boils and abscesses, the contents of the infection must be evacuated, or they may be reabsorbed. Evacuation occurs when a boil bursts or an abscess is surgically lanced and drained. Squeezing a boil or pimple may actually spread the infection by forcing germs into surrounding tissue.

General infections

When invading microorganisms overwhelm the body's defense

702

forces, or when some of them slip past the body's blockade, they are usually entrapped by the lymphatic system (see page 828). The lymph (tissue fluid), together with the invading germs, is carried by tiny vessels to the lymph nodes, where the invaders must run the gauntlet of additional defense cells. The lymph nodes may enlarge as additional forces are brought in to fight the enemy.

Despite these efforts, germs frequently do enter the bloodstream (**bacteremia, septicemia**—the presence of hostile microorganisms in the blood). These meet additional "lines of defense" in the cells of the liver, spleen (reticulo-endothelial), and lungs (phagocytic) that attack and destroy the invaders. Germs may enter the blood during the treatment of local infections, such as the extraction of an infected tooth or the draining of an abscess. On very rare occasions invaders from these sources can cause serious infections such as endocarditis, osteomyelitis, and brain abscess. To avoid this danger, the physician may prescribe antibiotics.

Infectious and contagious diseases

An **infectious disease** is a disease caused by a germ or virus that enters the body. Malaria, caused by a parasite, is an example of an infectious disease. By contrast, atherosclerosis is not caused by a microorganism and is not an infectious disease. A **contagious disease** is an infectious disease that can be easily transmitted from a sick person to a well person,

usually by close contact. Syphilis is an example of such a disease. Sometimes contagious diseases are spoken of as **communicable diseases.**

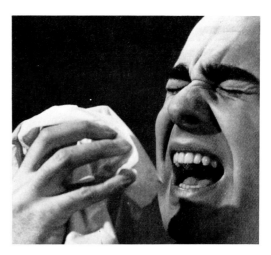

Many infectious diseases are spread by droplets carrying germs and viruses that are discharged into the air by sneezing and coughing.

Responses to infections

Toxins from an infection, circulated through the body, may prompt chills (ague) and fever. This occurs, for instance, when the malarial parasite is released from the red blood cells during one phase of the disease. Fever is a uniform accompaniment of many serious infectious diseases. In some cases the rise in body temperature aids the body's defenses in combating the infection.

Infection and other diseases may alter the "thermostat" setting in the brain, impairing its effectiveness, and causing the body temperature to rise. When this happens we say that the patient has a fever. Delirium may result anytime the temperature rises above 105°F. In infants and young children high temperatures may precipitate convulsions, making it necessary to take steps to lower the temperature. This can include tepid baths, with or without medication.

Another response to infection is the rise in the number and type of certain white blood cells in the blood, and also in the immediate vicinity of the source of the infection, as in septic sore throat.

Infections that the body can overcome if given enough time are called **self-limited.** Should the body's defenses prove inadequate, the illness may be prolonged, or the outcome may be fatal. When the defense is adequate, the organisms are overcome, the disease is terminated, and health is restored.

Therapy for infections

Two principles underline the treatment of infections: (1) reinforcement and augmentation of the body's own defense mechanisms and (2) weakening or destroying the invaders by physical or chemical means.

The body must ultimately heal itself. Providing adequate rest and sleep, simple diet, abundant fluids (often provided intravenously), a quiet environment, and certain physical therapy procedures (see page 589) aid the body's defenses. Sometimes antibodies (immune globulins) and antitoxins (in tetanus) greatly accelerate recovery.

Anti-infective agents attack the invaders by making them more vulnerable to the body's defenses by killing them. The antibiotic penicillin weakens the cell wall surrounding the pneumococci bacteria (which causes one form of pneumonia), causing it to die. Quinine is directly toxic to the malarial parasite.

Prevention

Maintaining health by means of a healthful lifestyle (see page 117) is the most effective and cheapest protection against infectious diseases. Life is such that we cannot live in a sealed environment that does not allow us to be exposed to germs and viruses. These would-be villains envelop us and are but waiting for an opportunity to strike. Health, good health, is best maintained by having a high regard for nature's laws. Such a lifestyle will maximize our resistance to infectious germs and minimize our risk of disease.

CHAPTER 25

Bacterial infections

Bacteria are minute organisms, observed only under a microscope, which contain both RNA and DNA (the two forms of nucleic acid) and are capable of active reproduction. Bacteria are widely distributed in nature and perform useful functions, such as withdrawing nitrogen from the air for use in growing plants. Many harmless bacteria inhabit the human intestinal tract and even synthesize certain vitamins the body needs. However, there are also harmful bacteria which, on entering the body, cause illness and disease. Many of these bacterial diseases have been described under the diseases of the various organ systems. Others will be discussed here.

Actinomycosis (lumpy jaw)

A rod-shaped bacteria, actinomycetes are normal inhabitants of the mouth, decayed teeth, tonsils, and intestines. Following a break in the mucous membranes of these areas (or of the lungs), these organisms establish an inflammation in the tissues and form abscesses. The disease displays itself as abscesses that drain through tunnels called sinuses. These sinuses drain to the surface of the body: in the neck; in the lungs, where the disease resembles tuberculosis; in the intestine, where it may cause partial obstruction; and occasionally as a generalized infection involving other organs of the body.

Another form of actinomycete is Anthrax (malignant pustule; woolsorter's disease) nocardia, which causes **nocardiosis**—a disease very similar to actinomycosis. The organism is present in the soil and may enter the skin through an injury, resulting in abscess formation. When inhaled, symptoms resemble tuberculosis, with cough and pussy sputum. Any organs of the body may be affected. The bacterial organisms are susceptible to sulfonamide.

What your physician can do. Certain antibiotics are effective in controlling this disease, but they must be continued for several weeks after apparent recovery. Sometimes surgery is required to eradicate the fistulas and sinuses.

705

Anthrax (malignant pustule; woolsorter's disease)

Anthrax is a serious inflammatory disease caused by the anthrax bacillus being transmitted to humans from diseased animals, either through the bacterial form or through spores (seedlike latent form). It can affect the skin, lungs, and intestine. The spores adhere to the skin and hair of animals and can enter the body through a break in the skin, through being inhaled in the air, or by eating contaminated meat. When contracted in the lungs or intestines, the disease is more serious than that of the skin. Even when the skin is involved, the mortality rate for untreated cases is 20 percent.

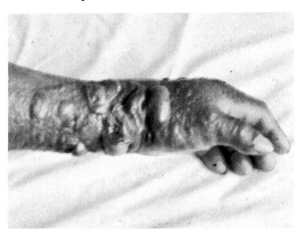

A typical case of anthrax.

Anthrax starts in the skin as a small, red, slightly raised spot. The lesion soon blisters, ulcerates, and spreads by forming large blisters that, in turn, break and ulcerate. The surrounding tissue is swollen, and the lesions itch, but little pain is felt.

Human anthrax can be prevented by a vaccine, strongly recommended for those at high risk in endemic areas. Antibiotics are effective in treating the disease.

Brucellosis (undulant fever)

Undulant fever, as its name suggests, is a disease that is characterized by a fever that rises and falls. The germ is transmitted to humans from infected domestic animals (cattle, sheep, pigs, and goats). It enters the body by way of breaks in the skin, by inhaling contaminated dust from the animals' excretions, or from consuming contaminated meat, milk, or milk products.

The incubation period is usually about two weeks (though it may be anywhere from one to seven), and typical symptoms include intermittent fever (high each evening), profuse sweating, headache, and muscle and joint pains. Symptoms gradually disappear, only to reappear in a few weeks, such episodes occurring one or more times.

What you can do. You can prevent the disease by treating or eliminating the infected animals; by wearing a face mask when handling their manure; by pasteurizing their milk and thoroughly cooking their meat; and by wearing gloves when handling infected animals or their carcasses. Should you have the disease, you should rest in bed during the acute phase, drink plenty of water, and eat easily digested, nutritious food.

What your physician can do. Your doctor will first make a precise diagnosis by means of laboratory tests, and then he will prescribe antibiotics that are effective against the disease.

Cat-scratch disease

This infection is caused by a small gram-negative bacillus that is usually conveyed by the scratch of a kitten, sometimes a bite, and more rarely by a thorn in the skin. It is seen most often in children. A scabbed ulcer of the skin develops at the site of a scratch, along with an enlarged lymph node (or nodes) in the affected area—the armpit, groin, or neck. General symptoms are loss of appetite, weakness, fever, and nausea.

There is no specific remedy, and recovery is usually in a few weeks or months. Heat over the infected nodes may provide relief. Antibiotics are ineffective.

Cholera

Cholera is one of the five major pestilences of the world, having caused millions of deaths in India, Southeast Asia, China, Africa, and southern Europe. The cholera germ, *vibrio cholera*, lives only in humans. It enters the body through contaminated food and drink and takes up residence in the upper small intestine. The stools of infected individuals are filled with germs, and thus unsanitary conditions contribute to the spread of the disease.

The germs manufacture a toxin that causes an extremely severe diarrhea. The incubation period is short—six to forty-eight hours. Symptoms begin abruptly with a watery, painless diarrhea in which as much as a quart (slightly less than one liter) of fluid can be lost within an hour. Effortless vomiting causes further water loss. This rapid depletion of fluids and minerals brings on profound shock. When untreated, the mortality rate is 50 percent. Death may occur within hours if replacement fluids containing minerals are not given promptly by mouth or vein.

A vaccine is available that provides partial protection for four to six months. Those travelling in areas where cholera is prevalent should be vaccinated in advance.

What your physician can do. Your doctor will immediately replace lost fluids with electrolyte (mineral-containing) solutions given by mouth or vein.

Diphtheria

Diphtheria is a dreaded disease which in the past has caused thousands of deaths, and is still prevalent in less developed areas of the world. Survivors may suffer paralysis of certain muscles and permanent damage to the heart and kidneys. Children from one to ten are most susceptible. The organisms are spread by inhaled secretions from the nose and mouth of an infected person, from contaminated fingers or towels, and from contaminated milk.

Diphtheria germs invade the membranes of the upper air passages (pharynx, larynx, and trachea) causing sore throat, fever, difficulty in breathing and swallowing, a discharge from the nose and throat, and severe prostration. The lymph glands in the neck become enlarged and tender. A thick membrane forms over the back of the throat and may cause difficulty in breathing or, if dislodged, obstruct the air passageway and cause asphyxiation. An opening in the windpipe (tracheotomy) may be necessary to save life.

Germs in the throat produce a very potent toxin that is circulated in the blood. Except from the danger of asphyxiation mentioned above, most deaths result from the damage this toxin produces in the heart and kidneys. Nerve damage causes paralysis of certain muscles, especially in the area of the throat and face.

In 1923 a diphtheria toxoid was developed which stimulates the body to produce a long-term immunity against the disease. A booster injection should be given every ten years. This program has virtually eliminated the disease from the major developed areas of the world. The occasional cases that occur are usually individuals who have not been immunized.

What your physician can do. As soon as possible, your doctor will administer an antitoxin that effectively neutralizes the toxin produced by the bacteria, and that, if given early enough, may prevent damage to your heart, kidneys, and nerves. He will also prescribe antibiotics to kill the diphtheria germs, and he will recommend bed rest, adequate fluids, nutritious food, and a gradual return to full activity. If you were not immunized, hospital care with close observation is essential.

Leprosy (Hansen's disease)

Leprosy is a chronic, mildly contagious disease that is caused by a germ resembling the germ of tuberculosis. The disease is most common in tropical countries, with ten to twenty million persons suffering from the malady worldwide. In the United States, approximately 500 new cases are diagnosed each year, occurring mainly among immigrants.

It is believed that the germs enter the body through the nasal mem-

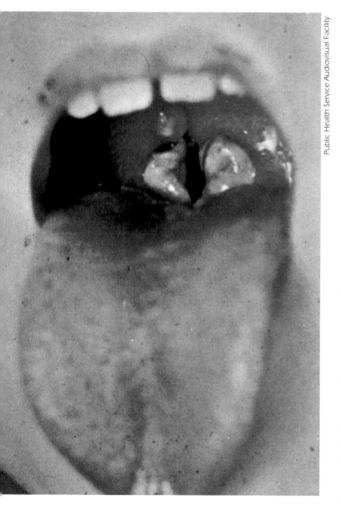

Public Health Service Audiovisual Facility

Inflammation of the throat in diptheria.

brane and through breaks in the skin. The incubation period is two to five years or longer. The first sign of leprosy is usually a light-colored (depigmented) patch of skin that is accompanied by the loss of the sensation of touch and temperature. There are two well-defined forms of leprosy: lepromatous and tuberculoid.

Lepromatous leprosy, in which the sufferer shows no resistance to the disease, exhibits nodules and dispersed infiltration of the skin. Nodules are especially abundant on the face. The cheeks, brows, and ears are swollen and irregular, giving the face a "lionlike" appearance. The nodules may ulcerate, breaking down the adjoining tissues. Fingers, toes, ears, and nose may be destroyed. Nerves in the limbs are affected, occasionally causing pain (neuritis) before losing all sensation. Much of the damage to extremities results from the lack of sensitivity to pain, and the resulting lack of care given to even minor injuries. The function of muscles may be lost.

Tuberculoid leprosy is less severe, progresses slowly, and principally affects the skin, causing discoloration and insensitivity. Damage to nerves may be considerable.

What you can do. During acute phases of leprosy in others, avoid contact with body discharges from their lesions as well as food, clothing, and other objects that may have been contaminated. Protect your eyes, hands, and feet. If you have the disease, remain as active as possible, eat a wholesome diet, and maintain a courageous outlook. Follow the

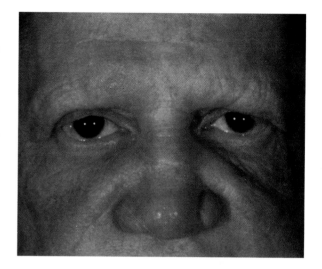

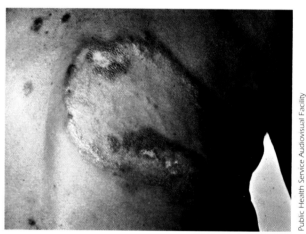

Public Health Service Audiovisual Facility

Upper: lepromatous leprosy; the eyebrows are lost. Lower: tuberculoid leprosy; the skin and sensory nerves are affected.

counsel of your physician.

What your physician can do. Initial care is best provided in a clinic or institution designed for the treatment and education of those afflicted with leprosy. Your physician will prescribe medications (antibiotics and sulfones) that effectively suppress the disease, permitting you to resume normal activities. Treatment is prolonged and may last five or more years. Tissue loss and major deformities may not be restored, but surgical procedures will allow a considerable return of function.

Plague (bubonic plague)

A highly infectious disease, bubonic plague—also known as "the plague"—is another of the five great pestilences of all time. It killed untold millions during the Middle Ages. Fortunately, the incidence and mortality of the disease have been greatly reduced through immunization and antibiotic therapy. The plague still exists in wild rodents in many parts of the world, even in the western United States. Other animals, such as rabbits, bobcats, coyotes, and domestic cats, dogs, and rats, may also harbor the germs. Australia is the only continent free from the disease. The germs are usually carried from an infected animal to humans through fleabites.

Following a bite from an infected flea, the incubation period is from a few hours to ten days. Symptoms begin suddenly with a high fever, great weakness, chills, severe headache, pains in the back and limbs, vomiting, and diarrhea. Lymph nodes that drain the area of the bite, such as those in the groin, armpit, and neck, become tender and swollen, and are called buboes. Abscesses form in these buboes and break through the skin. The germs travel largely in the lymphatic system, but may enter the bloodstream and affect any organ of the body.

Pneumonic plague is a serious complication of bubonic plague, and if untreated is almost uniformly fatal.

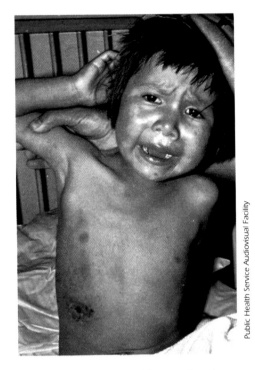

Public Health Service Audiovisual Facility

Bubonic plague. Note the large buboes or swellings under the arms.

The disease is transmitted through bacteria-laden droplets discharged from the sufferer's mouth and nose as he coughs, sneezes, or speaks forcibly.

A vaccine is available for immunizing persons at high risk, especially those caring for plague sufferers and for veterinarians.

What your physician can do. If you contract the plague, you will be hospitalized, and your doctor will promptly start appropriate antibiotic therapy. All precautions will be taken to limit the spread of the disease. He will prescribe bed rest, adequate fluid intake, and cooling measures for high fever. Ice bags applied intermittently over painful buboes will provide some relief.

Ratbite fever

Ratbite fever includes several uncommon infections transmitted by the bite of a rodent, usually a rat. Infection may be caused by a bacillus or spirochete. The general symptoms are the same for both forms and include chill, fever, headache, muscle pains, and weakness.

Bacillus form. The onset of symptoms occurs less than ten days after the bite. Joint pains commonly occur and persist for months. A rash develops on the limbs, involving even the palms and soles. The spleen and liver are sometimes enlarged. Infection of the heart lining (endocarditis) is the most serious complication. Untreated, the mortality rate is 10 percent.

Spirochete form. The incubation period is more than ten days. The infection at the site of the bite heals quickly, and as quickly becomes inflamed again. The lymph nodes in the area of the bite become tender and swollen. Some forms develop liver and kidney failure. The fever runs for periods of three to four days, followed by periods of no fever. This pattern lasts for months if the infection is untreated. The joints are seldom involved.

What your physician can do. The history of the bite, together with your symptoms, will help your doctor to determine the nature of the infection. He will prescribe large doses of antibiotics, especially if there is endocarditis, and this will usually terminate the illness. Recovery is generally assured if the therapy is started promptly.

Scarlet fever (scarlatina)

Scarlet fever is a complication of a streptococcus (beta-hemolytic) infection (that is, strep sore throat—see page 913). In an acutely ill child, it manifests as a red rash with fever. The bacteria in the throat produce a virulent toxin that injures the capillaries of the skin. The resulting rash first appears on the upper chest and back, later on the rest of the body, but frequently not on the face. Elevations like goose pimples develop and usually turn into tiny blisters. The skin peels as the rash fades, and large sections become loose, especially on the palms of the hands and soles of the feet. The lymph nodes of the neck enlarge. If untreated, complications may include sinusitis, middle-ear infection, and mastoiditis. Other strep toxins may damage the heart, causing acute rheumatic fever, or the kidneys may be affected, causing acute nephritis.

Children in poor health who have been exposed to scarlet fever or strep sore throat may be protected from the extreme results of the disease by the prompt administration of penicillin.

What your physician can do. Your doctor will administer an appropriate antibiotic to minimize the risk of complications. He may recommend bed rest, plenty of fluids, and nourishing food. Heating compresses to the neck help to relieve the sore throat. A lotion may be soothing as the skin peels. Complications may require hospitalization.

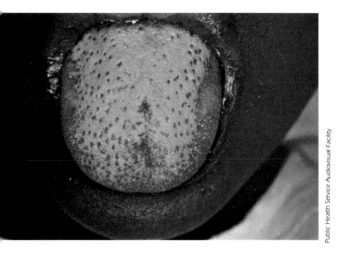

Public Health Service Audiovisual Facility

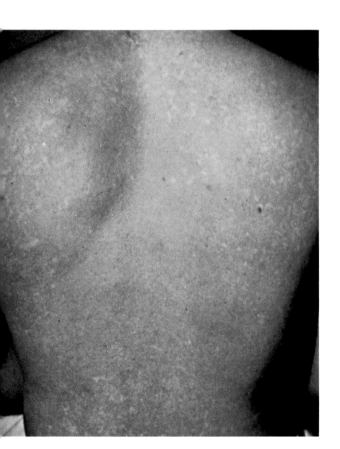

Scarlet fever. Note the coated tongue and skin rash.

Shigellosis (bacillary dysentary)

This is an acute infection of the bowel, caused by the bacillus shigella that occurs in all parts of the world, especially the tropics. However, it is rarely the organism responsible for "travelers's diarrhea." It is prevalent in areas without sanitary food and water. Little children are especially susceptible.

During the incubation period the germs invade the lining of the colon. One to three days after exposure there is an abrupt onset of fever, with loss of appetite, drowsiness, a desire to vomit, abdominal pain, and frequent passage of stools (as many as 100 a day, sometimes more) containing mucus, blood, and pus. The danger to life, especially in children, is due to marked loss of fluid.

In healthy adults who develop bacillary dysentery, the fever will cease in about four days, while the diarrhea and abdominal cramps usually continue a few days longer. It is extremely important to replace fluids, especially in infants, children, and those who are frail, even if this must be done intravenously in a clinic or hospital.

What you can do. If you live where this disease is commonplace, you must adopt the principles of good sanitation: control flies, handle sewage appropriately, use safe food and water, and keep your hands clean.

What your physician can do. Your doctor will provide appropriate antibiotic medication to shorten the duration of the illness. He will also determine the need for intravenous fluids.

Salmonella infection (salmonellosis)

Each year some two million cases of salmonella infection occur in the United States. The incidence is highest during the summer and fall and is associated with outbreaks of food poisoning. It is most frequently seen in infants. The bacteria causing the infection in industrialized societies are nontyphoid salmonellas, while those seen in less developed countries are the salmonella that cause typhoid fever.

Farm animals and poultry commonly harbor the bacteria. It is spread by infected poultry, eggs, raw milk, and meat. The organisms are not killed by freezing, but are de-stroyed by cooking. Hands that handle foods carrying the bacteria (including frozen foods) may contaminate other foods and kitchen utensils. Varying sizes of groups may become infected, depending on how many people eat the contaminated food. Groups likely to become victims are members of one family, picnic partiers, diners at restaurants, and patients in retirement homes. The organisms may also spread person to person because of unwashed hands. More recently, some sources of marijuana have become contaminated, infecting users over widespread areas.

The infection can take one of four forms: gastroenteritis, enteric fever (typhoidlike), bacteremia (germs in the blood), and the human carrier. Two-thirds of all salmonella infec-

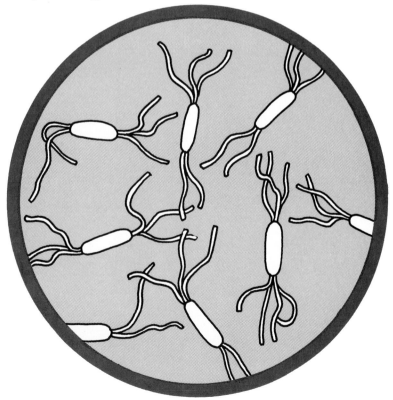

Salmonella organisms under magnification.

713

tions cause gastroenteritis.

Gastroenteritis occurs about forty-eight hours after exposure with the onset of nausea, vomiting, abdominal cramps, and diarrhea. The infection is generally self-limited and ends in three or four days, but may last a week. The severe form is associated with fever (102°F or higher), tenderness in the abdomen, a severe choleralike disease, or a dysentery with bloody stools. The infection may enter the bloodstream and cause pockets of infection.

Enteric fevers resembling typhoid develop more slowly, having an incubation period of one or two weeks. The symptoms, which are similar to those associated with the flu, include prolonged fever, loss of appetite, pains in the muscles and joints, cough, sore throat, and headache. These symptoms gradually increase in severity for about a week, after which the symptoms of true typhoid fever will be seen—those mentioned above plus nausea, vomiting, mental confusion, and abdominal tenderness. A rose-colored, slightly raised rash, with discrete spots on the chest, will appear and fade after three to four days. In untreated cases the symptoms begin to subside after a week. For details, see page 718.

Bacteremia means the presence of bacteria in the blood. A mild, short-lived form of bacteremia may accompany gastroenteritis. However, sustained blood infections may cause localized infections in the lining of the large arteries and heart (endocarditis). Infections may develop in the bones (osteomyelitis) and joints (pussy arthritis). Meningitis may also develop, especially in infants.

Human carrier state. In this form of the disease, the person feels healthy but passes the salmonella organism in his or her stool, and thus transmits the disease and becomes a carrier. It is quite common for people with nontyphoid salmonella to develop carrier status (5 percent). Less than 1 percent of those infected become permanent carriers. In the typhoid-type, about 3 percent of infected persons become permanent carriers.

What you can do. If you develop a diarrhea with several of the symptoms mentioned above that persists for more than two or three days, or if you suffer from severe thirst or have a fever of more than 101°, see your physician.

What your physician can do. Using laboratory tests, your doctor will attempt to isolate the infecting organism. Blood tests available for certain types of salmonella are not practical to use. The gastroenteritis infection is treated with restoration of fluids and the relief of pain. Antibiotics are used only if the patient has the enteric form or bacteremia. In other disturbances, your physician will employ the appropriate antibiotic, depending on the offending organism.

Tetanus (lockjaw)

Tetanus is a life-threatening and often fatal disease caused by the toxin of a germ. Because of immunization, this disease is rare in industrialized nations, but worldwide, each year some one million deaths occur from tetanus, almost half of them in newborn infants.

The organisms and their spores are abundant in garden and barnyard soil, in dust on the roadside and in playgrounds, and especially in soil and dust mixed with horse manure. Spores enter a deep wound from a nail, thorn, bite, or deep laceration, and, excluded from oxygen, multiply and produce a toxin. In many parts of the world cow and horse manure are used to cover the navel of newborns in order to reduce bleeding. This increases the exposure to tetanus spores, and, of course, the occurrence of tetanus.

The incubation period varies, but is usually five to fourteen days. The toxin alters nerve conduction.

The original wound may begin to heal when symptoms appear. Symptoms include restlessness and concern, stiffness of the muscles of the face with difficulty in opening and closing the mouth—hence the popular name **lockjaw.** Other muscles of the body gradually become involved. The stronger muscles out-pull the weaker, drawing the face, extremities, and body into unusual positions.

Mass contractions of muscles may occur, accompanied by intense pain, fever, sweating, and exhaustion. Contractions of the back muscles may result in fractures of the vertebrae. Spasm of the muscles of respiration not infrequently causes death by asphyxiation. Untreated, the mortality rate is between 50 and 60 percent.

The disease can be prevented by immunization with tetanus toxoid. Infants and children should be immunized at an early age and given a booster shot every ten years.

What you can do. If you or your children have not been immunized, go to your physician immediately for immunization. If you have received a dirty injury, clean it thoroughly with soap and water. If it is a penetrating wound, see your physician. If your last immunization was more than ten years ago, have your physician give you a booster.

What your physician can do. If symptoms have developed, your doctor will admit you to the intensive care unit of a hospital and treat you with an antitoxin from a human source. This will not alter the toxin already attached to your nerves, but will neutralize any circulating toxin. Muscle relaxants will relieve the spasms in your muscles and may safeguard you against possible fractures. A respirator may be needed if your breathing becomes impaired. Your wound will be opened and cleaned to remove the possibility of additional toxin being formed.

Tuberculosis (TB)

Tuberculosis is a mildly contagious disease caused by bacteria. It most commonly affects the lungs and is spread by an infected person through contact with his sputum or through inhalation of droplets released by his coughing or sneezing. A hundred years ago, one out of five deaths in the United States was caused by tuberculosis. Today it is only a minor threat and then only to those who are old, poor, and malnourished. Worldwide, however, tuberculosis takes the lives of some three million people each year, especially in crowded, poverty-ridden countries.

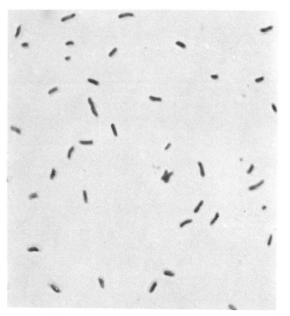

Tuberculous germs (bacilli) may enter the lungs from germ-laden air, or they may enter the intestines from contaminated food.

The first breakthrough in handling the disease came from Edward Trodeau, a young physician who himself had contracted and overcome the disease. In 1885 he established an institution for the treatment of tuberculosis by means of a program that provided **P**ure **A**ir, **M**aximum **S**unshine, **E**quitable **T**emperature, **G**ood **A**ccommodations, and **A**bundant **F**ood—a sequence of words that forms the acronym PAMSETGAAF. Trodeau's method was to build up his patients' resistance, and his efforts brought considerable success.

The bacteria that cause TB may enter the lungs from bacteria-laden air, or they may enter the intestines through contaminated food—usually milk from infected cows. The disease has two phases. In the **first phase** the body usually develops the ability to attack and contain the germs, whether they remain in the lungs or are carried in the lymph or blood to other locations. Those that survive are entrapped and walled off by a fibrous capsule called a granuloma. Here they may remain alive for a lifetime. It is estimated that some fifteen million people in the United States have experienced such a primary infection. Some people are unable to successfully contain the TB bacteria, and in these people the germs spread, attacking the patient. Unless properly treated with antibiotics, these patients will die in the first phase.

The **second phase** is usually seen in the lungs. The defenses no longer restrain the organisms in the granulomas. The initial inflammation

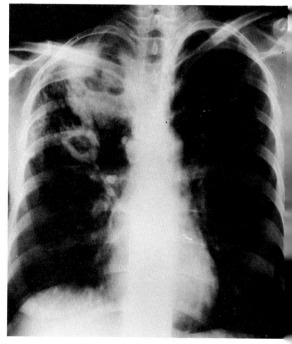

An X-ray of the chest reveals the presence of tuberculosis.

grows or the once entrapped bacteria break loose. This usually occurs insidiously and may involve any site in the body where granulomas have formed. The symptoms depend on the particular organ involved. While any organ can be infected, the lungs are the most likely. The kidneys and bones are the next most frequently involved. Even the brain is not exempt.

In the lungs, for example, as tissue damage increases, the disease manifests itself with loss of appetite, loss of body weight for no other reason, night sweats, low-grade fever, cough, and the production of sputum that may contain blood. This is commonly called "consumption" or "the white plague." The sufferer becomes short of breath and may experience chest pain. If untreated, the course is progressively downhill with the development of anemia, hemorrhages, pneumonia, and death. In the past, those who survived built up their resistance following the measures recommended by Dr. Trodeau.

Occasionally, when the natural defenses are completely inadequate, the infection, carried in the blood, is spread throughout the body, and is called **miliary tuberculosis.** The disease is not localized anywhere, and is uniformly fatal if untreated. Today, even with combined treatment, the mortality rate for this form of the disease is still 35 percent.

The **tuberculin skin test** is a most effective way to determine whether a person has been infected by the tuberculosis germ. Once infected, the test will remain positive, since it cannot differentiate between an active or latent infection. It is an excellent guide for both prevention and treatment.

Prevention of this disease takes many forms. A healthful lifestyle to maintain adequate resistance is the most important. Obviously, it is wise to avoid unnecessary exposure. If you or those close to you have been exposed, ask your physician for a

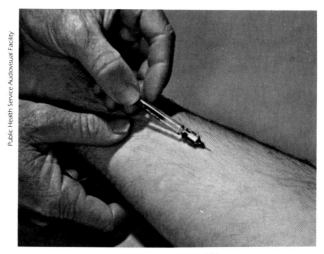

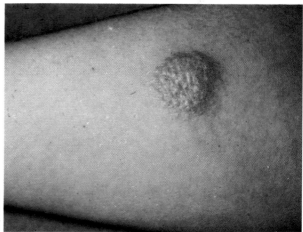

A positive tuberculin test indicates that germs causing tuberculosis have entered the body and preventive treatment may be needed.

tuberculin test. He may recommend taking one of the medications used for treating the disease, since this has also been found to prevent its development in those at high risk. BCG vaccine, once believed to prevent tuberculosis, is now used only where there is high exposure.

What you can do. If you have tuberculosis, you should be under the care of your physician. If you are at high risk, seek his advice. Maintaining your resistance by a healthful lifestyle is most important.

What your physician can do. There are now some ten medications, including antibiotics, that alone or in combination have been found to effectively combat the vast majority of tubercular infections. In severe forms of the disease it may be necessary to surgically remove part or all of an organ in order to rid the body of a potent source of germs. Your physician can best advise you after examining you and using X-rays and other procedures in his diagnosis.

Tularemia (rabbit fever)

Tularemia is an infectious disease acquired by contact with infected animals and birds, by inhaling the bacteria from feathers or fur, by eating poorly cooked meat, and from the bites of ticks and other insects. The cottontail rabbit is the most common source. At high risk are hunters, butchers, and housewives.

The infection enters the body through a break in the skin, through membranes, or by swallowing or inhalation. The resulting illness may follow various patterns, depending on where the germs gained entrance

to the body. Three to seven days after the entry of organisms, an ulcer of the skin or membrane develops with enlargement and later breakdown of lymph nodes in the area. This is accompanied with high fever, severe headache, and enlargement of the liver and spleen. Less commonly, the disease may affect the lungs, digestive organs, or the membranes of the eyes.

Prevention. A vaccine to protect against this infection is available and should be especially useful to those at high risk.

What your physician can do. Following diagnosis, your doctor will prescribe appropriate antibiotics, put you to bed, and require you to drink plenty of water. An ice bag applied to the swollen lymph glands every ten minutes at half-hour intervals should provide relief. Special treatment is required when one or both eyes are affected.

Typhoid fever and paratyphoid fevers

Typhoid fever is an acute, dangerous, highly infectious disease. With improved sanitary conditions the occurrence of this disease has been greatly reduced. Some four hundred cases are reported each year in the United States, half of which acquired the infection while traveling abroad.

The germs of typhoid fever enter the body through food or drink that has been contaminated by bowel or kidney discharges from a person sick with the disease or from "carriers"—persons who carry the bacteria and infect others but do not have the disease themselves. Salads, sauces, and polluted water are the most common sources of infection. The housefly can transfer the bacteria to food.

Symptoms develop gradually, usually within one or two weeks, though the onset may at times be delayed as long as sixty days after exposure. They include headache, loss of appetite, increasing weakness, vomiting, and fever that rises steadily to 104°F (40°C) or higher, and lasts up to three weeks. Lethargy or delirium may also be associated with the disease. Diarrhea is common, but there may also be constipation. About the end of the first week a rash will appear, then gradually fade away. The rash consists of rose-colored spots on the skin, chiefly on the abdomen, but also on the back. The inflammatory process of the disease mainly involves the small intestines, and as it progresses may result in hemorrhage and perforation of the bowel.

If untreated, the fever begins to fall gradually around the third week. Even in mild infections, the danger of intestinal complications is always present. When hemorrhaging occurs, the pulse becomes weak and rapid. Perforation causes sudden pain in one part of the abdomen which spreads to the entire abdomen.

Prevention. The occurrence of this disease has been greatly reduced in all but the developing countries through food inspection, frequent hand washing by those who prepare food, pasteurization of milk, and increased sanitary conditions in the environment—water purification and sewage disposal. Those traveling in areas where the disease is prevalent should be vaccinated (a vaccine is available with a booster given yearly). In many areas of the world food handlers must periodically undergo examinations to detect if they are typhoid carriers. The organisms sometimes take up residence in the gallbladder. Treatment with antibiotics may eliminate the infection, though in some cases surgical removal of the organ is necessary.

What your physician can do. He will recommend that you be hospitalized. He will make a precise diagnosis by means of blood tests, culturing the blood, and stool samples, following which he will select the appropriate antibiotic or some other agent. Some organisms have developed resistance to certain medications. Your physician will observe you carefully for possible complications. During the illness, adequate fluid intake must be assured. Every precaution should be taken to avoid spreading the disease to others. Good nursing care is essential.

Paratyphoid fevers. The paratyphoid fevers are caused by germs much like those that cause typhoid fever. The disease caused by these bacteria tends to run a shorter course and be less severe than regular typhoid fever. The sufferer should receive similar care, with the same precautions against the spread of infection to others. The treatment is the same as for typhoid fever.

Spirochetal diseases

Spirochetes are spiral-shaped bacteria. The diseases which these organisms cause include **syphilis** (the only one that is sexually transmitted—see page 1117), **yaws, endemic syphilis (bejel),** and **pinta**. Except for syphilis, which is found worldwide, the other three are seen only where people are crowded together under poor hygienic conditions. Other spirochetal diseases include **Lyme disease, leptospirosis, relapsing fever,** and **ratbite fever.**

Lyme disease. This spirochetal disease is carried by a tick and has three clinical stages.

Stage one. A skin lesion appears about two weeks following the tick bite. Starting as a papule, it enlarges to form a large red ring or series of rings. The person feels ill, tired, and has chills, with fever, headache, stiff neck, muscle pains, and backache. There may be nausea, vomiting, and sore throat, and adjacent lymph glands may enlarge. The skin lesion fades within about a month, and in the majority of cases, recovery is complete.

Stage two. Some people are not affected beyond stage one, especially if treatment is prompt. However, others show involvement of the heart and nervous system some days to months after the skin lesion appears. Heart irregularities include palpitations, shortness of breath, chest pain, and dizziness with possible pericarditis. The neurological symptoms are commonly headache, stiff neck, and sensitivity to light (photophobia). There may also be encephalitis and inflammation of the nerves of the face and limbs (neuritis).

Stage three. Days to months after the initial lesion, approximately half the patients develop an arthritis that generally affects a single large joint, most frequently the knee.

You can avoid Lyme disease by carefully checking yourself for ticks after moving about in a tick-infested area. Remove any attached ticks as described on page 534. Pregnant women should avoid going into areas infested with ticks that carry Lyme disease because the fetus is usually adversely affected.

Report a tick bite to your physician. He can detect the presence of Lyme disease by the characteristic skin lesion, by other symptoms which occur, and by a laboratory test of your blood. He will select an antibiotic to which the organism may respond. He should monitor your progress for several years.

Yaws. Yaws, the most common of the nonvenereal treponema diseases, is a chronic infection of the skin and bones, mainly of young children living in the tropics of Asia, Africa, and Latin America. The spirochetes, which cannot penetrate the intact skin, enter through abrasions in the skin that come in direct contact with matter discharged from infected lesions, or possibly from the bites of insects. The disease passes through three states.

Primary. After about four weeks the initial lesion appears at the site of infection, usually on the leg, and is called the "mother yaw." It soon develops into a large itching sore whose discharged matter is filled with infective spirochetes. It heals in about six months.

Secondary. Outgrowths occur anywhere on the skin or at a junction of skin and mucous membranes, and the overgrowths on the palms and soles of the feet are painful. The coverings of the bones (periosteum) become inflamed, especially of the legs, hands, and feet. There is pain, and there may be deformity. Healing takes place gradually.

Tertiary. This stage develops five or more years after the infection started. There is fever associated with destructive lesions of the skin, bones, and joints. Chronic ulcers that heal and then recur leave scars and changes in the color of the skin. Destruction of the nose, palate, and facial bones (upper jaw) is not uncommon.

The disease responds to large doses of antibiotics. If more than 10 percent of the population has yaws, the entire population should be treated. If less than 10 percent, then children under fifteen years of age and those known to be in contact with the infection should receive medication. Improved hygiene must accompany such therapy to be successful.

Endemic syphilis (bejel). Endemic syphilis is a chronic infectious disease affecting the skin, mucous membranes, and bones. It occurs in parts of Africa, Arabia, central Asia, and Australia, and is spread by direct contact or from using contaminated utensils used for eating and drinking. The period of incubation is about three weeks. The initial lesion is seen on the membrane lining the mouth (mucous patch). The lymph nodes of the neck become enlarged and tender. Later there often develops an inflammation of the outer covering of the leg bones (periosteum), and in the skin of the trunk and extremities. Late in the disease, the skin, membrane, and underlying cartilage or bone of the nose and pharynx are destroyed. Treatment is the same as for yaws.

Pinta (carate; azul). Pinta is an infection of the skin affecting adolescents and adults and is seen in the tropics of Central and South America. Its spread is believed to be contracted from intimate contact with an infected person. The incubation period is from one to four weeks. The initial red, raised lesion usually develops on an exposed area of the face, arms, or legs, and is a small papule that gradually increases in size. The lymph nodes of the area are tender and swollen. In weeks or months other satellite lesions (pintides) develop and fuse with the original lesion.

One or more years later, during the secondary stage of the infection, there is a generalized enlargement of lymph nodes, and many new lesions develop on the face, neck, and limbs. The lesions are red at first, changing to brown when exposed to the sun, gradually becoming dark (slate-blue), and finally turning white. These permanent white blotches cause disfigurement. The treatment is the same as for yaws.

Leptospirosis. This is a systemic infectious disease that occurs worldwide, but most commonly in the tropics. The disease exists in and is perpetuated by animals such as cattle, pigs, sheep, raccoons, and

721

dogs. It is spread to humans from an infected animal, the leptospira gaining entrance to the body through an abrasion in the skin or through the mucous membranes of the eye or mouth. The period of incubation is one to three weeks.

The symptoms vary depending on the severity of the disease, and resemble those of a viral infection. They may include chills, fever, headache, muscle pains, vomiting, abdominal pain, diarrhea, chest pain, cough, and stiff neck. There may be a skin rash. In more serious cases, when the liver is affected, jaundice develops. Involvement of the kidneys may result in renal failure. There may be enlargement of the spleen and lymph nodes. Mortality is 5 or 6 percent, but higher in the elderly, especially those developing jaundice.

The diagnosis is confirmed by identifying the organisms in blood, spinal fluid, and urine, or from an antibody response to leptospira. Antibiotics are quite effective if given during the first four days of the infection. Beyond that, good nursing care and specific attention to recognizing and treating complications are very important.

Relapsing fever. This is an acute infectious spirochetal disease seen in two forms: louse and tick. In the epidemics that follow natural disasters such as wars and famines it is transmitted by the louse. In sporadic cases it is caused by the bite of a tick.

The louse-borne type is not seen in the United States, but persists in Ethiopia, South America, and the Far East. The tick-borne type occurs in the summer in the mountainous areas of the western United States, and also in areas of Africa, Asia, and South America.

The louse-borne and tick-borne fevers are clinically similar. The symptoms begin abruptly with chills, high fever, severe headache, muscle pains, nausea, vomiting, diarrhea, abdominal pain, cough, and prostration. A mild skin rash sometimes develops. Jaundice may be seen late in an attack. The fever lasts three to six days and ends in a "crisis," when the temperature abruptly drops, accompanied by profuse sweating. An interval of about a week passes without fever, and then a relapse occurs. There are from two to ten attacks in a series, with each attack a little shorter than the one before, and the fever-free interval a little longer.

The mortality rate from the louse-borne type is high, probably due to the malnutrition and other illnesses (such as typhus) that are associated with its occurrence. The treatment of both types is antibiotic therapy that prevents future recurrences. When the medication acts too rapidly, the patient's condition is made worse. To avoid this, antibiotics are given or administered during fever-free periods. Bed rest, adequate fluid intake, and good nursing care aid recovery.

CHAPTER 26

Viral infections

Viruses are tiny particles that exist inside of living plant and animal cells. Most are too small to be seen through an ordinary microscope. More than 600 viruses have been isolated from animals and humans. Some are harmless, but many cause serious disease. The cores of viruses contain a form of nucleic acid, either DNA or RNA. This distinguishes them from bacteria and other disease-producing agents that have both.

Thus viruses lack the cellular constituents necessary for self-existence. They live within cells like minute parasites, each cell being specific for a particular virus (nerve cell, liver cell, skin cell, and others). When active, they invade cells, taking over the cells' reproductive processes so that the cells then produce thousands of viruses. The cells are usually destroyed in the process, and the process is repeated.

Great progress has been made in preventing virus-induced diseases through vaccination, which stimulates the body to produce antibodies against the particular virus. Small-pox, which has killed millions throughout the world, has now been eradicated. Effective immunizations have been prepared against measles, German measles (rubella), poliomyelitis, mumps, yellow fever, rabies, and certain forms of influenza and hepatitis.

Unfortunately, viruses are not killed by antibiotics, so viral diseases are difficult to treat. Some progress has been made in finding certain substances that adversely affect some viruses (acyclovir, amantadine, vidarabine, and interferons), but it is hoped that better antiviral medications will soon become available.

After entering the body, some viruses may lie **latent** (inactive) for long periods of time, sometimes years. Others multiply, but in insufficient numbers to cause symptoms. The time between the entry of the virus and the outbreak of the disease is called the **incubation period.**

Chickenpox (varicella)

Chickenpox is a usually mild, highly contagious viral disease that occurs throughout the world and typically appears in children under nine years of age. It is caught from some other sufferer, who can spread the disease for three or four days before the rash appears. The incubation period is one to three weeks.

General symptoms are a slight

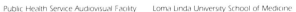

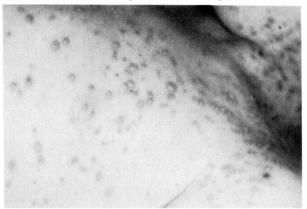

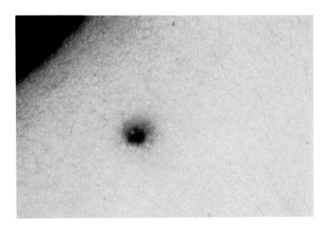

Chickenpox. Red papules on the skin (upper); small crusted blister (lower).

fever (in severe cases, it may be high), feeling of chilliness, aching back and limbs, and vomiting. The rash begins as small red spots that become bumps, then blisters. These break and form scabs. The rash, which itches intensely, appears in

"crops," first on the scalp and face, and later on the chest and back. The lesions, as they heal, rarely leave scars. Children recover in about two weeks, and immunity is for life.

What you can do. The general symptoms are worse while the rash is erupting. If the fever is high, tepid baths will help. Avoid aspirin because of the complication of Reye's syndrome (see page 467). Children's nails should be cut short or their hands placed in gloves to reduce scratching and to minimize infection of the open blisters. A soothing cream or lotion (calamine) and antiseptic baths will relieve itching. See your physician if lesions become infected or develop around the eyes, in the mouth, or in the vagina.

What your physician can do. He may decide that an antibiotic is required because the lesions are infected. Occasionally an antihistamine will prove beneficial. Adults who contract chickenpox should place themselves under the care of a physician because of possible serious complications, such as pneumonia or encephalitis.

The common cold (acute rhinitis)

See under "respiratory diseases of the lung," page 909.

Dengue (breakbone fever)

This epidemic disease, which occurs in tropical areas, is caused by a virus that is usually transmitted by a mosquito *(aedes aegypti)*. It is rarely seen in the United States. After an incubation period of five to seven days, symptoms appear suddenly with high fever up to 106°F (41°C), flushed face, headache, painful eyeballs, sore throat, nervousness, disturbed sleep, and severe pain in the head, back, and joints (hence the term breakbone). Prostration may be great.

About the third or fourth day the temperature usually drops to normal, only to recur after about three days. The second wave of illness is usually less severe and shorter in duration, and is accompanied with a rash on the hands and feet that spreads to arms, legs, and body. The acute symptoms soon end. Usually the disease is self-limited, but convalescence is slow.

What you can do. There is no specific treatment, and deaths from the disease are almost unknown. Good nursing is important. Bed rest and drinking an abundance of water are essential. Cool enemas and tepid baths will lower the temperature should it rise above 104°F (40°C). An ice bag to the head usually feels good.

Influenza (flu)

Influenza is an acute, contagious, viral disease of the upper respiratory tract. It should not be confused with a severe attack of the common cold that is often called the "flu." True influenza is of short duration and is caused by either A, B, or C type influenza viruses. Type A viruses are associated with epidemics, Type B with more sporadic diseases, while Type C viruses are milder and outbreaks are rare. Influenza viruses are carried in droplets, so the disease is spread by coughing and sneezing. It

has an incubation period of one to three days.

The symptoms consist of a feeling of chilliness followed by fever,

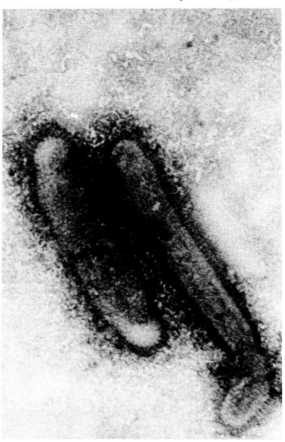

Influenza virus (Imai strain) magnified 166,400 times.

general weakness, loss of appetite, inflammation of the membranes of the bronchi with cough and sputum that may be bloody, and aches and pains, including headache and pain in the muscles. The bronchial membranes, weakened by the viruses, may allow the ever-present bacteria to invade the tissues and produce complications such as sinusitis, ear infections, and the more serious

725

bacterial pneumonia.

Except for complications, influenza is usually self-limited, lasting about a week, with weakness remaining for several days after symptoms have disappeared. Persons at high risk—those with chronic heart disease, chronic pulmonary disease, diabetes, and anyone older than sixty-five years of age—should take a vaccine in the late fall to early spring when influenza tends to be prevalent. The strains of virus keep changing, so immunity is not permanent, and thus vaccination should be repeated annually.

What you can do. Remember that flu is more serious than a cold. Rest in bed, drink plenty of water, and use a vaporizer to ease the irritation in your nose, throat, and possibly your bronchi. Cigarette smoking irritates the respiratory tract and thus increases coughing. Alcohol lowers your resistance and predisposes to pneumonia. Do not give aspirin to children for any viral infections, as it may cause Reye's syndrome (see page 467). Should you develop any complications, see your physician.

What your physician can do. Most complications are bacterial in origin. Your doctor will give you a physical examination, and, if necessary, order X-rays and a laboratory test to determine the organism involved. Physical therapy measures or an antibiotic may be prescribed.

Measles (rubeola)

Measles, which occurs worldwide, is possibly the most serious of the infectious childhood diseases. It is highly contagious and is easily trans-

Public Health Service Audiovisual Facility

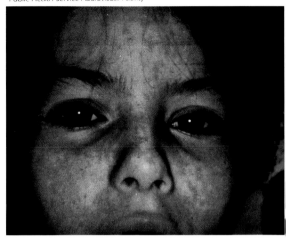

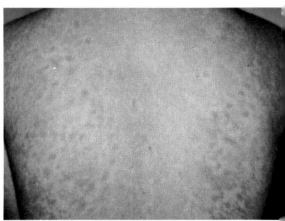

The pink spots of measles (rubeola) appear first on the face and later spread to the trunk and limbs.

mitted by invisible discharges from the nose or mouth of someone who has the disease. It is caused by a virus and has an incubation period of one to two weeks.

The first symptoms are a runny nose; low-grade fever; a hoarse, dry cough; pain in the chest, and redness of the eyes, with sensitivity to bright light. The fever gradually rises day by day and may reach 105°F (40.5°C). After about three days pink spots are seen behind the ears and on the neck, scalp, and forehead. From here the rash spreads to the trunk and limbs. The spots run together and look blotchy. White spots appear on the lining of the mouth. In severe cases there may be high fever, delirium, rapid pulse, and even unconsciousness. For a day or two the child looks gravely ill, but usually improves abruptly.

Unless there are complications, recovery generally occurs in seven to ten days. Serious complications, seen more frequently in adults, are pneumonia and encephalitis, and, more rarely, inflammations of the heart, liver, eyes, and middle ear.

What you can do. Measles can now be prevented by vaccination during infancy and early childhood, so be sure your child is immunized. Bed rest, plenty of fluids, subdued light in the room, a steam inhalator, and a soothing lotion (calamine) on the skin, should provide comfort and relief. Should you suspect a complication, see your physician immediately.

What your physician can do. Antibiotics are not effective against viruses, but may be employed against bacterial pneumonia or other bacterial complications. He may recommend that vaccinated people who have not had measles, but who have been exposed, be given gamma globulin (antibodies) as a preventive measure.

Measles, German (rubella)

This is a mild, contagious viral disease with an incubation period of one to two weeks. Its symptoms are similar to those of the common cold, with

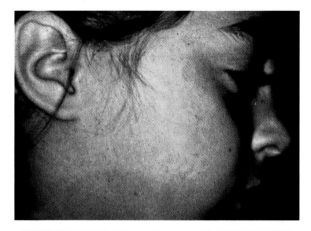

The German measles (rubella) rash first appears on the face and neck, and spreads rapidly to the trunk and limbs.

sore throat and cough. Some people develop a fever, generally feel ill, have a headache, their muscles ache, and their lymph nodes enlarge, especially behind the ear and sides of the neck. On the second day a skin rash usually appears on the face and neck and quickly spreads to the trunk and limbs. The rash is a faint blotchy redness of the skin and lasts about two days.

Anyone above six months of age may get rubella. The virus is transmitted from one person to another through the respiratory secretions. The disease is usually mild and is self-limited, being over in four or five days. To prevent the disease, children should be routinely vaccinated along with other vaccinations.

German measles may cause serious damage to the baby of a pregnant woman, especially during the first three months of pregnancy. Possible congenital defects include abnormalities of the heart, eyes (blindness), brain (mental retardation), and bones. Since the vaccination against rubella might affect the fetus, women should be vaccinated at least three months before they anticipate becoming pregnant. Many authorities believe that all girls should be vaccinated at age ten, even if they were vaccinated in infancy. This immunity should safeguard them against any problems during pregnancy.

What you can do. Since there is no specific treatment for rubella, you should stay at home and get plenty of rest. Do not expose others to the disease. If the lymph nodes are tender, an ice bag applied periodically will give relief. If you are pregnant, see your physician immediately. He will advise you regarding the hazards of continuing your pregnancy.

Mononucleosis (infectious mononucleosis or "mono")

"Mono," once called glandular fever or "kissing disease," is a worldwide infectious disease that is caused by the Epstein-Barr virus. It appears in young adults (ages fifteen to thirty) and is probably transmitted by contaminated oral secretions.

After an incubation period of thirty to sixty days, the patient becomes

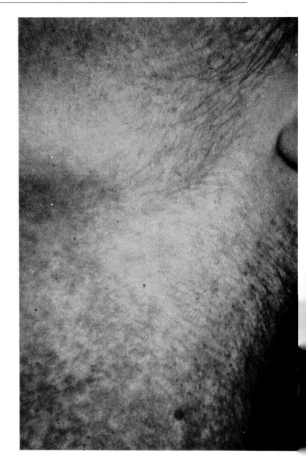

In mononucleosis, enlarged lymph nodes typically develop in the armpit and groin.

feverish, and enlarged lymph nodes appear in the armpit and groin. Sore throat, weakness, muscle pains, loss of appetite, and loss of weight are accompanying symptoms. The ·spleen and liver frequently enlarge. Jaundice and a skin rash are uncommon. An injury is more likely to rupture the spleen. Many of these symptoms are similar to those of acute leukemia or infectious hepatitis.

The major symptoms disappear in about three weeks, but weakness and lassitude may continue for three months or more. The disease is self-limited, and there is no specific treatment.

What you can do. You should stay indoors, drink plenty of fluids (water and fruit juices), get adequate rest, and refrain from vigorous exercise and contact sports till your strength returns. Rest when you are tired.

What your physician can do. Your doctor will make a precise diagnosis that requires special laboratory tests—a distinctive antibody, and a characteristic lymphocyte seen in the bloodstream. Antibiotics are ineffective. He will watch for complications.

Mumps

Mumps is a contagious viral disease that causes enlargement of one or more of the salivary glands. It usually occurs in childhood, but when developing in teenagers and adults it can cause serious complications.

The incubation period is two to three weeks, following which chilliness, headache, lack of appetite, and moderate fever are seen. One or more of the salivary glands becomes painful and swollen. The parotid gland, in front and below the ear, is most commonly affected. External pressure, swallowing, and eating sour foods increases the pain.

Complications, most often observed in youth and adults, are involvement of the testes (orchitis) and ovaries. Orchitis of at least one testicle occurs in some 25 percent of older sufferers. The testicle is swollen and very painful, and the disease may cause destruction (atrophy) of the male sex cells. Sterility may occur if both testicles are involved.

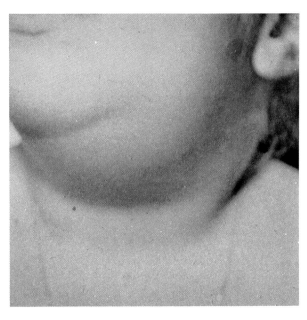

In mumps, the salivary glands are swollen and tender.

The production of male sex hormones is unaffected. The ovaries are affected less often, and the infection is less serious.

Encephalitis develops in about 10 percent of all cases of mumps, with severe headache, drowsiness, and vomiting. Pancreatitis also occurs, with severe nausea, vomiting, and abdominal pain. Usually these problems heal spontaneously without residual problems.

What you can do. Mumps can be prevented by early vaccination of the child. Bed rest or at least confinement to the home is desirable during the early phases of the disease. This will prevent further spread of the disease to other children and adults. Warm, bland soups and easily eaten foods can be encouraged. A hot-water bottle or ice bag, whichever provides greater relief, can be ap-

729

plied to the swollen glands. Recovery should be complete within a week. Older persons should stay in bed. Should complications develop, call your physician.

What your physician can do. Your doctor will advise therapy for any complication. Cradling the swollen scrotum and applying an ice bag may provide some relief.

Poliomyelitis (polio)

Polio is an acute viral infection that in 85 percent of cases produces a mild illness lasting two or three days, causing headache, sore throat, and fever. Half the sufferers recover without any permanent damage.

In the other half, these symptoms may be followed by a stiff neck and pain in the muscles of the neck and back. The virus seriously damages the nerve cells that control the muscles of the body, and the muscles the damaged nerve cells control are paralyzed. Half of these have minor disabilities from muscle loss, while the other half are seriously disabled. When the breathing muscles are affected, mechanical respirators (iron lungs) may be lifesaving.

In the United States the disease has all but been eliminated because of the use of the anti-polio vaccine (given orally or by injection) to both infants, children, and adults. If you have not been vaccinated, see your physician immediately. The virus is still widespread. If you are traveling abroad, it may be wise to have a booster.

What your physician can do. In mild cases bed rest and plenty of

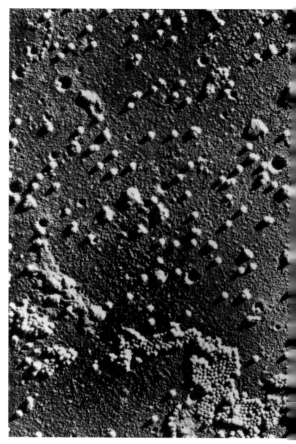

Photomicrograph of poliovirus, enlarged 77,000 times actual size.

fluids are all that is needed. In severe cases you will be hospitalized. Fomentations (Kenny packs) applied to the affected muscles will relieve the painful muscle spasms. Should the muscles of respiration be involved a respirator may be required. Well-directed physical therapy is essential for good rehabilitation.

Rabies (hydrophobia)

Rabies is a fatal viral disease which can occur in man and animals. Once the virus enters the body through a break in the skin, it travels by way of the nerves to the brain and salivary glands, so the saliva carries the virus. The incubation period is ten days to one year after exposure, the average being four to seven weeks. The period is shorter if the wound through which the virus enters is in the neck, face, or head.

In the brain the virus causes an inflammation, with fever, a feeling of illness, mental depression, and increasing restlessness. In two or three days the person becomes extremely excited, irrational, and has painful spasms of the mouth and throat. The spasms are triggered by an effort to drink water. This causes a fear of drinking, hence the term *hydrophobia,* meaning "fear of water." The disease is usually fatal in about five days.

The virus is harbored in wild animals, such as skunks, foxes, coyotes, badgers, raccoons, squirrels, rats, bats, and domestic cats. A dog that has become rabid may infect other mammals and man. The virus is transmitted from a carrier by a bite or from saliva entering a break in the

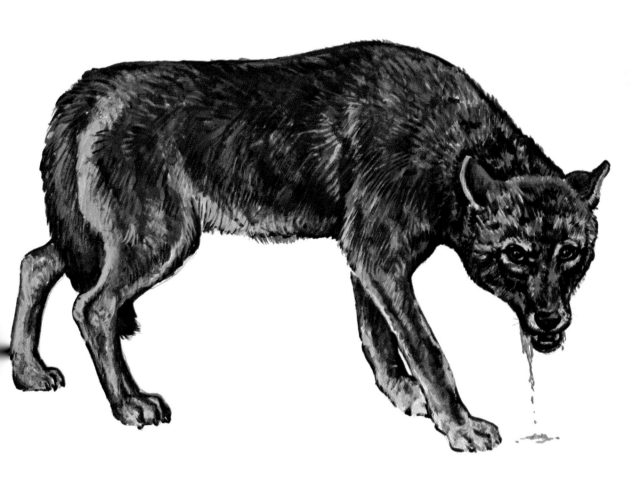

Rabies is usually transmitted by the bite of a rabid animal.

skin or mucous membrane. A rabid animal sometimes becomes furious and bites other animals and humans without provocation. The wound, laden with viruses, becomes infected.

What you can do. If you have a dog, see that it is immunized against rabies. If you are bitten or otherwise possibly exposed to the rabies virus (saliva from a possibly rabid animal) report it to your physician immediately. Try to have the animal captured. The local authorities will observe it for a few days to see whether it is actually infected with rabies.

What your physician can do. He will carefully clean your wound and report the matter to the local board of health. If the animal either develops rabies or cannot be found, you will receive a single dose of rabies-immune globulin and five injections of rabies (diploid cell) vaccine. (This replaces the older method of having one milligram of rabies vaccine injected daily for twenty-eight days.)

Reye's syndrome

This disease develops suddenly a few days following a viral infection such as chickenpox or influenza. The onset is sudden, and the brain and liver are involved. There is severe vomiting, which may be followed by lethargy, coma, and sometimes convulsions. The liver is enlarged, and the disease is often fatal. The treatment is supportive. While the cause is unknown, **it is strongly advised by the surgeon general of the United States and the American Academy of Pediatrics that salicylates (aspiring and aspirin-con-**taining compounds) not be given to children with chickenpox or influenza.** For additional discussion, see page 467.

Sandfly fever (phlebotomus fever; pappataci fever)

Sandfly fever is a viral, relatively mild self-limited disease, which occurs in certain parts of Europe and Africa, in the Middle East, in central Asia, in southern China, and, occasionally, in Central America and Brazil. It is transmitted by bites of infected sandflies—flies so small they can penetrate ordinary window screens.

The onset of symptoms, which last four or five days, is sudden, with moderately high fever, severe headache, dizziness, general itching, and pain behind the eyes.

Prevention of the disease requires eradication of sandflies, which hide during the day in weeds and shrubbery and lay their eggs in dark, damp places. Using insect repellent, sleeping under fine bed nets, and wearing close-woven clothing helps to avoid being bitten by sandflies.

What you can do. There is no remedy for the fever. Rubbing alcohol or a soothing lotion on the skin relieves the discomfort.

Smallpox

Smallpox was a serious, acute, highly communicable viral disease, with sudden onset of severe illness, high fever, a progressive skin rash followed, after recovery, by blemished, scarred, and pitted skin.

Prior to coordinated worldwide

vaccination to prevent smallpox, thousands died in severe epidemics. The virus has now been eradicated except that it exists in a few medical laboratories where the virus is controlled and used for research—surely an encouraging example of what general immunization can accomplish.

Yellow fever (yellow jack)

Yellow fever is a frequently fatal, epidemic disease. The virus is transmitted by the bite of a mosquito (*Aëdes aegypti* or closely related species). Once present in the eastern and southern United States, it is still a problem in South America and in sub-Sahara Africa, and certain other areas of the world.

The onset is abrupt, coming three to six days after being bitten by an infected mosquito, with a rapid rise in temperature to 103°F (39.4°C) or more. The face is flushed and swollen, and the eyes bloodshot. Vomiting, first of mucus, then of bile, appears early. By the fourth day the kidneys are affected with large losses of albumin in the urine. A unique finding is that despite the high fever, which is higher in the evening than the morning, the pulse remains slow.

As the temperature declines, acute symptoms improve. However, the sufferer becomes increasingly toxic due to involvement of the liver, showing the typical signs of yellow fever—jaundice and hemorrhage. Jaundice (yellow color) is seen in the white of the eyes and in the skin. Hemorrhages occur under the skin (black-and-blue spots) and in the stomach and intestines (brown vomitus and black stools).

Sometimes liver damage is extreme, and severe yellow fever may be fatal. If the sufferer survives nine days, recovery usually follows. This is signaled by the temperature returning to normal.

What you can do. An effective yellow-fever vaccine (17D) is available, and anyone traveling to areas of risk should be vaccinated at least ten days earlier for immunity to develop. A booster should be taken every ten years. Vaccines should not be given to pregnant women. Persons living in the vicinity of someone with yellow fever should be vaccinated as a precautionary measure. Mosquito eradication, by spraying and elimination of breeding areas (standing water and damp, dark hiding places), is a wise procedure.

What your physician can do. Anyone with yellow fever should be under the care of a physician and preferably in a hospital. There is no specific remedy, but good nursing care is essential. Your physician will keep you in bed and well hydrated with fluids, by vein if necessary, to restore water losses caused by vomiting and diarrhea.

CHAPTER 27

Rickettsial and chlamydial infections

Rickettsia are bacteria that must live within living cells to grow. They contain both RNA and DNA, and are susceptible to some of the antibacterial drugs.

The rickettsial diseases include (1) the spotted fevers, (2) the typhus fevers, and (3) Q fever. The rickettsia live within the bodies of animals and are transmitted to humans by biting insects, lice, flying squirrels, and contaminated dust.

Spotted fevers

Rocky Mountain spotted fever

In this disease the rickettsia are introduced into the body by the bite of an infected tick, which may be unnoticed. Three to six days after the tick bites the sufferer, he experiences severe headache, chills, severe pains in the muscles, and high fever—104° F (39°C) or more. The eyes also find bright light very uncomfortable, and there are sore throat, vomiting, and prostration.

After the third day, a bluish-purple, blotchy rash appears, first on the palms and soles, then the wrist and ankles, and finally the arms, legs, and trunk. In severe infections, sleeplessness, delirium, and stupor or coma may develop. The kidneys, liver, lungs, and blood are damaged. If untreated, the mortality rate is alarmingly high, though the death rate is now as low as 3 percent, and largely involves those who received therapy late. The disease is prevalent throughout most of the United States, but more especially in the southwestern part of the country, and in Canada, Mexico, Columbia, and Brazil. A vaccine has been developed, but it is currently under trial.

What you can do. During the tick season, avoid tick-infested areas, wear protective clothing, and repeatedly check your body for ticks. If you have had high exposure in a high-risk area, ask your physician about vaccination.

What your physician can do. Your doctor can make a clinical diagnosis and verify it by means of an antibody test. Since the test does not become positive until the tenth to the fourteenth day, treatment should be started earlier. Antibiotics are effective, and delay in instituting treatment is dangerous.

Rickettsialpox

This is a mild, nonfatal, self-limited disease transmitted by mites from mice to humans. It occurs in Russia and infrequently in the United States. After about twenty days, at the site where the mite penetrated the skin, a single initial skin lesion develops, which enlarges and blisters. Soon thereafter the sufferer experiences chills, fever, sweating, loss of appetite, and muscle pains. A generalized skin rash appears, similar to chickenpox, and lasts about a week. The treatment is the same as for Rocky Mountain spotted fever.

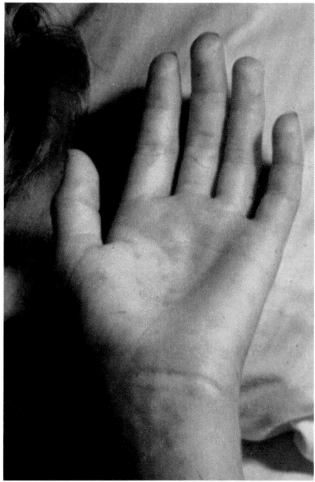

Public Health Service Audiovisual Facility

The skin rash typical of Rocky Mountain spotted fever.

Typhus group

Epidemic typhus (louse typhus)

Epidemic typhus is one of the "five great pestilences" which caused the loss of millions of lives before these diseases were brought under control by modern medical science. The other four are smallpox, yellow fever, plague, and cholera. During World War I an estimated thirty million cases of epidemic typhus occurred in Russia and eastern Poland, with three million deaths. Because of the

735

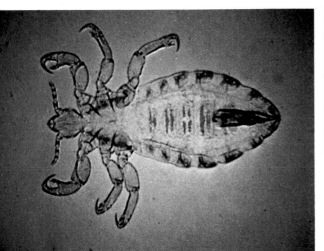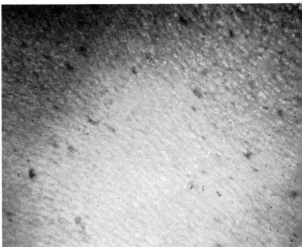

Epidemic typhus fever transmitted by body lice. Note the rash (pink spots) on the skin.

therapy that is now available this disease is of minor importance in the United States and many other countries.

The disease is spread from person to person by the body louse (the germs may remain alive in dried louse feces). The first symptoms are similar to those of the common cold and appear about two weeks after infection, followed by sudden chills, high fever, headache, general aches and pains, nausea, vomiting, diarrhea or constipation, prostration, and possible delirium or stupor. After about four days a pinkish rash (which turns red, purple, and then brown) spreads over the limbs and body, but not the face. Commonly there is a severe bronchitis with a productive cough. The disease is most serious among the elderly, and untreated the mortality is from 10 to 50 percent.

What you can do. The most effective means of preventing epidemic typhus is eliminating lice infestations.

These develop where people live crowded together in unhygienic conditions, the lice being spread by clothing or close contact. Personal cleanliness and sterilizing of clothing (heating in an oven), together with dusting powders, have proved very effective.

What your physician can do. Your doctor will prescribe fluids and appropriate antibiotic therapy which should clear symptoms in about forty-eight hours. Also, a vaccine is available which will prevent or greatly reduce the severity of the disease.

Murine typhus (endemic typhus)

This mild form of typhus is caused by a rickettsia that is harbored by rats and mice and transmitted by the bite of the rat flea. The symptoms develop after an incubation period of eight to sixteen days and include chills, fever, and headache, followed in about five days with a generalized blotchy, dull red rash. Symptoms last about twelve days. The disease is seldom fatal. Elimination of rats and mice and the extermination of fleas are the best preventive measures. Treatment is the same as for epidemic typhus.

Scrub typhus

The rickettsia causing scrub typhus are transmitted by a number of species of mites. Rodents possibly act as reservoirs of infection.

Typically a papule appears in some part of the body that is usually covered by clothing, and enlarges to form an ulcer which, on healing, leaves a scar. Adjacent lymph nodes become swollen and tender. The symptoms, which steadily worsen, include fever, headache, loss of appetite, vomiting, muscular twitching, difficult breathing, cough, deep prostration, and delirium. Symptoms subside in about two weeks. Without specific treatment, one in five sufferers will likely die.

No vaccine is available to prevent scrub typhus. The best form of prevention is extermination of mites through the application of substances such as dibutyl phthalate or benzyl benzoate to the skin and clothing. The treatment of the disease is the same as for epidemic typhus.

Q fever

Q fever, first identified in Queensland, Australia (hence the name), is a nonfatal, self-limited rickettsial disease which occurs worldwide except in Scandinavia. It differs from other rickettsial diseases in that it exhibits no skin rash and is transmitted by inhaling contaminated dust rather than by the bites of insects. People who are in close contact with cattle, sheep, and goats are at highest risk.

The lungs develop an atypical pneumonia, probably from dust inhalation. The symptoms, which develop abruptly, include fever, headache, pain behind the eyes, and pain in the chest. Only rarely are the heart and liver involved. The disease runs its course in one to two weeks.

No vaccine is available for those at high risk, such as dairy workers, slaughterhouse workers, woolsorters, and tanners. When antibiotics are given early, prompt recovery occurs. Rest in bed, plenty of fluids, a light diet, and cool cloths to the head will provide comfort and relief.

Chlamydial disease

Chlamydia are disease-producing bacteria that are generally transmitted by close contact with humans and birds.

Psittacosis (parrot fever)

Psittacosis is transmitted by close contact with several birds, including parrots, parakeets, pigeons, finches,

737

chickens, pheasants, and turkeys. The bird usually shows no sign of illness, but chlamydia are present in its nasal secretions, feathers, and excreta. Symptoms develop seven to fourteen days after the organisms are inhaled, and may be similar to a mild case of influenza or a severe atypical pneumonia.

In mild infections, recovery is in about ten days. In severe illnesses, the fever may continue for three or more weeks. If untreated, the mortality is about 5 percent, but with antibiotic therapy, less than 1 percent.

In cases of severe pneumonia see your physician. With his approval, bed rest, plenty of fluids, oxygen inhalation, and fomentations to the chest and back (see page 590) will bring relief and aid recovery.

Trachoma

Trachoma is a highly contagious chlamydial disease affecting the membrane lining of the eyelids and the "white of the eye" (conjunctiva). It is a major cause of blindness in humans, and is common in Africa, the Middle East, and Asia. It is also present in the southwestern United States. It is mainly seen in areas where poor hygiene and overcrowding prevail. While the organism is usually carried from eye to hand to eye, it may also be spread from the genital tract to the eye.

Initially the membranes are red, itch mildly, and produce a watery discharge. The lids swell, and the eyes are sensitive to light. Once the disease becomes chronic, scarring of the membrane lining the lids occurs. The scar tissue scratches the cornea,

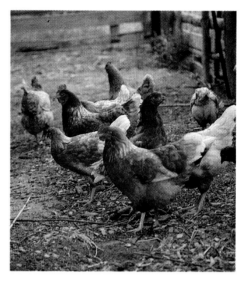

The organism that causes psittacosis is present in the nasal secretions, feathers, and excreta of a number of birds, including chickens.

causing keratitis and sometimes blindness.

Once the disease has become well established, it is difficult to treat. Anti-infectives (antibiotics, sulphas) are given for four to eight weeks, and often must be repeated. Sexual partners of sufferers must also be treated. Tetracycline-containing ointments are helpful. Surgical repair of the scarred lids may be necessary.

Prevention includes improving the general hygiene, and the daily use of tetracycline ointments by those in close contact with infected persons.

Other chlamydial diseases

Chlamydial vaginitis, see page 1108.

Lymphogranuloma venereum, see page 1120.

Nongonococcal urethritis, see pages 1081, 1120.

CHAPTER 28

Systemic fungal infections

Fungus (plural = fungi) is an organism that is largely parasitic or saprophytic, meaning that it derives most of its sustenance from plant or animal tissues or from decaying matter. There are numerous species of fungi, but only a few cause systemic diseases (mycoses). Those that cause skin infections are described elsewhere (see page 977).

Systemic fungal diseases are not transmitted from person to person, but are acquired by inhaling spores or seeds (dormant state) of the fungus. These diseases tend to run a chronic course, with symptoms that typically include chills, fever, loss of weight, night sweats, indisposition, and mental depression. When spread throughout the body in the bloodstream, they cause serious complications. The diseases are often self-limited, that is, even without treatment recovery occurs.

Blastomycosis

This disease is seen primarily in central and southeastern areas of the United States, scattered parts of Africa, and in a slightly different form among coffee growers in Brazil. It is caused by inhaling a fungus, and the symptoms vary from mild to severe. In its severe form the disease imitates a viral infection. In the majority of cases blastomycosis is a benign, self-limited disease. Areas where serious infection may occur are in the lungs, skin, bones, kidney, bladder, and the female genital tract. Antibiotic therapy effectively controls the infection, especially when begun early.

Coccidiomycosis (valley fever)

This disease enters the body by inhaling the spores of the fungus along with dust. It is present in the soil of the southwestern United States and in several sites in Central and South America. The usual infection is of the lungs, with flulike symptoms that develop in one to four weeks after exposure. There may be chest pain and pleurisy. Recovery is usually spontaneous. However, serious complications can develop in the lungs.

In a small percentage of cases the organisms are carried by the blood from the lungs to other parts of the body (disseminated form). Sometimes the meninges that cover the brain are involved. The mortality with this complication is as high as 60 percent. The organisms can be microscopically observed in the laboratory in sputum or pus. A skin test is positive after the infection is established.

Therapy is not required for the usual infection. However, because the disseminated form is life threatening, intensive antibiotic treatment is given.

Cryptococcosis (torulosis)

This fungus enters the lungs from inhaling dust contaminated with the droppings of chickens and pigeons. It occurs in various parts of the world, including the southeastern United States. The lungs are initially involved, but the most serious infections occur in the central nervous system and its covering (meninges). The skin, bones, and other organs may be affected. If untreated, the disease progresses slowly with remissions and relapses over several years. In untreated cases where the brain is involved, the outcome is usually fatal in a few months. Antibiotic therapy is generally effective. When the central nervous system is infected, the antibiotic may be administered directly into the cerebrospinal fluid.

Histoplasmosis

The spores of this fungus enter through the lungs by breathing

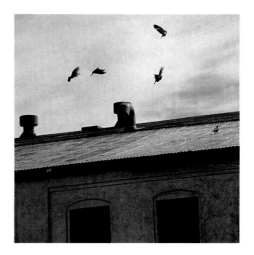

Cryptococcosis may be carried in the dust from the excreta of pigeons and other birds.

dust, particularly that which has been contaminated by the droppings of chickens, starlings, and bats. In the United States the fungus is prevalent in the Mississippi River valley and its tributaries. It occurs in the river valleys of South America, Africa, and the Far East. Activities that disturb the soil—farming, building construction, and cleanup campaigns—may increase the incidence of the disease.

When symptoms do develop, they resemble those of the common cold or flu. Persons with mild cases of lung infection generally recover without treatment. In a few cases the infection spreads through the body (disseminated form), especially in those with low resistance. The liver is often affected, but other organs may be involved, such as the adrenals. Such cases need intensive antibiotic therapy. Untreated, the death rate is 90 percent. With treatment it is less than 10 percent.

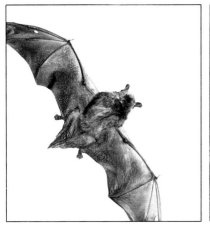
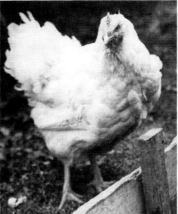
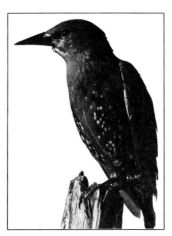

Histoplasmosis spores may be present in soil contaminated by fecal droppings of bats, chickens, or starlings.

Maduromycosis (madura foot; mycetoma)

This chronic fungus disease is most common in tropical areas, but does occur in the southern United States. It may be caused by a number of fungi, and also by Nocardia bacteria (see under "actinomycoses" and "nocardiosis," page 705).

The organism enters the body through a break in the skin, commonly of the foot or leg. A painless swelling develops at the site of infection, which in a few weeks ruptures, discharging blood-streaked pus. More swellings form and rupture, till the entire foot or limb is involved. All the tissues, including the bones, are destroyed. If untreated, the disease may persist for ten to twenty years. The fungus is controlled with appropriate therapy.

Sporotrichosis

This chronic infection occurs worldwide and is caused by a fungus that lives in decaying vegetation. The organism gains entrance through a scratch in the skin or from the prick of a thorn. In a week or two a firm nodule develops under the skin. As it enlarges, it becomes inflamed and then breaks through the skin, forming an ulcer.

Other nodules form along the lymph vessels, draining the area, and become inflamed and cordlike. If untreated, skin infections may persist for several years without impairing the sufferer's general health. The infection may become disseminated. Nodules may develop anywhere in the body, including bones, joints, muscles, and various organs. The lungs may be infected from inhaling the fungus.

The skin lesions respond to potassium iodide taken by mouth.

On occasion an appropriate antibiotic may also be used for the skin lesions and is the accepted treatment when internal organs are involved.

741

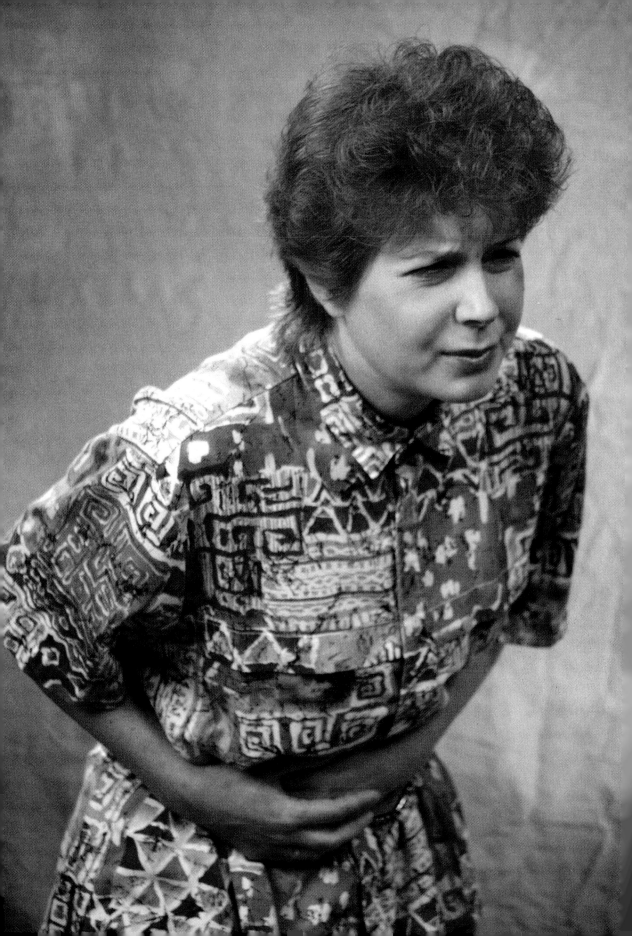

CHAPTER 29

Parasitic infections

Parasites are animal organisms of simple structure. Some invade the body and cause disease. Most are larger than bacteria and obtain their nourishment from human tissues, living either on or in the body. Those that inhabit the skin, such as lice and ticks, cause discomfort and can be carriers of disease. Others, that live within the body, may cause severe problems. Examples of these are malaria, tapeworms, and trichina.

Two groups of parasites are discussed in this chapter. The **protozoa,** which are considered among the simplest forms of life, consist of a single cell or a few cells loosely grouped together. The malarial parasite is the most important of these. **Worms,** which are larger multicellular organisms, cause a variety of problems.

Diseases caused by protozoa

African sleeping sickness (African trypanosomiasis)

This disease is caused by a protozoa (a trypanosome) that is larger than a red blood cell. It enters the body through the bite of the tsetse fly. The fly itself became infected from biting a person or an animal with the disease. Many species of wild and domestic animals harbor trypanosomes, which may or may not make them ill.

Two days following the bite of a tsetse fly, a red nodule develops at the site of the bite. The onset of fever typically begins in two or three weeks and may continue intermittently for months or years, or it may relapse with long periods between bouts. Headache, neuralgic pains, sleeplessness, and inability to concentrate are common symptoms. Pink or red patches may appear on the trunk and thighs from time to time, and the lymph nodes may enlarge anywhere in the body. Enlargements in the neck and behind the ear are characteristic of the disease.

In some cases the disease runs an

acute course that affects the brain, causing convulsions, seizures, and coma. In others the disease progresses slowly. The sufferer becomes mentally and physically feeble and is in a constant state of lethargy—a condition that has given rise to the popular name "sleeping sickness." If untreated, the outcome is fatal.

What you can do. Prevention is your best defense against African sleeping sickness: avoid being bitten by the tsetse fly in the first place. If you travel in an area where it lives, be sure to wear protective clothing, screen all living quarters, sleep under a mosquito net, and use insect repellent. An injection of the drug pentamidine will protect you for two to six months against the Gambian form of the disease, but is probably ineffective against the Rhodesian type. Some persons react unfavorably to the drug.

What your physician can do. Once they infect a person, trypanosomes are difficult to eradicate. Your physician will select the appropriate medication for the particular form of the disease. The medications carry considerable hazards in themselves. Relapses may occur after treatment, so the blood and cerebrospinal fluid may need to be examined for parasites at six- to twelve-month intervals.

American trypanosomiasis (Chagas' disease)

Chagas' disease occurs in South and Central America, Mexico, and occasionally in the southern United States. The protozoa are transmitted by the assassin or kissing bug (reduviid bug), which usually attacks at

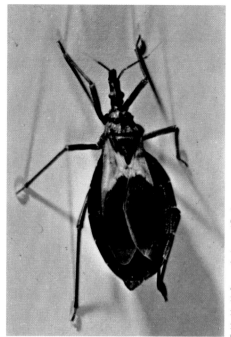

The kissing bug, vector of the parasite involved in Chagas' disease.

Public Health Service Audiovisual Facility

night. The bite, however, does not transmit the disease. The organisms are in the bug's feces, which it deposits at the site of the bite. Scratching and rubbing then pass the protozoa into the bite wound. Humans, cats, dogs, and wild animals such as the opossum and armadillo are the usual reservoirs of the infection.

The disease manifests itself as a high, continuous fever. The swelling of one side of the face and inflammation of the corresponding eye are characteristic signs. Additional symptoms include swelling of local lymph nodes, enlarged liver and spleen, nervous and mental disturbances, and rapid, irregular heartbeat.

The acute phase is relatively brief, with most sufferers recovering completely. The chronic phase appears one or more years later with damage to the heart, and often to the digestive organs. The disease becomes progressively worse and may end in death.

What you can do. You should avoid being bitten by the kissing bug by sleeping under a bed net. Since the bugs reside in the cracks in plaster walls, spraying with a residue insecticide (benzene hexachloride) is helpful. There is no satisfactory treatment for this disease. Damage to the organs is irreversible. Complications should be treated as the need arises. A drug (Lampit) has been used in the acute phase of the disease with some benefit.

Amebic dysentery (amebiasis; amebic colitis)

Amebic dysentery is an infection of the large intestine caused by a tiny one-celled parasite called ameba. It is estimated that 10 percent of the world's population is infected by ameba, the majority of whom have no symptoms, although they may excrete the cysts of the parasite by way of the feces and thus serve as carriers of the disease. The ameba gains entrance to the body through the mouth (fecal-oral spread), and is transmitted either between people through direct contact or through the use of contaminated food and water.

The ameba cause inflammation and ulcers in the lining of the colon and rectum. The symptoms, which develop gradually, include cramping abdominal pain with intermittent diarrhea or constipation. The stools contain pus, mucus, and blood. The diagnosis is made by identifying the ameba through microscopic examination of several stools, or from a specimen of the mucosa obtained through a proctoscope. Liver abscesses are a complication that may develop when the ameba reaches the blood.

What you can do. You should protect all foods and drinks from contact with fecal or sewage matter as well as from unwashed hands. In areas where the disease is prevalent you should boil your drinking water and cook all fruits and vegetables that cannot be peeled or disinfected.

What your physician can do. Your physician will give you a course of treatment lasting approximately ten days, which should clear up the problem. Follow-up stool examinations will determine whether the parasite has been eradicated.

Balantidial dysentery (balantidiasis)

The dysentery caused by this protozoa is similar to amebiasis but is less common and less severe, though more widespread geographically. The majority of infected individuals have no symptoms and are healthy carriers. This or a similar strain is a common parasite of swine, and those in close contact with these animals have a higher rate of infection. Liver abscesses do not occur, or are extremely rare.

The organism is identified by the microscopic examination of stool specimens. Symptoms include abdominal pain, diarrhea, and dysentery. Recovery is typically followed

745

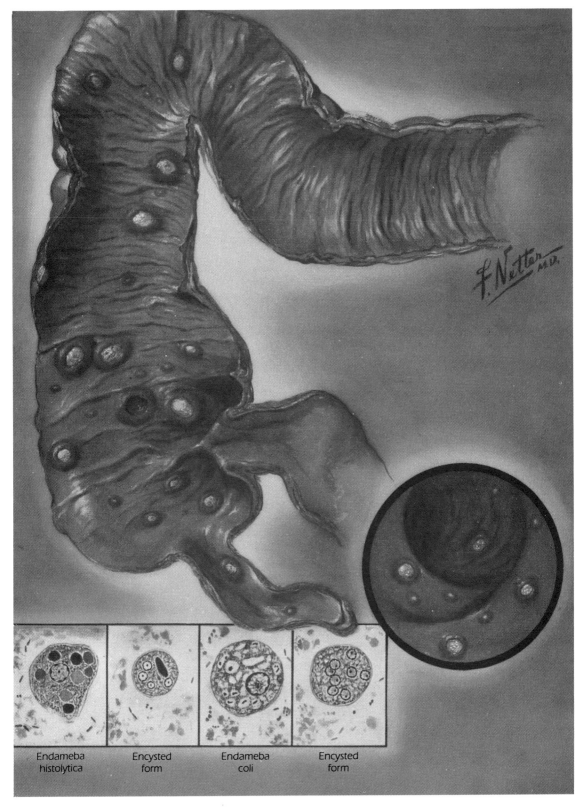

| Endameba histolytica | Encysted form | Endameba coli | Encysted form |

Amebic colitis (amebiasis).

within weeks or months by a recurrence. Your physician will give you a course of treatments with an antibiotic to which the organism is quite susceptible.

Giardiasis

This protozoan infection is one of the important causes of diarrhea, and has been recognized in approximately 100 countries in various parts of the world. Isolated cases and even epidemics of this illness have occurred in the United States. Beavers are the reservoir for this parasite, which is transmitted by water supplies contaminated with beaver feces. Cysts of this protozoa are removed by sand filters, but also require chlorination. They are also killed by heating to 122°F (50°C) or by chemicals that contain iodine.

The usual symptoms are diarrhea with watery, foul-smelling stools, abdominal distension and pain, and loss of weight. In most cases symptoms are mild to severe, lasting from several days to a period of weeks, though occasionally there are no symptoms at all. In many persons both parasites and symptoms disappear without treatment. The diagnosis is made by identifying the causative organism under the microscope. Your physician will prescribe an appropriate and effective medication which you can tolerate.

Leishmaniasis

Protozoa called leishmania cause several diseases scattered in various countries of the world. The protozoa are spread from animals to humans or humans to humans through the bite of various species of sandflies.

Espundia (American leishmaniasis). This disease occurs chiefly in forest workers in various parts of Central and South America, though an occasional case has been observed in Texas. Forest rodents and dogs harbor the tiny parasites. Ten or more days after a person has been bitten by an infected sandfly, a lesion develops on the skin at the site of the bite and gradually enlarges till it forms an ulcer. Secondary bacterial infections are common. Other lesions may develop on the face and ears. The ulcers usually heal spontaneously in about six months.

Lesions may spread to cause ulcers of the nose, mouth, and throat, with destruction of these structures, resulting in disfigurement and impairment of function. Neglected cases progress slowly toward a fatal outcome.

Diagnosis is made by identifying the protozoa in tissue taken from the edge of an ulcer or by growing the organisms in a culture. Your physician will give injections of an antimony preparation which will help to suppress the disease. Antibiotics are administered to control secondary infections.

Oriental sore (tropical sore; cutaneous leishmaniasis; Delhi sore). This skin infection, caused by a protozoan, is seen in parts of China, India, Asia, and West Africa. It is spread by the bite of sandflies and by direct contact with an ill person. After a long incubation period, the typical sore begins as a small, itchy, slightly raised spot on the skin. It enlarges slowly and becomes scaly.

747

When the crust is removed, a moist, bleeding ulcer is revealed. The lesion is usually solitary, but multiple bites can produce several ulcers, which may enlarge to an inch (2.5 cm) or more in diameter.

Healing, which begins after several months (even a year or more is not uncommon), leaves a scar. However, one attack usually protects against future infection. The sores are neither painful nor dangerous, serious consequences coming from secondary infection. Treatment is aimed toward preventing or controlling the secondary invaders. Your physician will administer an antimony preparation which usually helps to cure the protozoan infection. He may give antibiotics to prevent or treat secondary invaders.

Kala-azar (visceral leishmaniasis; dumdum fever). This disease occurs in India, China, Central and South America, East and West Africa, and the countries bordering the Mediterranean. It is spread by the bite of a sandfly. In India the reservoir of disease is an infected human, but in other regions animals such as dogs, foxes, and wild rodents are more often the carriers.

Kala-azar parasites multiply in the blood and the tissues of the spleen, liver, bone marrow, lymph nodes, skin, and small intestine. The symptoms include chronic irregular fever, emaciation, anemia, and enlargement of the liver and spleen. In women, menstruation ceases early in the disease. Untreated, 100 percent of all sufferers die. Peculiarly, despite the fever, weakness, and emaciation, the kala-azar victim does not feel seriously ill. Death comes from other infections, not from kala-azar itself.

Ninety-five percent or more of sufferers can be saved by antimony treatments given by a physician, together with antibiotics to control secondary infections, bed rest,

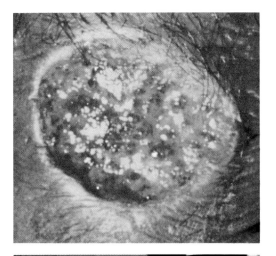
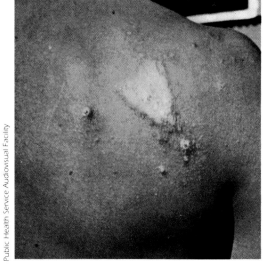

Public Health Service Audiovisual Facility

In one form, the parasites of leishmaniasis abound beneath the skin and give rise to sores.

nourishing food, and, on occasion, transfusions.

Malaria

Malaria is characterized by episodes of fever that are caused by one of four species of protozoa. These organisms are transmitted to man only by the bite of an infected female anopheles mosquito. The parasites travel to the liver, where they multiply. This phase of the disease is not associated with symptoms. The organisms reenter the bloodstream where they continue to develop and multiply within the red blood cells. Ultimately, the red blood cells burst, releasing a new generation of protozoa. Two of the four types of organisms (P. vivax and P. ovule) repeat the cycle at this point, and for all types, some parasites remain in the liver and periodically release new organisms into the bloodstream, causing repeated attacks unless treated.

The bursting of red blood cells begins some ten to forty days after the bite of the infected mosquito.

This releases hundreds of thousands of protozoa into the blood, triggering the typical chills and fever. Sudden attacks of chills and fever recur in two- or three-day cycles, depending on which species of parasite (commonly vivax) is involved. In the falciparum type, the most serious form of malaria, the fever is severe—105°F (40°C) or higher—and if not treated, may persist for ten or twelve cycles. Once the infection clears naturally or with treatment, there are no further episodes of fever unless the patient is reinfected. The symptoms of acute malaria include headache, muscle pains, increasing weakness, anemia, and enlargement of the spleen and liver. Victims of chronic malaria have few parasites in the blood, minimal symptoms, and a large spleen.

The *P. falciparum* **malarial infection** is the most serious, often being fatal. Unfortunately, in some important geographical areas of the world, strains of this species have become chloroquine resistant. Thus, the treatment has changed, and preven-

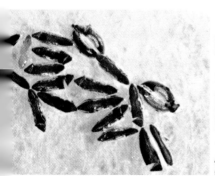
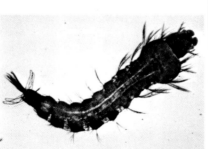
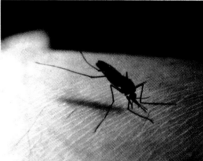

CNAS. Chas. Pfizer and Co., Inc. Public Health Service Audiovisual Facility

The three main stages in a mosquito's development: egg, larva, and adult.

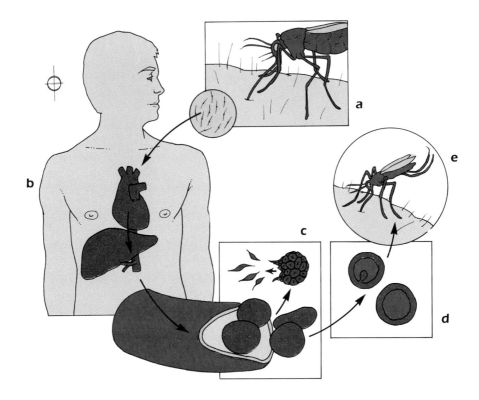

The life cycle of the malarial parasite. (A) An infected female mosquito, carrying malaria parasites (sporozoites) in its saliva, injects them into the bloodstream of a victim. (B) The parasites mature in the liver and enter the red blood cells, where the organisms asexually reproduce. (C) Eventually the cells burst, and the parasites are released, whereupon they enter other red blood cells. The parasites may also divide into male and female and reproduce sexually. Another mosquito bites an infected human and becomes infected with the male and female parasites, which reproduce within the mosquito. (D) The infected mosquito then passes these sporozoites on by biting another human. Thus the cycle is completed.

tive medication has become complicated. Fansidar (a combination of sulfadoxine and pyrimethamine) has been used successfully, but there are severe to fatal side effects. This medication is now available in the United States. Those planning to travel in a malarial area should check with a physician for information about the best preventive measures.

If at all possible, pregnant women should avoid traveling in areas that are infected with malaria.

Blackwater fever and **cerebral malaria** are serious complications of falciparum malaria. When red blood cells rupture, large quantities of hemoglobin (the red protein pigment) are released, damaging and plugging the small vessels in the kidneys. The result is kidney failure. In cerebral malaria the parasites block the small blood vessels of the brain, causing unconsciousness and convulsions. Death often occurs.

Prevention. The first rule of prevention for malaria is to avoid being bitten by mosquitos. You can do this by wearing appropriate clothing, using insect repellent, sleeping under a bed net, and removing stagnant pools of water from the environment, since these are breeding places for the mosquitoes that carry the disease. Travelers should take anti-malarials two weeks before entering a malarial zone and continue treatment for four to six weeks after leaving. Pregnant women should avoid, if possible, traveling in malaria-infected areas.

What your physician can do. Malaria is diagnosed by observing the parasites in the blood. The best time to obtain the blood sample is between attacks. Your physician will select the most appropriate medication from a number of effective agents. While relief will come within a few hours, the treatment may continue for several days. Bed rest during the acute episodes, adequate water intake, and cool sponges to reduce the fever will provide relief. Subsequently, a nutritious diet will hasten recovery. Even then, relapses can occur years later in two of the species (P. vivax and P. ovule). If only the blood forms are treated, the liver parasites can subsequently invade the blood and begin the process over again. Medication kills the live parasites.

Toxoplasmosis

This disease is caused by a protozoan that may affect the lymphatic system, the eye, the unborn child of an infected mother, or a person whose immunity mechanisms have been suppressed. The parasite is distributed worldwide, and the primary reservoir is the cat, though it may also be present in other domestic and wild animals. The illness only affects a minority of those who harbor the organism.

The cyst of the parasite enters the body through undercooked pork, mutton, or beef, or from swallowing contaminated material from the feces of infected cats. It may also be transmitted from an infected mother to her unborn child while the organisms are circulating in her blood. Once swallowed, the cysts change to a more active form and circulate briefly in the blood, soon reaching the body's organs, where they become encysted and remain latent through the lifetime of most people.

Three species of protozoan parasites play an important part in complicating the course of infection in patients with acquired immune deficiency syndrome (AIDS). In addition to the toxoplasmosis discussed above, a related form is called *cryptosporidium*. It undergoes its development in the lower bowel, causing severe diarrhea and life-threatening water loss. In healthy persons with a good immune system, the infection is not severe, and within five to seven days there is self-cure. Infection results from eating or drinking the fecally-contaminated materials. There

751

is no known treatment.

Pneumocystosis, which is caused by *pneumocystis cariniis,* is seen in more than half of all AIDS patients. Transmission appears to be both airborne and by person-to-person contact.

Lymphatic form. The enlargement of the lymph nodes, most commonly those in the neck, is the most frequent indication of the disease, and may persist for months. Accompanying symptoms include fever, pain in the muscles, fatigue, and weakness. Usually no specific treatment is required.

Ocular form. See under "eye diseases," page 1140.

Congenital form. The protozoa can be spread to the child only when the active form of the parasite is circulating in the mother's blood. If the mother was infected prior to pregnancy, she cannot transfer the protozoa to her unborn child. For-

tunately, only a few unborn children who are infected develop symptoms. Those who do develop symptoms suffer serious damage to the brain with a frequently fatal outcome. There is no effective treatment for congenital toxoplasmosis. Pregnant women should not eat undercooked meat, and should avoid cats.

Immune suppressed form. Should a person who has acquired the parasite undergo suppression of the immune system (such as for tissue or organ transplant), the latent cysts become active, causing encephalitis, infections of the brain and nerves, and frequently pneumonia. The parasite may be transmitted by an infected organ transplant. Toxoplasmosis is a serious problem in those with AIDS. If untreated, the outcome is usually fatal. Treatment is by the drug pyrimethamine in combination with sulfonamide.

Trichomoniasis. See page 1108.

Diseases caused by worms

Certain parasitic worms will take up residence in the body, and some of these are life threatening.

Hookworms (ground itch)

Hookworms are present in many parts of the world, including the southeastern part of the United States. Hookworms are small and slender—half an inch (0.75 cm) in length for males, the female being somewhat longer. When swallowed as larvae, hookworms attach themselves by their mouths to the wall of the small intestine, where they suck

blood from the capillaries.

The females produce great numbers of eggs which are expelled in the stool. Warm, moist soil favors the hatching of the eggs. The young embryos penetrate the skin of the feet and hands and are carried by the blood to the lungs. Here they enter the air passageways, and, after reaching the throat, are swallowed. Soon they arrive in the small intestine, and, attaching themselves to the wall, grow to maturity. Thus the cycle repeats itself.

The symptoms depend on the loca-

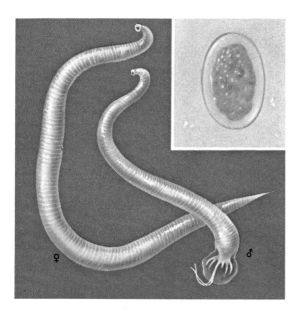

A hookworm (magnified 10 times) and an ovum (magnified 350 times).

tion of the parasites. At the site of entrance there is itching (hence, "ground itch") and burning of the skin, where a small raised blister develops. During the time they are in the air passages, the sufferer will experience spells of coughing, sore throat, and bloody sputum. After they attach themselves to the intestinal wall, the symptoms are diarrhea, bloating, and abdominal discomfort.

Fewer than 100 worms cause no symptoms. However, more than 4,000 have been found in a single individual. Large numbers of worms, constantly drawing the host's blood for their nourishment, cause weakness, pallor, fatigue, weight loss, and anemia. This is a serious problem in children, especially if they are malnourished to start with. In severe, untreated cases, the child's life is threatened.

Prevention. Proper handling of human waste is essential to prevent contamination of the soil. Where the organisms are present, hands should be kept out of the soil, and shoes should be worn.

What your physician can do. Diagnosis is made by identifying the organism's eggs in a stool specimen. Your physician can prescribe one of several effective medications. If you are severely anemic, he may order a transfusion. A good nutritious diet will restore you to health after the worms have been destroyed.

Threadworms (strongyloidiasis)

The threadworm is found in the same geographic areas as the hookworm. Although smaller, its mode of entry and life cycle are similar to that of the hookworm. One difference is that some of the larvae in the lower bowel may transform into the infective stage and penetrate the tissues, enter the bloodstream, and establish an internal or autoinfection. Thus the infection may persist for years, even without an external, skin-penetrating invasion such as occurred in the initial infection. An important clinical sign, of diagnostic value, is the presence of an elevated and persistent increase in the number of certain white blood cells (eosinophilia).

Usually there are no symptoms, though occasionally a watery diarrhea or an intestinal ulceration may develop. However, prompt treatment will prevent the potentially fatal complication of the larvae penetrating the intestinal wall due to the use of immunosuppressive drugs. Your physician will prescribe a course of

753

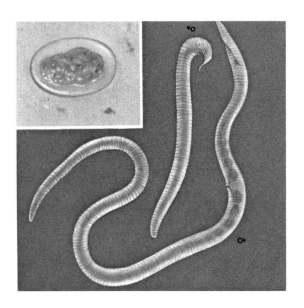

A threadworm (magnified 70 times) and an ovum (magnified 350 times).

antiparasitic therapy. Subsequent stool examinations should be made to make sure the parasites have been eliminated.

Pinworms

Pinworms are the most common parasitic infection among children. The worms are small and white, the female (larger than the male) being less than half an inch long (13 mm). The worms live in the lower colon, especially the rectum. At night the females crawl out through the anus to lay their eggs on the surrounding skin, causing intense itching. Apart from itching, there may be vague gastrointestinal discomfort, restlessness, and sleeplessness.

An infected child may reinfect himself by scratching himself and then handling food or putting his fingers in his mouth, and he can infect others who eat food that he has handled. The diagnosis is confirmed by placing a piece of cellophane tape near the anus to collect the eggs and identifying them under a microscope.

What your physician can do. Your physician will prescribe a medication that should eliminate up to 90 percent of the worms with a single dose. The entire family should be treated in order to abolish the infection completely. Clothes, bed linens, and toilet seats should be washed frequently to destroy the eggs or worms. Every effort should be made to prevent small children

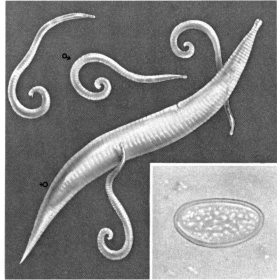

A pinworm (magnified 10 times) and ovum (magnified 300 times).

from scratching their anal area, and children and adults should keep their fingers out of their mouths.

Roundworms (ascariasis)

Roundworms are a worldwide problem, but are especially prevalent in warm, moist climates. It is estimated that 25 percent of the world's

754

population—one billion people, including more than one million in the United States—harbor the parasite. The worm is 6 to 14 inches (15 to 35 cm) long, the female being larger than the male. They live mainly in the upper small intestine, but may travel to other parts of the intestinal tract, even entering the stomach, from which they may be vomited.

The females lay large numbers of eggs, which abound in things contaminated with feces, such as leafy vegetables, drinking water, pets, and soil. Unwashed hands and dirty fingernails may also transport the eggs to the mouth. It takes several weeks for the embryo worms to develop in the eggs. After they hatch, the tiny embryos burrow through the intestinal wall and migrate to the lungs, where they undergo growth for two to three weeks. Initially they will cause a form of pneumonia. Breaking out of the lung tissue, they enter the air passages and travel upward to the throat, where they are swallowed. Arriving in the small intestine, they develop into adult male and female ascaris worms.

While the immature worms are migrating through the lungs there may be wheezing, cough, and fever. A few

worms in the intestine produce no symptoms. Large numbers, however, may cause abdominal pain, diarrhea, fever, restlessness, intestinal obstruction, nutritional deficiency, and even convulsions, especially in children. Occasionally adult worms may be passed in the stool or vomited. Otherwise their presence is determined by finding the eggs in the feces. Your physician will prescribe a medication that causes the worms to

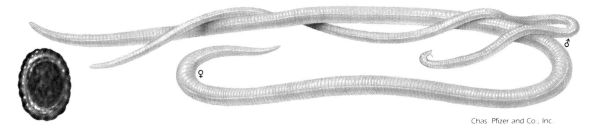

Chas. Pfizer and Co., Inc.

Roundworms (actual size) and ovum (magnified 400 times).

release their attachment within the intestine so they will be eliminated in the stool.

Tapeworms

Tapeworms are long, flat, thin worms with segmented bodies. Some grow to a length of 40 feet (12 meters), are a half inch in breadth (13 mm), and may have 3,000 or more segments. They lack digestive organs and absorb their food through their entire surface, attaching themselves to the lining of the intestine of a human or animal host. From time to time the terminal segments drop off, usually filled with eggs, while new segments form at the head. The eggs are eaten by some animal along with its food, and hatch in its stomach or intestine. The released larvae migrate into the muscles or other organs of the animal and become encysted. The cysts remain dormant until the infected flesh is eaten by a human or some other suitable host.

While there are some differences between the life cycles of the differ-

consumption of raw or undercooked beef or fish transmits these worms. Pike and yellow perch are common offenders. The fish tapeworm requires large amounts of vitamin B12 and thus competes with the host for this nutrient. Sufferers often develop B12 deficiency anemia (macrocytic).

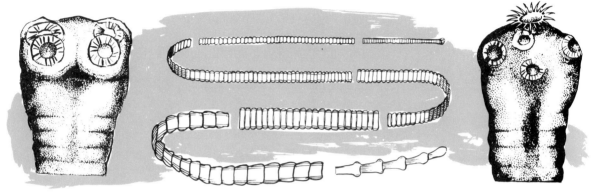

A beef tapeworm may grow up to 30 feet long (10 m). Note the sucking discs and hooklets (right) for holding onto the intestinal lining.

ent tapeworms, they all gain entrance to the human intestine by someone swallowing the eggs with larvae from contaminated food or fingers, or from the cysts entering the stomach and intestines from eating raw or undercooked beef, fish, or pork. In the majority of cases the symptoms are unnoticed. In others, they include abdominal discomfort, diarrhea, weight loss, nausea, and a greater-than-usual appetite.

Diagnosis can be made by observing a worm or a segment, or by microscopic identification of the eggs. Your physician will prescribe a medication which is generally effective against the beef, fish, dwarf, and adult pork tapeworms.

Beef and fish tapeworms. The

Dwarf tapeworm. This is the most common tapeworm in the southeastern United States, and is seen more frequently in children than in adults. The parasite is common in mice, which may contaminate cereals and grains. Eggs are readily transferred by unwashed fingers from the anal area to the mouth.

Pork tapeworm. Infection with this tapeworm may take two different forms, depending on whether the larvae or eggs transmit the parasite. The **larval form** is similar to other forms of tapeworm disease, the larvae being acquired by eating inadequately cooked, infected pork. The **cyst form** develops when the eggs of the tapeworm are swallowed, usually from consuming food con-

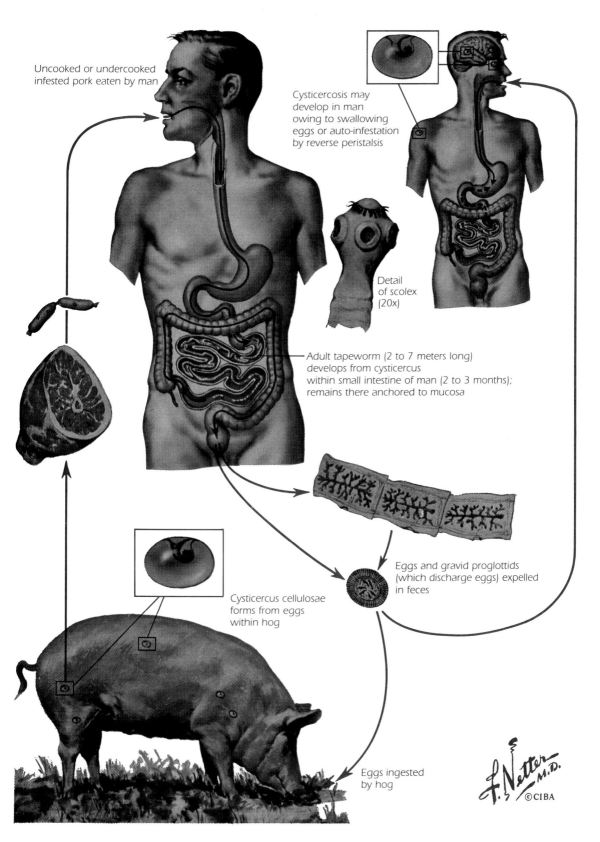

Uncooked or undercooked infested pork eaten by man

Cysticercosis may develop in man owing to swallowing eggs or auto-infestation by reverse peristalsis

Detail of scolex (20x)

Adult tapeworm (2 to 7 meters long) develops from cysticercus within small intestine of man (2 to 3 months); remains there anchored to mucosa

Eggs and gravid proglottids (which discharge eggs) expelled in feces

Cysticercus cellulosae forms from eggs within hog

Eggs ingested by hog

The life cycle of the pork tapeworm.

taminated by egg-containing human feces. Auto-infection is also possible.

The eggs hatch in the stomach and upper intestine, releasing larvae that penetrate the intestinal wall and are carried by the blood throughout the tissues and organs of the body, lodging beneath the skin, in the muscles (commonly of the tongue, neck, and trunk), and in the heart, liver, eye, lungs, and brain. Within two or three months the larvae become encysted (cysticercus) and may remain alive for years.

The usual symptoms of **cysticercosis** are muscle pains, weakness, and fever. When the brain is involved, the symptoms mimic brain tumor or encephalitis, and convulsions may occur. Diagnosis can be made by X-rays or by means of a chemical test. A new drug is available, but may be dangerous to use. Sometimes the cysts are removed by surgery.

Hydatid disease (echinococcosis) is caused by a tapeworm that involves sheep and sheep dogs. The adult tapeworms live in the intestines of dogs, foxes, and wolves, which become infected by eating sheep carcasses containing the tapeworm larvae. Humans acquire the infection by placing accidentally contaminated food or fingers containing or contaminated with eggs into the mouth.

On hatching in the intestine, the young worms burrow into the tissues, mainly lodging in the liver. A cyst develops, filled with fluid and worm heads. Cysts may also develop in the lungs, heart, bones, or brain. Some cysts act as malignant tumors

and produce a serious illness. Surgical removal of cysts is the treatment of choice. To prevent the disease, sheep dogs should be dewormed, and sheep carcasses should not be fed to dogs.

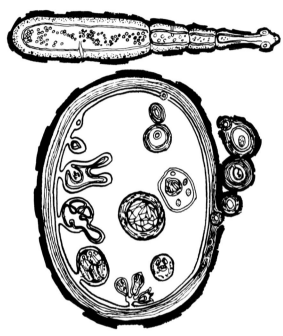

Echinococcosis granulosus (above), magnified 23 times, and a section through a hydatid cyst (below).

Whipworms

Whipworms occur mostly in tropical regions where sanitary conditions are poor. The worm is 1-1/2 to 2 inches (15 to 50 mm) long and resembles a whip with a slender lash and a thicker handle. Whipworm eggs enter the body by being swallowed in contaminated food or water. They live chiefly in the lower small intestine and rarely cause symptoms, though in large numbers they may produce intestinal distress, diarrhea, dysentery, bloody stools, and abdominal bloating. Your physician will pre-

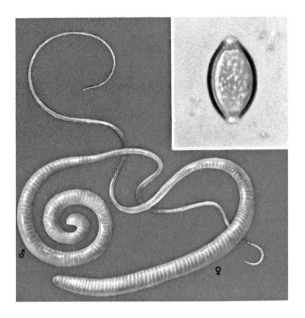

A whipworm (magnified 5 times) and an ovum (magnified 350 times).

scribe a medication that is uniformly successful in eliminating the worms.

Guinea worms

These worms infect about fifty million people in parts of India, Africa, the Middle East, northeastern South America, and the Caribbean Islands. Once consumed by drinking contaminated drinking water, the larvae penetrate the upper small intestine and migrate to the subcutaneous tissues, where, after several months to a year, they develop into adult worms 1 to 2 feet in length (30 to 60 cm). They are smooth, slender, and white.

After mating, the male dies, and the female worm migrates to the extremities, emerging through those parts of the skin most frequently in contact with water, usually the legs and feet. The worm secretes an irritating and toxic substance that

causes a blister to form. The blister ruptures, leaving a raw area with a hole in the center. When the extremities are placed in cool water, the worm discharges a milky cloud of coiled embryos through this hole. The embryos then enter water fleas, which act as an intermediate host. The infected water fleas are swallowed in drinking water where the embryos emerge and grow to the adult worm. The cycle is now complete, and ready to start again.

The worm's head may protrude from the hole. At the time of emergence there may be itching, vomiting, diarrhea, dizziness, and difficulty in breathing. Secondary infections commonly develop in the ulcerated area. Serious infection often occurs if the worm dies within the human tissue or is broken during attempts at removing it.

What you can do. The worm may be removed by several methods. A thread is tied around the head of the worm and, by gently pulling, the worm can be slowly extracted over a period of a week or two. Another procedure is to wind several centimeters of the worm around a stick each day until it is drawn out.

What your physician can do. Your physician may enlarge the opening through which the worm's head protrudes and loosen the tissues around the worm to make extraction easier. He may prescribe a drug that kills the worm, allowing it to be withdrawn quite readily.

Flukes

Flukes (trematodes) are flatworms, a number of which are parasitic in man and animals. The infections are prevalent in large areas of the world, including China, Southeast Asia, India, Africa, and Central and South America. The frequency of occurrence and the seriousness of symptoms will vary, depending on the fluke, its method of transmission, and the organs of the body in which it colonizes.

Blood flukes (schistosomiasis; bilharziasis). Three types of blood flukes, which look like small, slender worms, are responsible for schistosomiasis. The eggs of the flukes are discharged in body wastes (urine, feces) and find their way into water, where they hatch, and the tiny parasites swim until they find a suitable snail to harbor them.

After further development within the snail, the parasites escape into the water and await an opportunity either to penetrate the skin of some human or other warm-blooded animal, or to be swallowed when water is drunk.

Once inside the body, they congregate in the small veins of the bladder, intestine, and liver. They may also travel to the lungs, and even the brain. Eggs are laid, and because of a dissolving tissue enzyme, the eggs pass into the bladder and intestine and are expelled in the urine or feces.

The symptoms vary according to the location of the organisms. In the urinary bladder they cause bleeding and the formation of bladder stones and cancer. In the intestine there may be diarrhea containing mucus and blood, with fever, abdominal pain, loss of appetite, chills, cough, and enlargement of the liver and

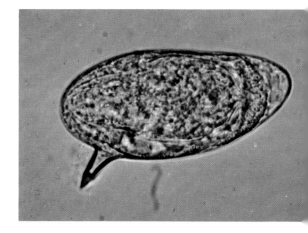

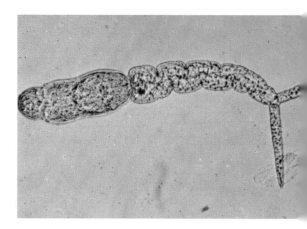

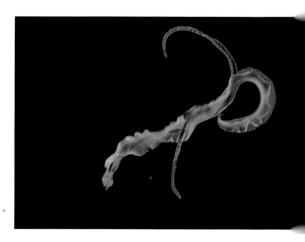

Schistosomiasis is caused by the blood fluke. Note its egg, young, and adult forms.

760

spleen. Collections of eggs form fibrotic lumps in the liver, lungs, and brain.

Sanitary disposal of human excreta is a must. You should boil all questionable drinking water. Avoid contact with water (rivers, ponds, rice fields) in the area in which blood flukes occur.

Diagnosis can be confirmed by identifying the eggs in stool and urine specimens, and from a biopsy of rectal mucosa. Your physician will determine the appropriate medication for the particular fluke involved. The remedial agents are toxic, so identification should be precise. Occasionally it may be necessary to surgically remove some of the affected tissues.

Liver flukes. In some parts of the Orient, half the population is infected with liver flukes, especially where raw fish forms part of the diet. In the vast majority no symptoms are observed, except perhaps indigestion. In severe cases, swelling of the liver and jaundice are typical.

Adult flukes live in the small bile ducts of the liver where eggs are laid. They then pass into the bile, on into the intestine, and out in the stool. On reaching a body of water, the eggs usually do not hatch unless they are swallowed by a freshwater snail. The next stage takes place in or on the body of a freshwater fish (especially carp). Humans become infected by eating raw or under-cooked fish, the infection persisting for several years.

To avoid liver flukes, you should dispose of bowel discharges carefully and avoid eating raw or insufficiently cooked fish.

Your physician can make a diagnosis of liver flukes by microscopic examination of a stool specimen. Agents used in therapy are toxic and no satisfactory medication is available. Adult worms may not be killed, but egg production can be reduced.

Liver rot. Primarily a disease of sheep, but also occurring in humans, liver rot is caused by a large liver fluke. The adult flukes live in the bile ducts. Eggs pass out in the stool, partially develop in snails, and become encysted on water plants such as watercress.

They become active when swallowed by sheep or humans, penetrate the wall of the intestine, and grow to maturity in the bile ducts. Although seldom fatal, some liver damage is produced, causing an irregular fever, vomiting, abdominal pain, itching, jaundice, and joint pains.

Your physician will confirm diagnosis by observing fluke eggs in a microscopic examination of a stool sample. He will then prescribe the best agent available for the problem.

Lung flukes. Lung flukes are found in parts of the Far East, West Africa, and Central and South America. The disease in humans results from eating cyst-infected raw, salted, or wine-soaked freshwater crabs or crayfishes. After being swallowed, the larvae develop in the intestine and then pass through the intestinal wall and diaphragm to reach the lungs.

The symptoms, which develop gradually, consist of chronic cough; discomfort in the chest; an abundant, sticky, blood-tinged sputum; and anemia.

Diagnosis is made by identifying the fluke's eggs in the sputum, but most frequently in the stool (since the eggs are coughed up and swallowed). Your doctor will prescribe a course of treatment with an appropriate agent.

Filariasis (elephantiasis)

Filariasis is a disease caused by small, extremely slender worms called filariae, usually 1 to 3 inches (2.5 to 7.5 cm) in length, but in one species reaching a length of 20 inches (50 cm). In some countries of southern Asia and the Far East, where the disease is prevalent, half the population is infected.

The filariae inhabit the lymphatic system in humans and discharge their offspring or microfilaria into the bloodstream. In the most important worm species they will be seen in the circulating blood only at night. Mosquitoes become carriers when they bite an infected person. When the infected mosquito bites another person, the parasites enter the victim's skin, find their way into the lymphatics, and grow to adult worms. Oddly, millions of microfilaria in the blood cause no distress. It is the adult worm that is the problem, irritating or blocking the lymph tissues and vessels.

In those who exhibit symptoms, following an incubation period of several months, there occur recurrent episodes of fever with pain in the lymph nodes and lymph vessels. This pain lasts seven to ten days, and then spontaneously disappears. Oc-

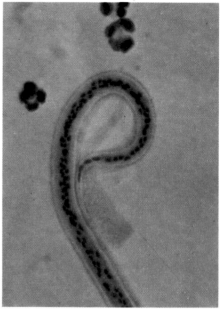

Public Health Service Audiovisual Facility

The parasite Wuchereria bancrofti is responsible for elephantiasis (lymphatic filariasis.

casionally the lymph nodes will abscess. Even after many years, a late development is the plugging of lymph vessels by adult worms, even when dead. The tissues gradually enlarge, hence the term *elephantiasis.* The legs are most commonly involved, but the feet, scrotum, vulva, breasts, and arms may be affected. The appearance is repulsive, the condition awkward. There is no cure for tissues once they have become enlarged.

What you can do. Use bed nets and insect repellant to avoid being bitten by infected mosquitoes. Keep infected persons from being bitten, and attempt to destroy the breeding places of mosquitoes. These efforts are not easy.

occurs in central Africa and in Central America. Mature parasites in the tissues cause itching, local inflammation, and some pain, with slowly growing nodules filled with microfilaria deep within the skin. After many years the tissues of the eye may be attacked, resulting in blindness.

What your physician can do. Where possible, your doctor will remove accessible nodules by minor surgery. A drug is available for therapy, but before administration your physician will determine if you can tolerate it, since it can cause kidney damage.

Trichinosis

Trichinosis is a worldwide disease caused by the larvae of a small worm *(Trichinella spiralis)*. It is transmitted by eating the raw or insufficiently cooked flesh of the hog (and occasionally other animals such as the bear), in which the encysted worm lies dormant. It has also been spread from chopping other meat on the same chopping block used to chop pork.

When infected meat is eaten, the embryo worms are liberated in the stomach and intestine, where, in four to six days, they grow to full size and are ready to migrate. Many lodge in the intestinal wall, but large numbers circulate throughout the body in the blood and lymph vessels. Ultimately they become encysted in the muscles, especially the diaphragm. During migration fever, chills, and abdominal and muscle pains are common. The muscles are tender and swollen. The nervous system can

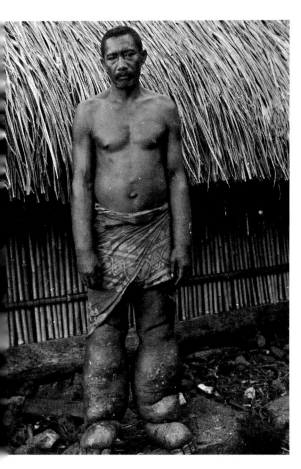

A man suffering from elephantiasis. Note the massive swelling of the legs.

What your physician can do. Your doctor will prescribe a course of therapy that will greatly reduce the number of microfilaria in the blood and will kill many of the adult worms. Antihistamines are given to lessen the severe allergic response that develops to the dying parasites.

River blindness (onchocerciasis)

This disease, which is caused by a filarial parasite, is transmitted by the bite of the black fly (buffalo gnat). It

763

be involved. The symptoms can be so severe as to cause death. Once encysted, the worms lie dormant and cause no symptoms. The mortality rate is less than 2 percent.

What you can do. If you eat pork or pork products, see that they are well cooked or have been frozen to low temperatures prior to cooking. Hot baths give relief for muscle pain.

What your physician can do. There is no satisfactory remedy for trichinosis. An experimental drug is available that may be used to kill the larvae in severe cases. Corticosteroids are sometimes used to alleviate inflammation when the nervous system is involved.

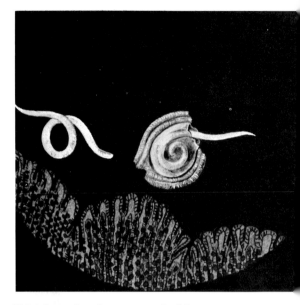

Trichinae in the stomach (the worm shown is much enlarged).

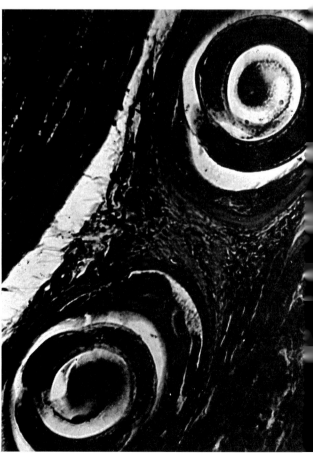

Trichinae encysted in a muscle.

764

General Index

Index

A

Abdomen
    Cramps in, **2**-611
    Distension of, **2**-611
    Masses in, **2**-612
    Rigidity of, **2**-612
    Tenderness in, **2**-612
Abdominal injuries, **2**-553
Abdominal pain, **3**-878
Abrasions, **2**-553
Abscess, **2**-702
Accidents
    As leading cause of death in children, **2**-443, **2**-452
Acclimatization to high altitudes
    Graded ascent, **1**-42
    Staging, **1**-42
Acetaminophen, **1**-330
Acid rain, **1**-65
Acne, **2**-489, **3**-982
Aquired immune deficiency syndrome
    See AIDS
Acromegaly, **3**-1006
Actinic keratoses, in the elderly, **2**-500
Actinomycosis (lumpy jaw), **2**-705
Acute epiglottis
    See Croup
Adam's apple
    See Larynx
Addiction
    See Drug abuse
Addison's disease, **3**-1007
Adenoiditis, **2**-470
Adenoids
    See Tonsils
Adenomyosis
    See Uterus, disorders of; Endometriosis
Adolescence, **2**-431, **2**-476
    Changes in female during, **2**-480
    Changes in male during, **2**-479
    Character formation in, **2**-477
    Physical development, **2**-478
    Sexual interaction during, **2**-482
Adrenal disorders
    Addison's disease, **3**-1007
    Adrenal virilism, **3**-1008
    Cushing's syndrome (and Cushing's disease), **3**-1007
    Hyperaldosteronism, **3**-1008
    Pheochromocytoma, **3**-1008
Adrenal gland hormones
    Aldosterone, **3**-1001
    Cortisone, **3**-1001

    Epinephrine, **3**-1001
    Glucocorticoids, **3**-1001
    Hydrocortisone (cortisol), **3**-1001
    Mineralocorticoids, **3**-1001
    Norepinephrine, **3**-1001
    Sex hormones, **3**-1001
Adrenal glands, **3**-1001
Adrenaline, **3**-1001
Adventist health studies
    Comparisons among Adventists, **1**-123
    Health habits of Adventists, **1**-122
    Observed health advantages, **1**-122
    Studies done outside the United States, **1**-123
Aerobic exercise, **1**-38
African sleeping sickness (trypanosomiasis), **2**-743
Age
    As risk factor in heart disease, **3**-779
AIDS, **3**-830, **3**-831
    Kaposi's sarcoma and, **3**-831
    Pneumocystis carinii and, **2**-752, **3**-831
    Toxoplasmosis and, **2**-752
    Treatment of, **3**-831
Air
    Composition of, **1**-62
    Ions, positive and negative, **1**-66
    Pollution in, **1**-64
Albinism, **3**-986
Alcohol
    As risk factor in diabetes, **3**-1018
    Content of, in standard alcoholic beverages, **1**-287
    Dependence, **1**-293
    Delirium tremens (DT's), **1**-293
    Tolerance for, **1**-292
    Use of that develops cross-tolerance, **1**-293
    Withdrawal from, **1**-293
Alcohol, effects of
    On digestive system, **1**-288
    On heart and blood vessels, **1**-290
    On nervous system, **1**-289
    On other drugs, **1**-292
    On sexual behavior, **1**-291
    On the unborn (fetal alcohol syndrome) **1**-292
Alcohol rub, **2**-577, **2**-598
Alcoholic
    Rehabilitation of, **1**-293
Alcoholic beverages
    Economic and social impact of, **1**-286
    Incidence of, **1**-286
    Why people drink, **1**-287
Alcoholics Anonymous, **1**-294
Alkalosis, from hyperventilation, **2**-617
Allergens, **2**-673, **3**-921
    "Germ," **2**-675
    "Injected," **2**-674
    Additives and preservatives, **2**-674
    Drugs, **2**-674

(4)

See Cardiovascular disease
Corpuscles
See Blood cells
Cortisone, **3**-1001
Cough, **2**-453, **2**-618, **2**-648
Coughing, **3**-905
Cowper's glands, **3**-1084
CPR
See Cardiopulmonary resuscitation
Cramps, muscle
See Muscles, disorders of
Cretinism, **2**-423, **3**-1010
Crohn's disease (regional ileitis), **3**-859
Cross-eye (Squint), **3**-1140
In children, **2**-469
Croup, **2**-458
Cryptococcosis (torulosis), **2**-740
CT scan
See CAT scan
Cushing's disease
See Cushing's syndrome
Cushing's syndrome, **3**-1007
Cutaneous leishmaniasis
See Leishmaniasis: Oriental sore
Cuts, **2**-554
Cyanosis, **2**-619
Cystic fibrosis, **2**-461, **3**-922

D

D&C
See Dilation and curettage
Dandruff, **3**-974
Deafness (hearing loss), **2**-620, **3**-1152 Conductive deafness, **3**-1153
In children, **2**-469
In the elderly, **2**-503
Nerve deafness, **3**-1153
Death, process of accepting
Acceptance, **3**-1058
Anger, **3**-1057
Bargaining, **3**-1057
Shock and denial, **3**-1057
Decision making
Discrimination, **1**-102
Judgment, **1**-103
Self-control, **1**-103
Willpower, **1**-103
Decompression sickness, **2**-559
Deformities
Congenital, **2**-426
Dehydration, **1**-80
Delhi sore
See Leishmaniasis
Delirium, **2**-558

Delirium tremens, **3**-1058
In alcohol withdrawal, **1**-293
Delivery
Date of, **2**-384
Signs of, **2**-399
See also Labor
Delivery, complications of, **2**-401
Abnormal presentations, **2**-403
Birth injuries, **2**-404
Caesarean section, **2**-402
Episiotomy, **2**-402
False labor, **2**-401
Forceps delivery, **2**-402
Hemorrhage following delivery, **2**-403
Multiple births, **2**-404
Premature birth, **2**-401
Premature rupture of the membranes, **2**-402
Respiratory distress syndrome, **2**-404
Retained placenta, **2**-403
Dementias
Alzheimer's dementia (disease), **3**-1041
Arteriosclerotic dementia, **3**-1041
Dengue (breakbone fever), **2**-724
Dental caries
See Tooth disorders
Dentist
Training of, **1**-9
Dentistry
Endodontics, **3**-890
History of, **3**-889, **3**-890
Orthodontics, **3**-890
Periodontics, **3**-890
Prosthodontics, **3**-896
Dentures, **3**-896, **3**-897
Deoxyribonucleic acid
See DNA
Depression, **3**-1055
In the elderly, **2**-502
Dermatitis
Allergic, **2**-464, **2**-678, **3**-973
Atopic, **2**-678, **3**-971
Atopic, in children, **2**-462
Atopic, in infants, **2**-421
Chronic, **3**-974
Contact, **3**-972
Contact, in children, **2**-470
Dyshidrosis, **3**-974
Irritant, **3**-972
Nummular, **3**-975
Seborrheic, **3**-974
Stasis, **3**-975
Xerotic eczema, **3**-974
DES therapy, and increased disease incidence, **3**-1109
Detached retina, **3**-1138
Diabetes, **3**-1013
Adult-onset (type II), **1**-6, **3**-1013

(11)

(14)

F

See Esophagus
Hiccup, **2**-560, **2**-624
High blood pressure
    See Hypertension
Histamine, **2**-675
Histoplasmosis, **2**-740
Hives (urticaria), **2**-676, **3**-989
    In children, **2**-471
Hoarseness, **2**-624, **3**-915
Hodgkin's disease, **3**-832
Home patient care, **2**-572
    Administering enemas, **2**-574
    Alcohol rub, **2**-598
    Bedsore prevention, **2**-577
    Counting respiration rate, **2**-574
    Determining pulse, **2**-573
    Food and drink, **2**-577
    For contagious diseases, **2**-580
    Giving baths, **2**-575
    Importance of good nursing in, **2**-582
    Medications, **2**-579
    Patient bowel movements, **2**-574
    Prevention of stiff joints, **2**-578
    Taking temperature, **2**-573
    Use of bedpan, **2**-574
Home treatments, **2**-585
    See also Dry heat applications
    See also Hydrotherapy
    See also Thermotherapy
Homeostasis, **1**-30, **2**-587
Homosexuality, **2**-483
Hookworms (ground itch), **2**-752
Hormones, **3**-999
"Hot flashes," **3**-1110
Hot-water bottle, **2**-599
Hunger, **1**-226
Huntington's chorea, **3**-1041
Hyaline membrane disease, **2**-404
Hydatid disease
    See Tapeworms
Hydatidiform mole
    See Trophoblastic disease
Hydrocephalus, **3**-1046
Hydrocortisone, **3**-1001
Hydrophobia
    See Rabies
Hydrotherapy, **2**-589
    Alcohol rub, **2**-598
    Cold compress, **2**-593
    Cold mitten friction, **2**-592
    Fomentations, **2**-590
    Heating compress, **2**-593
    Hot and cold to thc chest, **2**-592
    Hot foot bath, **2**-589
    Hot half-bath, **2**-597
    Hot mitten friction, **2**-593

Hot-and-cold immersion baths, **2**-589
Ice water or ice pack, **2**-597
Showers, **2**-595
Sitz bath, **2**-597
Sponge or rub, **2**-598
Steam inhalation, **2**-594
Tub bath, **2**-596
Hymen, **3**-1088
Hyperactive child, **2**-449
Hyperglycemia, **3**-1017
Hyperkinetic child
    See Hyperactive child
Hypertension, **1**-7, **1**-32, **1**-778, **3**-785
    In children, **2**-457
    In the elderly, **2**-496
Hyperthyroidism, **3**-1009
Hypochondria, **3**-1057
Hypoglycemia, **3**-1017
Hypotension, **1**-32, **3**-904
Hypothermia, **1**-32, **2**-555
Hypothyroidism, **3**-1010
Hysterectomy, **3**-1105
Hysteria, **3**-1055

I

Ichthyosis (fishskin), **3**-988
    In children, **2**-465
IgE
    See Immunoglobulin E
Illness, **2**-367
Illusionary drugs
    See Drugs of abuse
Immunity (defenses), **2**-605, **2**-760, **3**-828
Immunizations, **2**-407
Immunoglobulin E, **2**-675
Impetigo, **3**-975
    In infants and children, **2**-422, **2**-465
Impotence, male, **3**-1112
Incontinence, **2**-624
Indigestion (dyspepsia), **2**-621, **2**-625, **3**-853
Infancy, diseases and disorders of
    Atopic dermatitis (eczema), **2**-421
    Bronchiolitis, **2**-422
    Cerebral palsy, **2**-427
    Congenital deformities, **2**-426
    Congenital glaucoma, **2**-427
    Congenital rubella (German measles), **2**-421
    Down's syndrome (mongolism), **2**-428
    Hemolytic anemia of the newborn (Rh disease), **2**-426, **3**-818
    Hypothyroidism (cretinism), **2**-423
    Impetigo, **2**-422
    Infant colic, **2**-424
    Infectious diarrhea, **2**-424

L

Labor
    "Breaking of the bag of waters," **2**-399
    "Show," **2**-399
    False labor, **2**-401
    First stage, **2**-399
    Second stage, **2**-400
    Signs of, **2**-399
    Third stage, **2**-400
Lactose intolerance, **2**-454, **3**-858
    In teenagers, **2**-493
Large intestine, **3**-841
    Appendix, **3**-841
    Ascending colon, **3**-841
    Cecum, **3**-841
    Descending colon, **3**-841
    Sigmoid colon, **3**-841
    Transverse colon, **3**-841
Larynx, **3**-901
Larynx, diseases of, **3**-914
    Hoarseness, **3**-915
    Laryngitis, **3**-915
    Vocal cord damage, **3**-915
Leishmaniasis
    Espundia (American leishmaniasis), **2**-747
    Kala-azar (dumdum fever), **2**-748
    Oriental sore (tropical sore, Delhi sore), **2**-747
Lens, disorders of
    Aging eyes (presbyopia), **3**-1137
    Astigmatism, **3**-1137
    Blindness, **3**-1138
    Cataract, **3**-1136
    Double vision, **3**-1137
    Farsightedness, **3**-1137
    Nearsightedness, **3**-1136
    Refractive errors, **3**-1136
Leprosy (Hansen's disease), **2**-708
    Lepromatous leprosy, **2**-709
    Tuberculoid leprosy, **2**-709
Leptospirosis, **2**-721
Leukemia, **2**-682, **3**-823 - **3**-825
    Acute, **3**-824
    See also Blood, diseases of
    Chronic, **3**-825
    Granulocytic, **3**-824
    Lymphocytic, **3**-824
Leukoplakia, **3**-850, **3**-916
Lice
    Body, **3**-982
    Head, **3**-982
    In children, **2**-464
    Pubic (crab), **3**-982
Life
    Defined, **1**-23
    Relation of health to, **1**-23

Life expectancy, **1**-24
Life, dimensions of
    Breadth (quality), **1**-26
    Depth (love for God and man), **1**-27
    Length, **1**-25
    Length (life expectancy), **1**-24
Lifestyle
    As consideration in establishing a home, **2**-365
    Healthful, **1**-124, **1**-125
    Influence of on health and disease, **1**-117
    Westerner's, **1**-124
Lifestyle diseases, **1**-8, **1**-29
Lipids, blood
    See Cholesterol
Lipoproteins, **3**-777
Lips
    Cracking of (cheilosis), **3**-846
Lister, Dr. Joseph
    Control of wound infection pioneered by, **1**-5
Little's disease
    See Cerebral palsy
Liver, **3**-842
    Abscess of, **3**-873
    Cancer of, **3**-873
    Cirrhosis of, **3**-871
    Functions of, **3**-843
Liver rot
    See Flukes
Liver spots, **3**-987
Lobar pneumonia
    See Pneumonia
Lockjaw
    See Tetanus
Louse typhus
    See Typhus
Low blood pressure, **3**-804
Low blood sugar
    See Hypoglycemia
LSD (Iysergic acid diethylamide), **1**-302
Lump in the throat, **2**-628
Lumpy Jaw
    See Actinomycosis
"Lumpy breasts," **1**-262, **2**-616
Lung abscess, **3**-927
Lungs, **3**-902
    Covering of (pleura), **3**-905
Lupus (SLE), **3**-957
Lyme disease, **2**-720
Lymph, **3**-826
Lymph nodes
    Infection-fighting role of, **3**-827, **3**-828
    Lymphocytes, **3**-827
    Phagocytes, **3**-827
    Swollen (lymphadenopathy), **3**-831
Lymphatic system, **3**-826
    Lymph nodes, **3**-826

Pharynx, **3**-837, **3**-901
Phenacetin
    See Pain-relieving drugs: Tylenol
Phenylketonuria (PKU), **2**-406, **3**-1047
Phlebitis
    See Veins, diseases of
Phlebotomus fever
    See Sandfly fever
Phobias, **3**-1055
Physical examination
    General appearance, **1**-12
    The abdomen, **1**-13
    The chest, **1**-13
    The ears, **1**-12
    The eyes, **1**-12
    The larynx, **1**-13
    The neck, **1**-12
    The nose, **1**-12
    The pelvis, **1**-13
    The throat, **1**-13
Physician
    Training of, **1**-8
PID
    See Pelvic inflammatory disease
Piles
    See Hemorrhoids
Pimples
    See Acne
Pineal gland, **3**-1000
Pinta (carate, azul), **2**-721
Pinworms, **2**-754
Pituitary disorders
    Abnormal milk production (galactorrhea), **3**-1005
    Diabetes insipidus, **3**-1005
    Dwarfism, **3**-1006
    Gigantism and acromegaly, **3**-1006
    Hypopituitarism, **3**-1006
    Tumors, **3**-1007
Pituitary gland, **3**-1000
Pituitary hormones
    Corticotropin (ACTH), **3**-1000
    Follicle-stimulating hormone (FSH), **3**-1000
    Gonadotropin, **3**-1000
    Growth hormone, **3**-1000
    Luteinizing hormone (LH), **3**-1000
    Oxytocin, **3**-1000
    Prolactin, **3**-1000
    Thyrotropin, **3**-1000
    Vasopressin (ADH), **3**-1000
PKU
    See Phenylketonuria
Placebo
    Ethics of using, **1**-342
    Impure, **1**-342
    Pure, **1**-342
    Reasons for not using, **1**-346

    Reasons for using, **1**-346
Placebo effect, **1**-342
Placebo effect, factors contributing to, **1**-343
    Factors related to the patient, **1**-344
    Factors related to the placebo, **1**-345
    Factors related to the practitioner, **1**-344
    Miscellaneous factors affecting placebos, **1**-345
Placenta, **2**-381, **3**-1090
Plague
    See Bubonic plague
Plaque, arterial, **1**-275, **3**-780
Plaque, dental, **3**-886, **3**-891
    Calculus, **3**-886
Platelets, **3**-773
Pleura, disorders of
    Empyema, **3**-932
    Pleural effusion, **3**-932
    Pleurisy, **3**-932
    Pneumothorax, **3**-933
Pleurisy, **3**-932
PMS
    See Premenstrual syndrome
Pneumoconiosis, **3**-928, **3**-931
Pneumonia, **2**-459, **3**-923
    Bacterial, **3**-923
    Bronchopneumonia, **2**-459
    In children, **2**-459
    Legionnaires' disease, **3**-924
    Mycoplasmal, **3**-924
    Viral, **3**-923
Pneumonic plague, **2**-710
Poison oak, poison ivy, **2**-464, **3**-973
Poisoning
    First aid for, **2**-520
    Important procedures in responding to, **2**-521
    National poison control center phone number, **2**-520
    Rules for preventing, **2**-519
Poisoning, how to respond to, **2**-519
Poisoning, response to specific kinds of
    Alcohol (ethyl alcohol, beverage alcohol), **2**-522
    Alcohol (methyl alcohol, wood alcohol), **2**-523
    Antifreeze (ethylene glycol), **2**-523
    Arsenic, **2**-525
    Aspirin, **2**-524
    Carbon monoxide, **2**-527
    Corrosive agents—strong acids and alkalis, **2**-522
    Coumarins (Warfarin), **2**-526
    Cyanide, **2**-526
    Food, **2**-526
    Hair removers (depilatories), **2**-524
    Insecticides, **2**-525
    Iodine, **2**-524
    Iron, **2**-524
    Medicinal products and drugs of abuse, **2**-523
    Nicotine, **2**-525

Q

(26)

R

Rabbit fever
    See Tularemia
Rabies (hydrophobia), **2**-730
Radiation therapy in treatment of cancer, **2**-696
Rape, **2**-492
Rash (skin eruption), **2**-632
    From drugs, **2**-632
    From infectious diseases, **2**-632
    In diseases of the skin, **2**-632
    In infants, **2**-632
    Of pellagra, **2**-632
    Urticarial reactions (hives), **2**-632
Ratbite fever
    Bacillus form, **2**-711
    Spirochete form, **2**-711
Raynaud's disease
    See Arteries, diseases of
RDS (Respiratory Distress Syndrome)
    See Infancy, diseases and disorders of
Recipes, **1**-191
    Index of, **1**-225
Rectum, **3**-842
    Prolapse of, **2**-633
Refined grains, **1**-90
Reflex, **3**-1026
Relapsing fever, **2**-722
Relaxation, **1**-52
    Progressive, **2**-601
Religion
    In the home, **2**-367
Religious beliefs
    Negative, effects of on health, **1**-113
    Positive, effects of on health, **1**-112, **1**-113
Religious faith
    Benefits of, **1**-115, **2**-367
    Influence of on health, **1**-114
Religious responses to adversity
    Fatalism, **1**-114
    Legalism, **1**-114
    True belief, **1**-115
REM (rapid eye movement)
    See Sleep
Renal failure
    Acute, **3**-1070
    Acute pyelonephritis, **3**-1072
    Chronic, **3**-1071
    Chronic pyelonephritis, **3**-1073
    Kidney stones (renal calculi), **3**-1073
    Nephrosis (nephrotic syndrome), **3**-1071
Reproduction
    See Sex
Respiration, **2**-574, **3**-904
Respiratory arrest, **2**-508
Respiratory distress syndrome, **2**-404

Respiratory system, **1**-63, **3**-899
Rest
    State of, **1**-53
Retina, disorders of
    Macular degeneration, **3**-1139
    Retinal detachment, **3**-1138
    Retinal hemorrhages, **3**-1139
    Retinal vascular disorders, **3**-1139
Retinal vascular disorders
    Diabetic retinopathy, **3**-1139
    Retinal artery occlusion, **3**-1139
    Retinal vein occlusion, **3**-1139
Reye's syndrome, **2**-467, **2**-732
Rh disease
    See Anemia
Rh factor
    See Blood types
Rheumatic fever, **2**-474
Rheumatic heart disease, **3**-795
    Endocarditis, **3**-795
    In children, **2**-457
    In teenagers, **2**-489
    Myocarditis, **3**-795
    Pericarditis, **3**-795
Rhythms, biological, **3**-1001
Rickets, **2**-426, **3**-944
    In children, **2**-475
Rickettsialpox, **2**-735
Ringworm (dermatophytosis), **3**-977
    Athlete's foot, **3**-978
    In children, **2**-464
    Of the beard, **3**-978
    Of the body, **3**-978
    Of the groin, **3**-978
    Of the nails, **3**-978
    Of the scalp, **3**-978
River blindness (onchocerciasis), **2**-763
Rocky Mountain spotted fever, **2**-734
Rosacea (acne rosacea), **3**-984
Roseola infantum, **2**-473
Roundworms (ascariasis), **2**-754
Rubella
    See German measles
Rubeola
    See Measles
Ruddy complexion, as symptom of illness, **2**-618

S

Saint Vitus' dance
    See Sydenham's chorea
Salivary duct stone, **3**-850
Salivary glands, **3**-881
Salivary glands, disorders
    Inflammation of, **2**-729, **3**-849

(28)

T

U

Ulcerative colitis, **3**-865
Ulcers, **2**-637, **3**-975, **3**-986
Ulcers (stomach or duodenal), **3**-855
    Complications of, **3**-856
    In children, **2**-461
Ultrasound, **1**-14
Ultraviolet lamps
    See Sunlamps
Umbilical cord, **2**-381
Unconsciousness (coma), **2**-557, **2**-637
    Caused by diseased blood vessels, **2**-638
    Caused by reduced blood supply to brain, **2**-639
    Due to head injury, **2**-637
    From taking alcohol, drugs, or poisons, **2**-637
    In "diabetic coma," **2**-638
    In association with brain tumor or abscess, **2**-638
    In epilepsy, **2**-638
    In hepatic coma, **2**-638
    In hypoglycemic coma, **2**-638
    In hysteria, **2**-639
    In meningitis and encephalitis, **2**-638
    In uremic coma, **2**-638
Undulant fever (brucellosis), **2**-706
Uremia, **3**-1070
Ureter disorders
    See Bladder and ureter disorders
Ureters, **3**-1066
Urethra, diseases of
    Gonorrheal urethritis, **3**-1080
    Nongonococcal or nonspecific urethritis (NSU),
        3-1081
    Urethritis, **3**-1080
Urinal, **2**-574
Urinary system
    Bladder, **3**-1066
    Kidneys, **3**-1065
    Ureters, **3**-1066
    Urethra, **3**-1067
    Urine, **3**-1067
Urine, **3**-1067
    Analyses of, **1**-19
Urticaria
    See Hives
Uterine tubes
    See Fallopian tubes
Uterus (womb), **3**-1087
    "Uterine milk," **2**-381, **3**-1089, **3**-1090
    Cervix, **3**-1087
    Endometrium, **3**-1089
Uterus, disorders of
    Absence of periods (amenorrhea), **3**-1100
    Cancer, **3**-1105
    Displacements of the uterus, **3**-1102
    Endometriosis, **3**-1103
    Fibroid tumors, **3**-1104
    Heavy periods (menorrhagia), **3**-1101
    Infrequent periods (oligomenorrhea), **3**-1101
    Painful periods (dysmenorrhea, cramps), **3**-1101
    Premenstrual syndrome (PMS), **3**-1102
    Trophoblastic disease, **3**-1103

V

Vaccinations, **2**-407, **2**-728
    DTP (diphtheria, tetanus, pertussis), **2**-407
    MMR (measles, mumps, rubella), **2**-407
    Risks and side effects of, **2**-407
    TOPV (trivalent oral polio vaccine), **2**-407
Vaccines, **1**-335
Vagina, **3**-1087
    Hymen, **3**-1088
Vagina, disorders of
    Vaginal cysts, **3**-1109
    Vaginal discharge, **3**-1107
    Vaginal fistulas, **3**-1109
    Vaginitis, **3**-1108
Vaginal discharge, **3**-1107
Vaginitis
    Chlamydial infections, **3**-1108
    Leukorrhea, **3**-1108
    Nonspecific, **3**-1108
    Postmenopausal, **3**-1108
    Trichomoniasis, **3**-1108
    Yeast infections (candidiasis, moniliasis), **3**-1108
Valley fever
    See Coccidiomycosis
Varicella
    See Chickenpox
Varicose veins
    See Veins, diseases of
Vas deferens, **2**-480, **3**-1084
Vascular nevus
    See Birthmarks
Veins, **3**-769, **3**-770
Veins, diseases of, **3**-806
    Hemorrhoids, **3**-807
    Phlebitis, **3**-808
    Thrombophlebitis, **3**-808
    Varicose veins, **3**-806
Venipuncture (for blood analysis)
    Blood count, **1**-19
    Blood culture, **1**-19
    Chemical analyses, **1**-19
    Clotting time, **1**-19
Vertigo, **3**-1052
Vincent's infection
    Trench mouth, **3**-849
Viruses
    Viral diseases, **2**-723

W

Selective Atlas of Normal Anatomy

Special acknowledgment is due Lederle Laboratories for the series of color plates appearing in the section "Selective Atlas of Normal Anatomy," these being part of a larger series of paintings by Paul Peck, copyrighted by Lederle Laboratories Division, American Cyanamid Company, Pearl River, N.Y., and included in this volume by permission.

Anatomy of the Heart

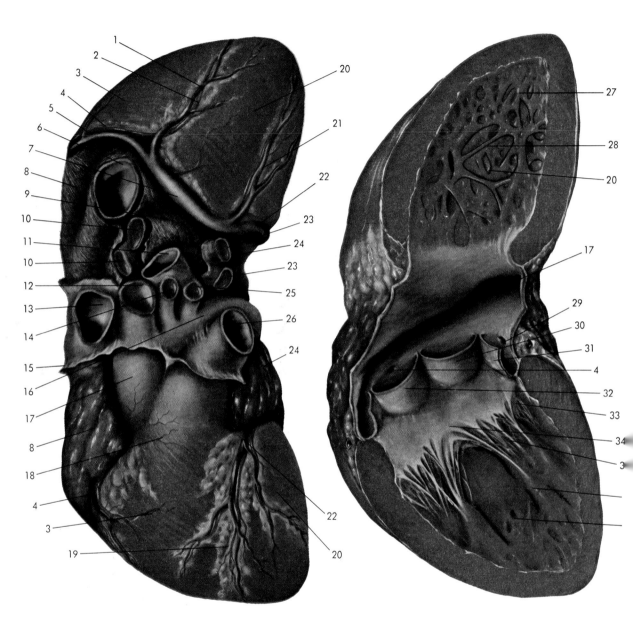

Anatomy of the Stomach

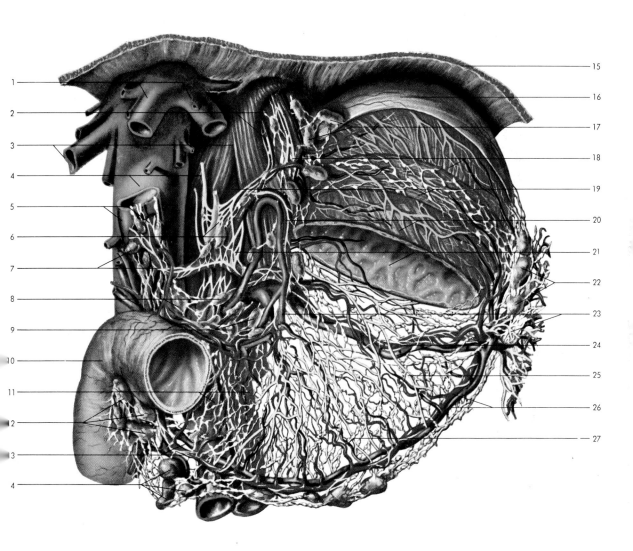

1 Middle and left hepatic veins
2 Right vagus nerve and esophagus
3 Right hepatic vein and crura of diaphragm
4 Inferior vena cava and greater splanchnic nerve
5 Portal vein and hepatic artery
6 Celiac plexus and celiac artery
7 Hepatic lymph node and hepatic rami of vagus nerve
8 Gastroduodenal artery and suprapyloric lymph nodes

9 Superior gastric lymph nodes
10 Duodenum
11 Superior mesenteric artery and vein
12 Subpyloric lymph nodes
13 Right gastroepiploic artery and vein
14 Inferior gastric lymph nodes
15 Diaphragm
16 Serosa
17 Paracardial lymph nodes
18 Left vagus nerve and longitudinal muscular layer

19 Abdominal aorta and circular muscular layer
20 Left gastric artery and oblique muscular layer
21 Celiac rami of vagus nerve and gastric mucosa
22 Splenic lymph nodes
23 Left gastric (coronary) vein and splenic rami of vagus nerve
24 Splenic artery and vein
25 Gastric rami of vagus nerve
26 Left gastroepiploic artery and vein
27 Gastric lymphatic plexus

The Sympathetic Nervous System

ABDOMINAL PORTION

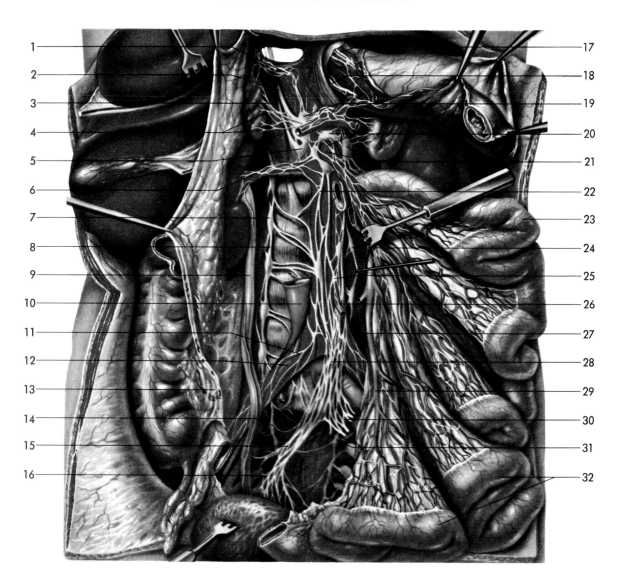

1 Phrenic ganglion and plexus
2 Greater splanchnic nerve
3 Lesser splanchnic nerve
4 Suprarenal plexus
5 Aorticorenal ganglion
6 Right renal artery and plexus
7 Right lumbar sympathetic ganglion
8 Right sympathetic trunk
9 Ureter
10 Vena cava
11 Iliac plexus

12 Right common iliac artery
13 Mesocolon (cut)
14 Right sacral sympathetic ganglion
15 Right pelvic plexus
16 Pudendal plexus
17 Left vagus nerve
18 Right vagus nerve
19 Celiac plexus and right celiac ganglion
20 Superior mesenteric ganglion and plexus
21 Left celiac ganglion; superior mesenteric artery

22 Abdominal aortic plexus
23 Jejunum
24 Left lumbar sympathetic ganglion
25 Inferior mesenteric ganglion
26 Inferior mesenteric plexus
27 Left sympathetic trunk
28 Hypogastric plexus
29 Branches of superior mesenteric artery and vein
30 Left pelvic plexus
31 Left sacral sympathetic ganglion
32 Ileum

The Sympathetic Nervous System

CEPHALIC, CERVICAL AND THORACIC PORTIONS

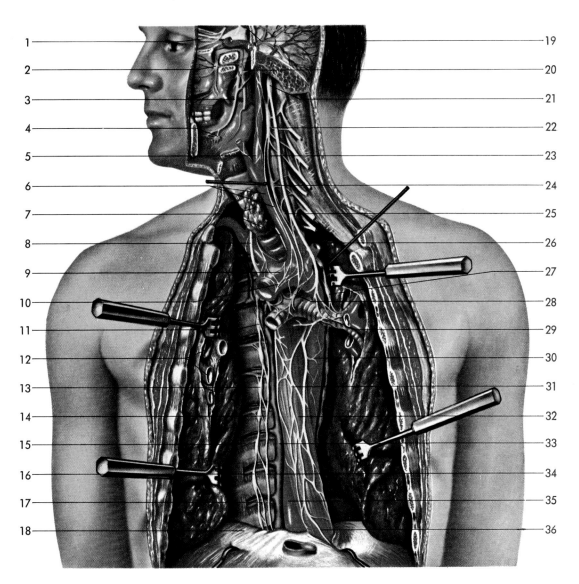

1 Ciliary ganglion
2 Sphenopalatine ganglion
3 Lingual nerve
4 Submandibular ganglion
5 Internal carotid artery
6 Common carotid artery; superior cardiac nerve
7 Thyroid gland; recurrent laryngeal nerve
8 Right vagus nerve
9 Aortic arch
10 Superficial cardiac plexus
11 Fifth thoracic sympathetic ganglion

12 Pulmonary artery and vein
13 Seventh thoracic sympathetic ganglion
14 Greater splanchnic nerve
15 Intercostal artery, vein and nerve
16 Tenth thoracic sympathetic ganglion
17 Lesser splanchnic nerve
18 Diaphragm
19 Trigeminal nerve
20 Otic ganglion
21 Nodose ganglion
22 Superior cervical sympathetic ganglion
23 Cervical sympathetic trunk
24 Middle cervical sympathetic ganglion

25 Inferior cervical sympathetic ganglion
26 Left vagus nerve
27 Fourth thoracic sympathetic ganglion
28 Cardiac ganglion
29 Anterior pulmonary plexus
30 Aortic plexus
31 Esophageal plexus
32 Esophagus
33 Azygos vein
34 Splanchnic ganglion
35 Aorta
36 Anterior gastric cord of vagus

The Coronary Arteries

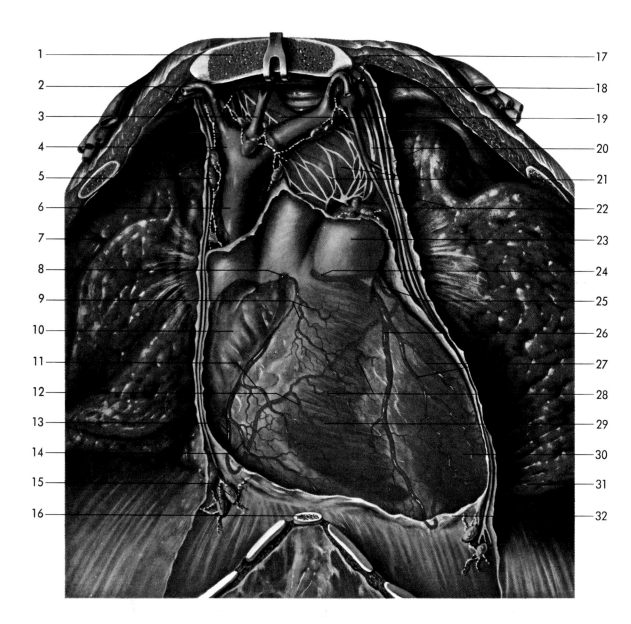

1 Manubrium
2 Right internal mammary artery and vein
3 Thyreoidea ima vein
4 Right brachiocephalic vein
5 Anterior superior mediastinal lymph nodes
6 Superior vena cava
7 Right lung
8 Right coronary artery
9 Preventricular arteries
10 Right atrium
11 Lateral branch of right coronary artery

12 Posterior descending branch of right circumflex artery
13 Right circumflex artery
14 Right marginal artery
15 Anterior inferior mediastinal lymph nodes
16 Xiphoid process
17 Left internal mammary artery and vein
18 Left brachiocephalic vein
19 Brachiocephalic trunk
20 Vagus nerve; mediastinal pleura (Cut)
21 Superficial cardiac plexus; arch of aorta

22 Pericardiacophrenic artery; phrenic nerve
23 Pulmonary artery
24 Left coronary artery
25 Left circumflex artery
26 Anterior descending branch of left coronary artery
27 Left marginal arteries
28 Left ventricular branches
29 Right ventricle
30 Left ventricle
31 Left lung
32 Pericardium (cut)

Anatomy of the Ear

FRONTAL SECTION SHOWING COMPONENT PARTS OF THE HUMAN EAR

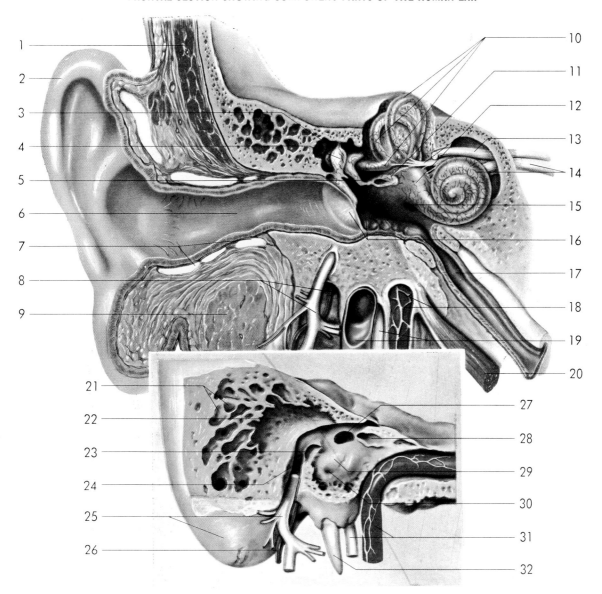

SECTION THROUGH RIGHT TEMPORAL BONE SHOWING RELATIONSHIP BETWEEN MASTOID CELLS AND TYMPANIC CAVITY

1 Temporal muscle
2 Helix
3 Epitympanic recess
4 Malleus
5 Incus
6 External acoustic meatus
7 Cartilaginous part of external acoustic meatus
8 Facial nerve and stylomastoid artery
9 Parotid gland
10 Semicircular canals
11 Stapes
12 Vestibule and vestibular nerve

13 Facial nerve
14 Cochlea and cochlear nerve
15 Cochlear (round) window
16 Tympanic membrane and tympanic cavity
17 Auditory (Eustachian) tube
18 Internal carotid artery and sympathetic nerve plexus
19 Glossopharyngeal nerve and internal jugular vein
20 Levator veli palatini muscle
21 Mastoid cells
22 Tympanic antrum

23 Cavity of the pyramidal eminence for the stapedius
24 Facial canal
25 Facial nerve and mastoid process
26 Stylomastoid artery
27 Vestibular (oval) window
28 Cochleariform process
29 Promontory
30 Cochlear fenestra
31 Internal carotid artery and glossopharyngeal nerve
32 Styloid process

Region of the Mouth

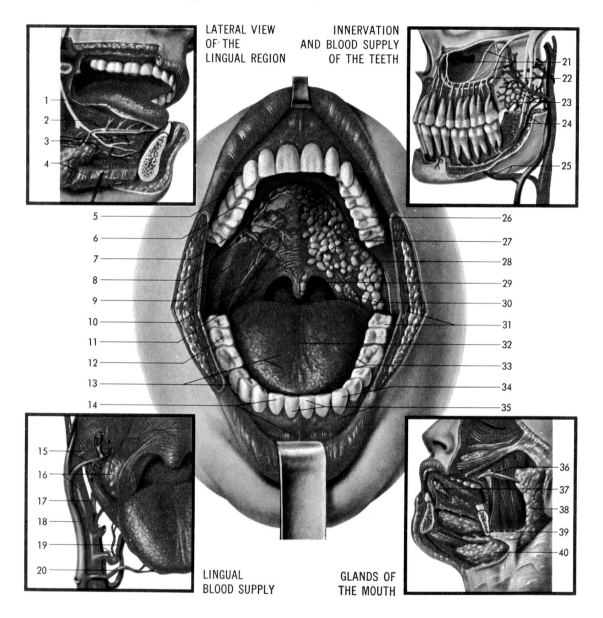

LATERAL VIEW OF THE LINGUAL REGION

INNERVATION AND BLOOD SUPPLY OF THE TEETH

LINGUAL BLOOD SUPPLY

GLANDS OF THE MOUTH

1 Lingual nerve
2 Submaxillary duct
3 Sublingual branches of lingual artery and vein
4 Submaxillary gland; mylohyoid muscle
5 First premolar
6 Second premolar
7 Greater palatine artery and nerve
8 Lesser palatine artery and nerve
9 Pterygomandibular raphe
10 Glossopalatine muscle
11 Pharyngopalatinus muscle
12 Second molar
13 Filiform papillae; second premolar
14 Lateral incisor; frenulum of lower lip

15 Internal maxillary artery and vein
16 External carotid artery; palatine tonsil
17 Internal jugular vein
18 Posterior facial vein
19 Lingual artery and vein
20 Ranine vein
21 Anterior, middle and posterior superior alveolar nerves
22 Posterior superior alveolar artery
23 Pterygoid venous plexus
24 Inferior alveolar nerve and artery
25 External maxillary artery; anterior facial vein
26 First molar
27 Palatine glands

28 Cut edge of mucous membrane
29 Uvula
30 Palatine tonsils
31 Third molar; buccinator muscle
32 Median sulcus of tongue
33 Fungiform papillae
34 Canine
35 Central incisors; gingiva
36 Parotid duct
37 Anterior lingual gland
38 Parotid gland
39 Sublingual gland
40 Submaxillary gland

Anatomy of the Lung

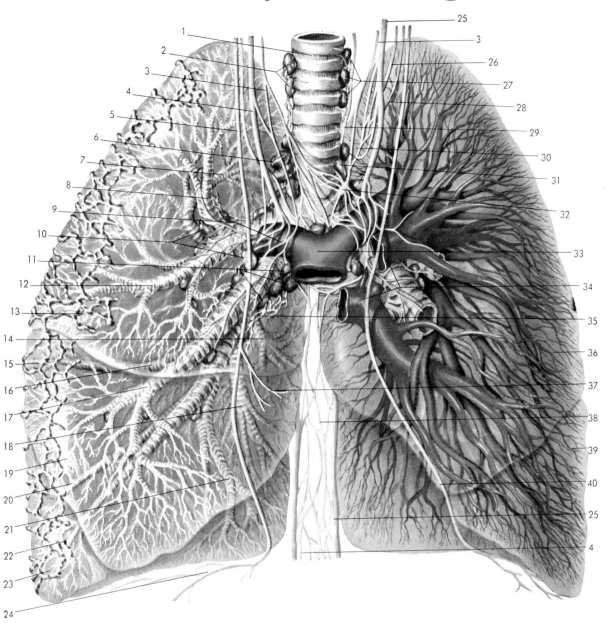

1 Trachea
2 Right tracheal lymph nodes
3 Superior cardiac nerve
4 Right vagus nerve
5 Right phrenic nerve
6 Right superior tracheobronchial lymph nodes
7 Posterior bronchial branch, upper lobe
8 Apical bronchial branch, upper lobe
9 Anterior pulmonary plexus
10 Interbronchial lymph nodes
11 Inferior tracheobronchial lymph nodes
12 Anterior bronchial branch, upper lobe
13 Upper lobe of right lung
14 Superior bronchial branch, lower lobe

15 Superficial lymphatic plexus
16 Lateral bronchial branch, middle lobe
17 Medial bronchial branch, middle lobe
18 Posterior basal bronchial branch, lower lobe
19 Middle lobe of right lung
20 Lateral basal bronchial branch, lower lobe
21 Medial basal bronchial branch, lower lobe
22 Anterior basal bronchial branch, lower lobe
23 Lower lobe of right lung
24 Phrenicoabdominal branch of phrenic nerve
25 Left vagus nerve
26 Middle cardiac nerve

27 Left tracheal lymph nodes
28 Inferior cardiac nerve
29 Recurrent laryngeal nerve
30 Superficial cardiac plexus
31 Left superior tracheobronchial lymph nodes
32 Inferior cardiac ganglion
33 Pulmonary artery
34 Left pulmonary veins
35 Deep lymphatic plexus
36 Upper lobe of left lung
37 Pericardial branch of phrenic nerve
38 Esophageal plexus
39 Lower lobe of left lung
40 Left phrenic nerve

The Intervertebral Disks

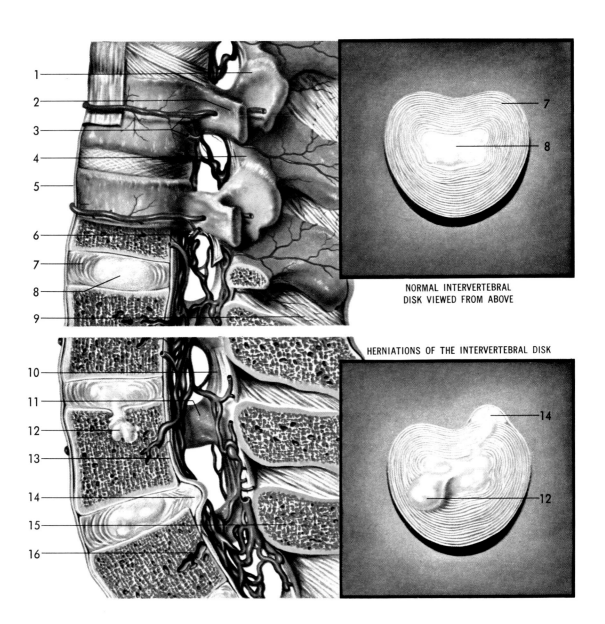

NORMAL INTERVERTEBRAL
DISK VIEWED FROM ABOVE

HERNIATIONS OF THE INTERVERTEBRAL DISK

1 Superior articular process
2 Transverse process
3 Lumbar artery and vein
4 Inferior articular process
5 Anterior longitudinal ligament
6 Internal vertebral venous plexus

7 Fibrous ring of intervertebral disk
8 Nucleus pulposus
9 Interspinous ligament
10 Ligamentum flavum
11 Lamina
12 Herniation of nucleus pulposus into
 the spongiosa (Schmorl lesion)

13 Posterior longitudinal ligament
14 Herniation of nucleus pulposus beneath
 the posterior longitudinal ligament
15 Spinous process
16 Basivertebral vein

Anatomy of the Brain

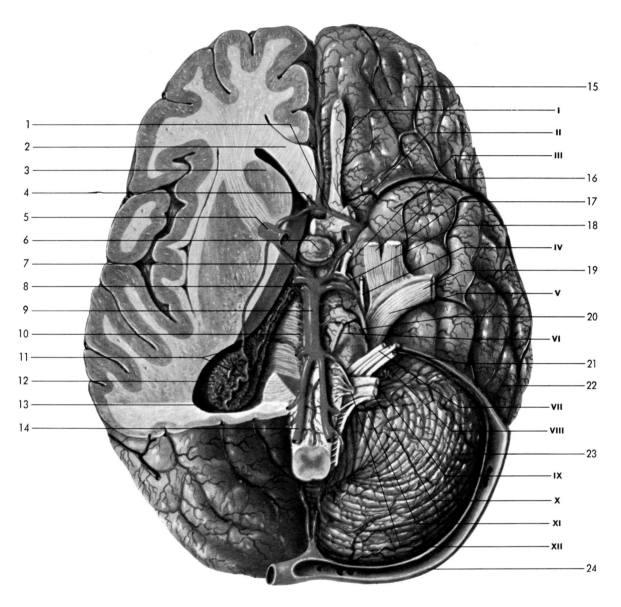

1 Anterior cerebral artery
2 Trunk of corpus callosum
3 Head of caudate nucleus
4 Anterior communicating artery
5 Middle cerebral artery
6 Hypophysis
7 Posterior communicating artery
8 Superior cerebellar artery
9 Basilar artery
10 Internal cerebral vein
11 Choroid artery and vein
12 Choroid plexus of lateral ventricle

13 Inferior cornu of lateral ventricle
14 Vertebral artery
15 Frontal lobe
16 Ophthalmic nerve
17 Maxillary nerve
18 Posterior cerebral artery
19 Mandibular nerve
20 Pons
21 Intermediate nerve
22 Temporal lobe
23 Cerebellum
24 Left transverse sinus

CRANIAL NERVES
   I. Olfactory nerve
  II. Optic nerve
 III. Oculomotor nerve
 IV. Trochlear nerve
  V. Trigeminal nerve
 VI. Abducens nerve
VII. Facial nerve
VIII. Acoustic nerve
 IX. Glossopharyngeal nerve
  X. Vagus nerve
 XI. Accessory nerve
XII. Hypoglossal nerve

Anatomy of the Ankle

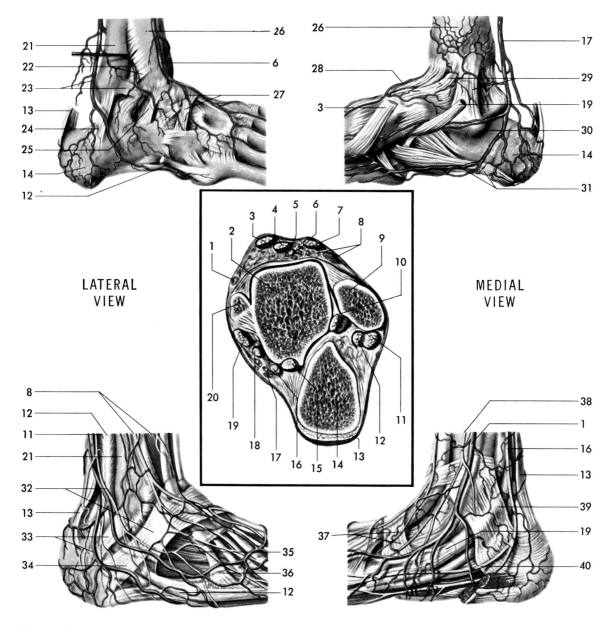

LATERAL VIEW

MEDIAL VIEW

1 Great saphenous vein
2 Talus
3 Tendon of tibialis anterior
4 Tendon of extensor hallucis longus
5 Deep peroneal nerve
6 Anterior tibial artery
7 Tendon of extensor digitorum longus
8 Peroneus tertius muscle and superficial peroneal nerve
9 Lateral malleolus
10 Posterior talofibular ligament
11 Tendon of peroneus longus
12 Tendon of peroneus brevis
13 Calcaneal tendon
14 Calcaneus
15 Tendon of flexor hallucis longus

16 Tibial nerve
17 Posterior tibial artery
18 Tendon of flexor digitorum longus
19 Tendon of tibialis posterior
20 Medial malleolus
21 Fibula
22 Perforating peroneal artery and anterior ligament of external malleolus
23 Peroneal artery and anterior talofibular ligament
24 Calcaneofibular ligament
25 External talocalcaneal ligament
26 Tibia
27 Lateral tarsal artery and dorsal cuboideo-navicular ligament
28 Dorsal pedis artery

29 Deltoid ligament
30 Sustentaculum tali
31 Long plantar ligament and lateral plantar artery
32 Sural nerve and cruciate ligament
33 Superior peroneal retinaculum and small saphenous vein
34 Inferior peroneal retinaculum
35 Extensor digitorum brevis muscle
36 Tendon of peroneus tertius
37 Medial dorsal cutaneous nerve and cruciate ligament
38 Saphenous nerve
39 Laciniate ligament
40 Medial plantar nerve

Pelvis and Hip Joint

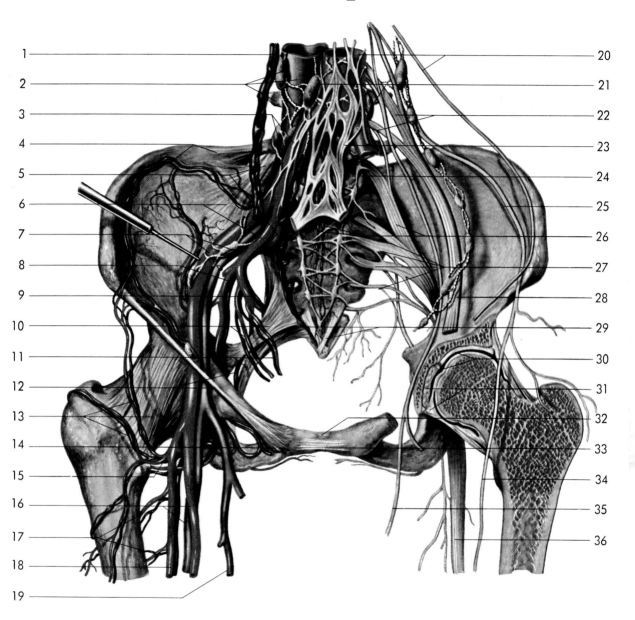

1 Ovarian artery and vein
2 Vena cava; lumbar lymph nodes
3 Right common iliac artery and vein
4 Iliolumbar ligament; branches of iliolumbar artery and vein
5 Lumbosacral ligament; superior gluteal artery and vein
6 Anterior sacroiliac ligament; internal iliac (hypogastric) artery
7 External iliac artery and vein
8 Obturator artery and vein
9 Inferior gluteal artery and vein
10 Sacrospinous ligament; uterine artery and vein
11 Sacrotuberous ligament; vaginal artery and vein

12 Inguinal ligament; internal pudendal artery
13 Iliofemoral ligament; branches of lateral femoral circumflex artery and vein
14 Lacunar ligament
15 Lateral femoral circumflex artery and vein
16 Femoral artery and vein
17 Perforating arteries and veins
18 Deep femoral artery and vein
19 Great saphenous vein
20 Aorta; ilioinguinal nerve
21 Lateral aortic lymph nodes
22 Lumbar nerves
23 Hypogastric sympathetic plexus
24 Sympathetic trunk

25 Lateral femoral cutaneous nerve
26 Middle sacral artery and vein; lumbosacral trunk
27 Sacral nerves
28 Femoral nerve
29 Lateral sacral artery and vein; anterior sacrococcygeal ligament
30 Lunate articular cartilage; joint cavity
31 Acetabular fat pad; ligamentum teres
32 Interpubic fibrocartilage
33 Superior pubic ligament
34 Anterior branch of lateral femoral cutaneous nerve
35 Obturator nerve
36 Great sciatic nerve

Anatomy of the Hand

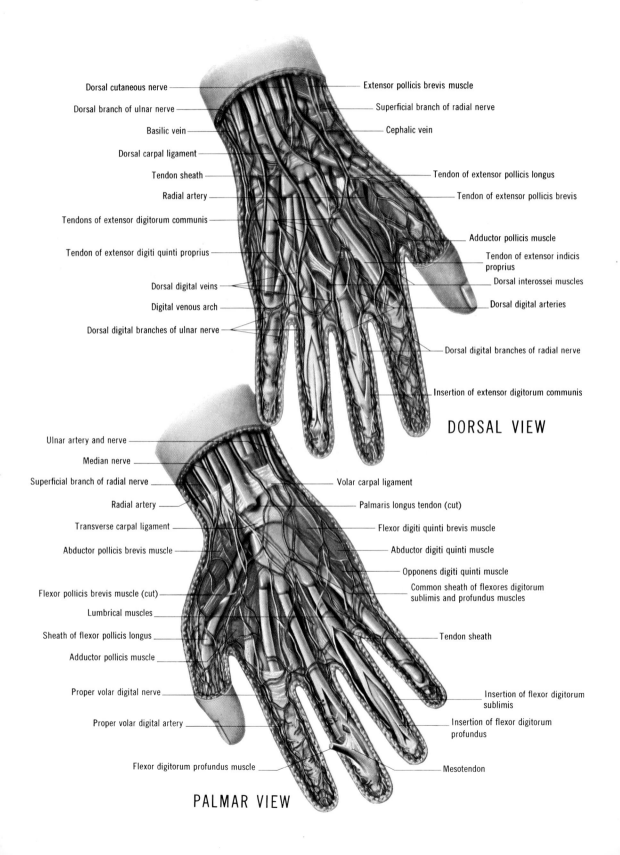

Dorsal cutaneous nerve

Dorsal branch of ulnar nerve

Basilic vein

Dorsal carpal ligament

Tendon sheath

Radial artery

Tendons of extensor digitorum communis

Tendon of extensor digiti quinti proprius

Dorsal digital veins

Digital venous arch

Dorsal digital branches of ulnar nerve

Extensor pollicis brevis muscle

Superficial branch of radial nerve

Cephalic vein

Tendon of extensor pollicis longus

Tendon of extensor pollicis brevis

Adductor pollicis muscle

Tendon of extensor indicis proprius

Dorsal interossei muscles

Dorsal digital arteries

Dorsal digital branches of radial nerve

Insertion of extensor digitorum communis

DORSAL VIEW

Ulnar artery and nerve

Median nerve

Superficial branch of radial nerve

Radial artery

Transverse carpal ligament

Abductor pollicis brevis muscle

Flexor pollicis brevis muscle (cut)

Lumbrical muscles

Sheath of flexor pollicis longus

Adductor pollicis muscle

Proper volar digital nerve

Proper volar digital artery

Flexor digitorum profundus muscle

Volar carpal ligament

Palmaris longus tendon (cut)

Flexor digiti quinti brevis muscle

Abductor digiti quinti muscle

Opponens digiti quinti muscle

Common sheath of flexores digitorum sublimis and profundus muscles

Tendon sheath

Insertion of flexor digitorum sublimis

Insertion of flexor digitorum profundus

Mesotendon

PALMAR VIEW

Anatomy of the Male Genitalia

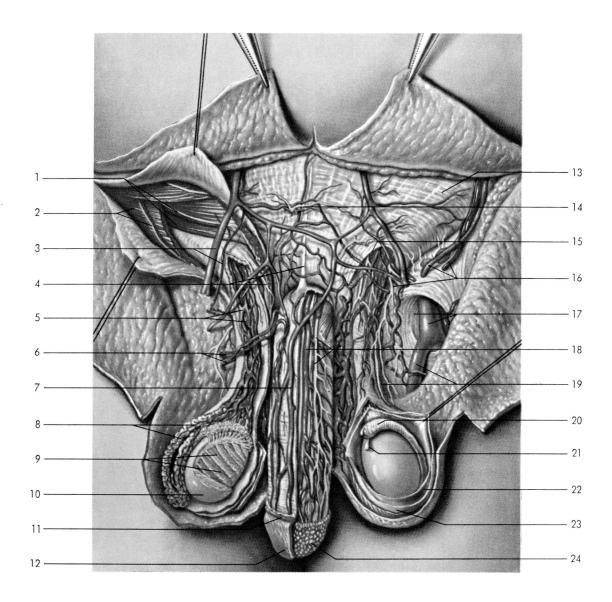

1 Transversus abdominis muscle and iliohypogastric nerve
2 Obliquus abdominis internus muscle and ilioinguinal nerve
3 Superficial epigastric artery and vein
4 Genital branch of genitofemoral nerve and suspensory ligament of penis
5 Internal spermatic artery and pampiniform plexus
6 External pudendal artery and vein
7 Superficial dorsal vein of penis
8 Vas deferens and deferential artery

9 Lobules of testis
10 Testis (covered by visceral tunica vaginalis)
11 Prepuce
12 Glans penis
13 Abdominal aponeurosis
14 Anterior cutaneous branch of subcostal nerve
15 Subcutaneous inguinal ring
16 Ilioinguinal nerve and superficial iliac circumflex artery and vein

17 Fossa ovalis and femoral artery and vein
18 Dorsal artery and nerve, and deep dorsal vein, of penis
19 Cremaster muscle and great saphenous vein
20 Head of epididymis
21 Appendix of testis
22 Parietal layer of tunica vaginalis
23 Infundibuliform fascia
24 Plexus cavernosus

Anatomy of the Female Genitalia

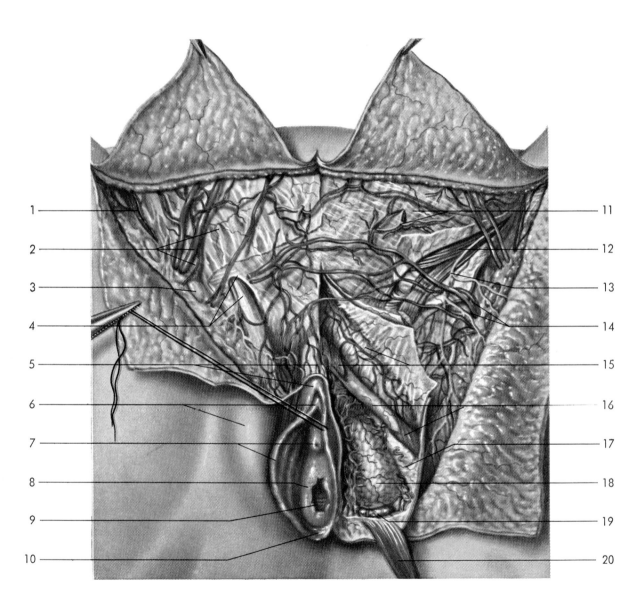

1 Superficial iliac circumflex artery and vein
2 Tela subcutanea and superficial epigastric artery and vein
3 Inguinal lymph node
4 Subcutaneous inguinal ring and round ligament of uterus
5 Prepuce and dorsal vein of clitoris
6 Clitoris and labium majus
7 External urethral orifice and labium minus
8 Hymen
9 Vaginal orifice
10 Navicular fossa
11 Abdominal aponeurosis and anterior cutaneous branch of subcostal nerve
12 Obliquus abdominis internus muscle
13 Ilioinguinal nerve
14 Superficial external pudendal artery and vein
15 Fascia lata and bulbocavernosus muscle
16 Ischiocavernosus muscle and crus of clitoris
17 Inferior fascia of the urogenital diaphragm
18 Vestibular bulb
19 Major vestibular (Bartholin's) gland
20 Bulbocavernosus muscle